**Revision Notes for the
MRCOG Part 1**

Revision Notes for the MRCOG Part 1

Arisudhan Anantharachagan
Specialist Registrar in Obstetrics and Gynaecology
London Deanery
London

Ippokratis Sarris
Specialist Registrar in Obstetrics and Gynaecology
London Deanery
London
and
Honorary Research Fellow
Nuffield Department of Obstetrics and Gynaecology
University of Oxford
Oxford

Austin Ugwumadu
Consultant Obstetrician and Gynaecologist
St George's Healthcare NHS Trust
and
Honorary Senior Lecturer
St George's University of London
London

Foreword by
Sabaratnam Arulkumaran
Professor and Head of Obstetrics and Gynaecology
St George's University of London
St George's Healthcare NHS Trust
London

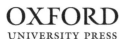
OXFORD
UNIVERSITY PRESS

OXFORD
UNIVERSITY PRESS

Great Clarendon Street, Oxford OX2 6DP

Oxford University Press is a department of the University of Oxford.
It furthers the University's objective of excellence
in research, scholarship, and education by publishing worldwide in

Oxford New York

Auckland Cape Town Dar es Salaam Hong Kong Karachi
Kuala Lumpur Madrid Melbourne Mexico City Nairobi
New Delhi Shanghai Taipei Toronto

With offices in

Argentina Austria Brazil Chile Czech Republic France Greece
Guatemala Hungary Italy Japan Poland Portugal Singapore
South Korea Switzerland Thailand Turkey Ukraine Vietnam

Oxford is a registered trade mark of Oxford University Press
in the UK and in certain other countries

Published in the United States
by Oxford University Press Inc., New York

© Oxford University Press, 2011

British Library Cataloguing in Publication Data
Data available

Library of Congress Cataloguing in Publication Data
Data available

Typeset in Gill Sans
by Glyph International Bangalore
Printed in Great Britain
on acid-free paper by
Ashford Colour Press Ltd, Gosport, Hampshire

ISBN 978–0–19–959233–3

Foreword

The MRCOG part 1 has long been a challenging exam for doctors because a large number of basic science topics need to be read and understood. This book consists of 13 chapters covering the basic sciences needed. The applied knowledge required to practice obstetrics and gynaecology is interwoven with the basics. Practice of obstetrics and gynaecology requires a sound knowledge of pathology, immunology, microbiology, pharmacology, intrapartum screening, medical physics and its applications, and research methodologies, and these subjects are comprehensively covered.

The chapters are well laid down with clear subdivisions explaining the essential topics in that particular field. The chapter on genetics starts with molecular biology, moves on to cellular division and replication, and finishes with chromosomal and genetic disorders. This complex subject is explained using tables and figures to help candidates to understand it without difficulty.

Knowledge of embryology is essential to understand congenital malformations. Embryo-genesis, and the formation of the placenta, foetal membranes, body cavities, and diaphragm are explained. The development of every system in the body is related to applied clinical knowledge. The chapter on anatomy deals with the relevant anatomy, i.e. the surface anatomy of trunk, abdomen, and pelvis, followed by that of the gastrointestinal, urinary, and genital tract. Vascular, lymphatic, and neural distribution for surgery is well-explained. Neuro-anatomy related to endocrine aspects and the relevant areas of the fetal skull is also explained. The chapter on physiology deals with acid base balance followed by the physiology of the various organs. Physiology of foetal and placental tissues and changes in pregnancy are discussed.

Hormones influence the biochemistry of an individual. The chapter on biochemistry deals with the structure of cells and the issues related to the metabolism of carbohydrates, fats, and proteins.

Endocrinology is intrinsically linked to the field of obstetrics and gynaecology and it has been dealt with in detail, from sex hormones to hormones from the hypothalamus, pituitary, thyroid, and adrenal glands. The others that play a role, such as the renin-angiotension system, pancreatic hormones, and placental hormones in pregnancy, labour, puerperium, and lactation, are also dealt with in detail.

Inflammation, cellular adaption, cellular injury, wound healing, neoplasia, and issues relating to the body in general, such as coagulation, sepsis, and shock are dealt with in the chapter on pathology followed by specific issues related to the genital tract and disorders of pregnancy. Infection has a major role to play in gynaecological diseases.

Microbiology has been dealt with in four sections: bacteria, fungi, protozoa, and viruses. Therapeutics related to pregnancy and gynaecology are dealt with, including specific medication of analgesics, antibiotics, anti-fungals, anti-virals, and anti-malarial drugs. Specific drugs used in pregnancy such as uterotonics, anti-hypertensives, anti-epileptics, and anticoagulants are dealt with in detail. Contraceptives are unique to our field and are explained in detail.

Intrapartum care is an area of major dissatisfaction and medical litigation. A basic understanding of labour and intrapartum surveillance of the foetus is explained. It is important to understand the basic physics related to ultrasound, ionizing radiation, and non-ionizing radiation, for the clinician's practice and to provide explanations for patients if they have concerns about the use of this technology during pregnancy. Today's research is the clinical practice of tomorrow. The clinician should understand research methodology and the medical statistics used to interpret the results. This is lifelong learning for good practice and is discussed in the final chapter.

It is credit to the authors of this book that they have condensed this vast area of knowledge into what is necessary, leaving out non-essential reading. I would recommend this book to those preparing for the MRCOG part 1 and for practicing clinicians as it presents the knowledge that forms the basis of our clinical practice.

Sir Sabaratnam Arulkumaran
Professor & Head of Obstetrics & Gynaecology
St George's University of London
18.4.11

Preface

Never regard study as a duty, but as the enviable opportunity to learn ... for your own personal joy and to the profit of the community to which your later work belongs.

Albert Einstein, theoretical physicist (1879 –1955)

Learn, revise, practise; the triad of exam preparation. There are no shortcuts to knowledge and the principles for success in any exam are the same. Royal College membership examinations are no exception.

Most textbooks tend, by nature and out of necessity, to be verbose. Put simply, for one to understand a topic it needs to be explained. For revision purposes, however, it is necessary only for the key knowledge points to be present. This is where notes come in handy. Notes serve as a map of information that needs to be remembered. The effectiveness and quality of note-taking methods are highly variable. Inevitably some facts will not be identified during revision. This leads to lost points in the exam and can make the difference between passing and failing. This book offers a backbone for revision; 'the perfect notes that one would make if they had all the necessary information and time available to do so'. With the curriculum at its core (found at www.rcog.org.uk) it will provide you with a guide to your revision. It is a high yield revision book that includes the knowledge and facts needed to pass the MRCOG part 1 exam and brings together the required fundamentals of all the basic sciences. Nevertheless, we would encourage you to annotate and draw in the margins of the book, thus personalizing your 'revision notes' to suit your own needs and learning style. Effectively, we would like you to turn it in to your very own 'perfect' *aide memoire*.

The book aims to be 'user friendly', making the task of finding and revising information easy. There are sections covering each of the basic sciences required. Information is concise with facts presented in visually easy to remember formats, such as boxes, flow diagrams, figures, and lists. Every piece of information in the book can essentially be viewed as the equivalent of the answer to a potential exam question. The dimensions of the book have been chosen specifically to allow it to be carried easily, helping with revision even in the most unlikely places (such as a quiet on-call, in between patients in theatre, on the train, or even the sofa!). Knowledge of the basic scientific principles that underpin clinical conditions is a prerequisite to attaining true understanding of our specialty. To demonstrate the relevance and applicability of the basic science knowledge, interspersed throughout the text are cross-references to clinical practice that can be found in the next book of the series, *Training in Obstetrics and Gynaecology*. Although not necessary for the MRCOG part 1 exam, this aims to encourage readers to retain the knowledge they have strived to acquire. This holistic approach will help with the next stage: application of basic science to pathological processes, both in everyday clinical practice and for the more pragmatic goal of passing the MRCOG part 2 exam in the future.

Our vision was to produce the book that we wished we had when we were revising for the MRCOG part 1 exam. The team of authors has been especially assembled for the complementary strengths and expertise that each brings. Arisudhan has extensive experience as a candidate passing college membership exams (he holds MRCOG, MRCS and MRCGP qualifications, all of which require thorough basic science knowledge and a good exam technique). Ippokratis is the lead editor of the successful and award-winning Oxford University Press title *Training in Obstetrics and Gynaecology* and as such brings his experience in presenting information in a fresh and easy to assimilate manner. Austin has a keen interest and breadth of knowledge with regards to basic sciences relevant to obstetrics and gynaecology, and ran a popular and successful MRCOG part 1 course for some time. Along with co-authoring this work, he is also the editor of the upcoming larger Oxford University Press book *Basic Science in Obstetrics and Gynaecology*.

All of the authors love the specialty and we find particular interest in understanding and solving problems from basic principles. We hope we can pass on some of that enthusiasm through these pages. Although we aspired to deliver a faultless book, we appreciate that perfection is unattainable and subjective. Any mistakes found lie with us. We encourage and would greatly appreciate readers to write to us with any suggestions, corrections, and feedback for the future.

How to use this book

The book has a simple layout, with numbered and bulleted points, figures, boxes, and tables. Interspersed throughout the book you will find in the margin of the pages two types of cross-reference. The first one, denoted by the symbol ⊞ and followed by a chapter number, is a cross-reference to a chapter within this book. To avoid repetition, you are being directed to a chapter with information relevant to the section next to which the cross-referencing symbol lies. The second type of cross-reference, denoted by the symbol T. in Obs Gyn and followed by a chapter number, links the basic science information found in this book to clinical practice that can be found in the next book of the series, *Training in Obstetrics and Gynaecology*. Although this is not necessary information for the MRCOG part 1 exam, you might find it a useful link between basic sciences and clinical practice for your future career. Finally, this book contains a large amount of information and, as is inevitable in medicine, abbreviations. A complete list of these can be found at the front of the book, which will help refresh your memory if needed. We hope that you enjoy the book, and good luck with the exam!

Acknowledgements

We would like to thank Fiona Goodgame and Christopher Reid for believing in our vision and commissioning the book, Katy Loftus, Sian Jenkins, and Lotika Singha for tirelessly helping with the preparation and production of the manuscript, the reviewers for helping improve the final content, the countless corridor consultations with our colleagues and students, and finally our families and friends for their selfless encouragement and support.

Arisudhan, Ippokratis, Austin

Contents

List of abbreviations

1,25(OH)₂D₃ calcitriol/1,25-dihydroxycholecalciferol

17β-HSD 17β-hydroxysteroid dehydrogenase

1° primary

2,3-DPG 2,3-diphosphoglycerate

25(OH)D₃ 25-hydroxycholecalciferol

2° secondary

3° tertiary

5-HT receptors 5-hydroxytryptamine receptors

β-hCG β subunit of human chorionic gonadotropin

λ wavelength

μm micrometre

μg microgram

μGy microgray

μmol micromole

AA amino acid

Ab antibody

ACE angiotensin converting enzyme

ACEi angiotensin converting enzyme inhibitor

Acetyl CoA acetyl coenzyme A

Ach acetylcholine

ACTH adrenocorticotropic hormone

ADEK vitamins A, D, E, and K

ADH antidiuretic hormone

ADMA asymmetrical dimethylarginine

ADP adenosine diphosphate

AF atrial fibrillation

AFI amniotic fluid index

AFP α-fetoprotein

Ag antigen

AIDS acquired immune deficiency syndrome

ALP alkaline phosphatase

ANA antinuclear antibody

ANOVA analysis of variance

ANP atrial natriuretic peptide

ANS autonomic nervous system

APS antiphospholipid syndrome

APTT activated partial thromboplastin time

AR absolute risk

ARDS acute respiratory distress syndrome

ART antiretroviral therapy

ASD atrial septal defect

ASIS anterior superior iliac spine

ATP adenosine-5′-triphosphate

AV alveolar ventilation

AV atrioventricular

AVN atrioventricular node

b.d. *bis die* (two times a day)

BAD Bcl-2-associated death promoter

BₐHP arterial blood hydrostatic pressure

BCG Bacillus Calmette Guérin

Bcl-2 B-cell lymphoma 2

BHP blood hydrostatic pressure

BMD bone mineral density

BMI body mass index

BOP blood oncotic pressure

BP blood pressure

BPD biparietal diameter

BPH benign prostatic hypertrophy

bpm beats per minute

Bq becquerel

BRCA breast cancer

BV bacterial vaginosis

BᵥHP venous blood hydrostatic pressure

c carbon atom

C coulomb

c speed of sound

CA carbohydrate antigen

Ca²⁺ calcium ion

CAH congenital adrenal hyperplasia

CAIS complete androgen insensitivity syndrome

cAMP cyclic adenosine monophosphate

CARS	compensatory anti-inflammatory response	**DPG**	2,3-diphosphoglycerate
cat.	category	**DPP**	dipeptidyl peptidase-4
CBG	corticosteroid binding globulin	**DPPC**	dipalmitoylphosphatidylcholine
CCK	cholecystokinin	**DSV**	dead space volume
CEA	carcinoembryonic antigen	**DVT**	deep vein thrombosis
CF	cystic fibrosis		
CFTR	cystic fibrosis transmembrane conductance regulator	**e.g.**	*exempli gratia*
		E1	oestrone
CGIN	cervical glandular intraepithelial neoplasia	**E2**	oestradiol
		E3	oestriol
cGMP	cyclic guanosine monophosphate	**EBV**	Epstein–Barr virus
CI	confidence interval	**ECF**	extracellular fluid
Ci	curie	**ECG**	electrocardiogram/ electrocardiography
CIN	cervical intraepithelial neoplasia	**EDTA**	ethylenediaminetetraacetic acid
Cl⁻	chloride ion	**EDV**	end-diastolic volume
cmH₂O	centimeter of water	**EF**	ejection fraction
CMV	Cytomegalovirus	**EGF**	epidermal growth factor
CNS	central nervous system	**EHF**	extremely high frequency
CO	carbon monoxide	**ENA**	extractable nuclear antigens
CO	cardiac output	**eNOS**	endothelial nitric oxide synthase
CO₂	carbon dioxide	**EPO**	erythropoietin
COCP	combined oral contraceptive pill	**ER**	endoplasmic reticulum
COMT	catechol-O-methyl transferase	**ERV**	expiratory reserve volume
COX1	cyclo-oxygenase 1	**ESR**	erythrocyte sedimentation rate
COX2	cyclo-oxygenase 2	**ESV**	end-systolic volume
CPAP	continuous positive airway pressure		
		f	frequency
CRH	corticotrophin-releasing hormone	**Fab**	fragment antigen binding
CRL	crown–rump length	**FAD**	flavin adenine dinucleotide
CRP	C-reactive protein	**FADH₂**	reduced flavin adenine dinucleotide
CSCC	cholesterol side chain cleavage		
CSF	cerebrospinal fluid	**Fc**	fragment crystallizable region
CT	computed tomography	**FDA**	Food and Drug Administration
CTG	cardiotocography	**FDPs**	fibrin degradation products
CTPA	computed tomography pulmonary angiogram	**FEV₁**	forced expiratory volume in 1 s
		FFA	free fatty acids
CV	coefficient of variation	**FFP**	fresh frozen plasma
CVP	central venous pressure	**FGF**	fibroblast growth factor
CXR	Chest X-ray	**FGR**	fetal growth restriction
		FIL	feedback inhibitor of lactation
DAG	diacylglycerol	**FIGO**	Fédération Internationale de Gynécologie et d'Obstétrique
DCDA	dichorionic diamniotic		
DCT	distal convoluted tubule	**FN**	false negative
DDT	dichlorodiphenyltrichloroethane	**FNR**	false negative rate
DEET	N, N-diethyl-*meta*-toluamide	**FP**	false positive
DEXA	dual energy X-ray absorptiometry	**FPR**	false positive rate
DHEA	dehydroepiandrosterone	**FRC**	functional residual capacity
DHEAS	dehydroepiandrosterone sulphate	**FSH**	follicle stimulating hormone
DHT	dihydrotestosterone	**FTA-ABS**	fluorescent treponemal antibody-absorption
DI	diabetes insipidus		
DIC	disseminated intravascular coagulation	**FVC**	forced vital capacity
DIT	diiodotyrosine	**g**	gram
dL	decilitre	**G6PD**	glucose 6-phosphate dehydrogenase deficiency
DNA	deoxyribonucleic acid		

GABA	γ-aminobutyric acid	**I⁻**	Iodide ion
GBS	group B streptococcus	**i.e.**	*id est*
GDP	guanosine diphosphate	**i.m.**	intramuscular
GFR	glomerular filtration rate	**i.u.**	international units
GH	growth hormone	**i.v.**	intravenous
GHRH	growth-hormone-releasing hormone	**I₂**	iodine
GHz	giga hertz	**IC**	inspiratory capacity
GIP	gastric inhibitory peptide	**IFN**	interferon
GIT	gastrointestinal tract	**Ig**	immunoglobulin
GM-CSF	granulocyte-macrophage colony-stimulating factor	**IGF**	insulin-like growth factor
		IHC	immunohistochemistry
GnRH	gonadotrophin-releasing hormone	**IHP**	interstitial hydrostatic pressure
		IL	interleukin
GTP	guanosine-5′-triphosphate	**iNOS**	inflammatory nitric oxide synthase
Gy	gray	**IOP**	interstitial oncotic pressure
		IP	intrapleural pressure
h	hour(s)	**IP₃**	inositol triphosphate
H⁺	hydrogen ion	**IRR**	Ionising Radiation Regulations
H₂O	water	**IRV**	inspiratory reserve volume
H₂O₂	hydrogen peroxide	**ISA**	intrinsic sympathomimetic activity
HAART	highly active antiretroviral therapy	**ITP**	idiopathic thrombocytopenic purpura
Hb	haemoglobin	**IUCD**	intrauterine contraceptive device
HBcAg	hepatitis B core antigen	**IUS**	intrauterine system
HBeAg	hepatitis B e-antigen	**IVC**	inferior vena cava
HBsAg	hepatitis B surface antigen	**IVF**	*in vitro* fertilization
hCG	human chorionic gonadotropin	**IVU**	intravenous urogram
HCL	hydrochloric acid		
HCO₃⁻	bicarbonate ion	**K⁺**	potassium ion
H₂CO₃	carbonic acid	**kcal**	kilocalorie
HDL	high density lipoprotein	**kDa**	kilodalton
HDS	hydroxysteroid dehydrogenase	**kg**	kilogram
HELLP	haemolysis, elevated liver enzymes, low platelets	**KHz**	kilohertz
		KOH	potassium hydroxide
Hep	hepatitis virus	**kPa**	kilopascal
HER2	human epidermal growth factor receptor 2		
		l	length
HIV	human immunodeficiency virus	**L**	litre
HLA	human leucocyte antigen	**L**	lumbar vertebral level
HMG-CoA	3-hydroxy-3-methyl-glutaryl-coenzyme A	**LASER**	light amplification by stimulated emission of radiation
HNPCC	hereditary non-polyposis colorectal cancer	**LDH**	lactate dehydrogenase
		LDL	low-density lipoprotein
hPL	human placental lactogen	**LH**	luteinizing hormone
HPO₄²⁻	hydrogen phosphate anion	**LLETZ**	large loop excision of the transformation zone
HPV	human papillomavirus		
HR	heart rate	**LMWH**	low molecular weight heparin
HRT	hormone replacement therapy	**log₁₀**	logarithm with base 10
HSD	hydroxysteroid dehydrogenase	**LPS**	lipopolysaccharide
HSP	heat-shock protein	**LR**	likelihood ratio
HTLV	human T-cell lymphotrophic virus	**LSD**	lysergic acid diethylamide
HUS	haemolytic uraemic syndrome	**m²**	square metre
Hyper-PTH	hyperparathyroidism	**MAC**	membrane attack complex
Hz	hertz	**MAO**	monoamine oxidase

MAOI	monoamine oxidase inhibitor	**NNRTI**	non-nucleoside reverse
MAP	mean arterial pressure		transcriptase inhibitor
MCA	middle cerebral artery	**NNT**	Number needed to treat
MCDA	monochorionic diamniotic	**NO**	Nitric oxide
MCMA	monochorionic monoamniotic	**NOS**	Nitric oxide synthase
MEN	multiple endocrine neoplasia	**NPV**	Negative predictive value
mEq	milliequivalent	**NRTI**	Nucleoside reverse transcriptase
mg	milligram		inhibitor
Mg²⁺	magnesium ion	**NSAID**	Non-steroidal anti-inflammatory
mGy	milligray		drug
MHC	major histocompatibility complex	**NTD**	Neural tube defect
MHz	megahertz	**NtRTI**	Nucleotide reverse transcriptase
min	minute(s)		inhibitor
MIS	Mullerian inhibiting substance		
MIT	monoiodotyrosine	**O₂**	oxygen
mL	millilitre	**o.d.**	*omni die* (once a day)
mIU	milli-international unit	**OR**	odds ratio
mM	millimole	**Osm**	osmole
mm³	cubic millimetre		
mmHg	millimetres of mercury	**π**	mathematical constant pi
MODS	multiple organ dysfunction	**P**	pressure
	syndrome	**PA**	plasminogen activator
mol	mole	**PAI**	plasminogen activator inhibitor
MOSF	multiple organ system failure	**PAIS**	partial androgen insensitivity
mOsm	milliosmole		syndrome
MRI	magnetic resonance imaging	**PAP**	prostatic acid phosphatase
mRNA	messenger ribonucleic acid	**PBR**	peripheral benzodiazepine
MRSA	meticillin-resistant *Staphylococcus*		receptor
	aureus	**pCO₂**	partial pressure of carbon dioxide
ms⁻¹	metres per second	**PCOS**	polycystic ovary syndrome
MS	multiple sclerosis	**PCR**	polymerase chain reaction
MSH	melanocyte stimulating hormone	**PCT**	proximal convoluted tubule
mSv	milliSievert	**PDA**	patent ductus arteriosus
mV	millivolt	**PDGF**	platelet-derived growth factor
MV	minute ventilation	**PDS**	physiological dead space
		PE	pulmonary embolism
n	number of observations in a	**PEFR**	peak expiratory flow rate
	sample	**PET**	pre-eclampsia
N₂	nitrogen molecule	**PG**	prostaglandin
Na⁺	sodium ion	**PGD**	prostaglandin D
NAD⁺	nicotinamide adenine	**PGDH**	prostaglandin dehydrogenase
	dinucleotide	**PGE₂**	prostaglandin E₂
NADH	reduced nicotinamide adenine	**PGF₂**	prostaglandin F₂
	dinucleotide	**PGI₂**	prostacyclin
Nd : YAG	neodymium-doped yttrium	**pH**	negative logarithm (base 10) of
	aluminium garnet		hydrogen ion concentration
NEC	necrotizing enterocolitis	**PI**	protease inhibitor
NFP	net filtration pressure	**PID**	pelvic inflammatory disease
ng	nanogram	**PI**	pulsatility index
NH₃	ammonia	**pK**	negative logarithm (base 10) of
NH₄⁺	ammonium ion		an equilibrium constant K
NICE	National Institute for Health and	**PNS**	peripheral nervous system
	Clinical Excellence	**pO₂**	partial pressure of oxygen
NK	natural killer	**PO₄³⁻**	phosphate ion
nm	nanometers	**POMC**	pro-opiomelanocortin
NMDA	N-methyl-D-aspartic acid	**POP**	progesterone-only pill

PPAR	peroxisome proliferator-activated receptors	**SPRM**	selective progesterone receptor modulator
PPH	postpartum haemorrhage	**SROM**	spontaneous rupture of membranes
PPI	proton pump inhibitor		
PPV	positive predictive value	**SRY**	sex determining region Y
PSA	prostate-specific antigen	**SSRIs**	selective serotonin reuptake inhibitors
PT	partial thromboplastin time		
PTH	parathyroid hormone	**STAN**	ST analysis
PTHrP	parathyroid hormone-related peptide	**STAR**	steroidogenesis acute regulatory
		START	short-term antiretroviral therapy
PTT	partial thromboplastin time	**STEAR**	selective tissue oestrogenic activity regulator
PTU	propylthiouracil		
PVN	paraventricular nucleus	**Sv**	sievert
PVR	pulmonary vascular resistance	**SV**	stroke volume
		SVC	superior vena cava
Q	quartile	**SVR**	systemic vascular resistance
q.d.s.	*quater die sumendus* (four times a day)		
		t-PA	tissue-type plasminogen activator
		T	tension
r	radius	**T**	tesla
R	resistance	**T**	thoracic vertebral level
RBC	red blood cell	**t.d.s.**	*ter die sumendum* (three times a day)
RDS	respiratory distress syndrome		
rem	roentgen equivalent man	T_3	triiodothyronine
RI	resistance index	T_4	tetraiodothyronine/thyroxine
RNA	ribonucleic acid	**TAG**	triacylglycerol/triglyceride
ROC	receiver operator characteristic	**TB**	tuberculosis
RPF	renal plasma flow	**TBG**	thyroid-binding globulin
RPR	rapid plasma reagin	**TCA**	tricarboxylic acid cycle
RR	relative risk	**TD**	tidal volume
RR	respiratory rate	**TGF**	transforming growth factor
rRNA	ribosomal ribonucleic acid	**Th-1**	T-cell helper 1
rT3	reverse triiodothyronine	**Th-2**	T-cell helper 2
RV	residual volume	**TIBC**	total iron-binding capacity
		TLV	total lung volume
s	second(s)	**TN**	true negative
S	sacral vertebral level	**TNF**	tumour necrosis factor
σ	standard deviation	**TNR**	true negative rate
SAH	subarachnoid haemorrhage	**TP**	true positive
SAN	sinoatrial node	**TPHA**	*Treponema pallidum* haemagglutination assay
SD	Standard deviation		
SE	standard error of the mean	**TPPA**	*Treponema pallidum* particle agglutination assay
SERM	selective oestrogen receptor modulator		
		TPR	true positive rate
SHBG	sex hormone-binding globulin	**TRAP**	tartrate reabsorption alkaline phosphatase
SI	Système international d'unités (International system of units)	**TRH**	thyrotrophin-releasing hormone
SIADH	syndrome of inappropriate antidiuretic hormone hypersecretion	**tRNA**	transfer ribonucleic acid
		TRPV6	transient receptor potential cation channel, subfamily v, member 6
SIRS	systemic inflammatory response syndrome		
		TSC	tuberous sclerosis complex
SLE	systemic lupus erythematosus	**TSH**	thyroid-stimulating hormone
SNS	somatic nervous system	**TTP**	thrombotic thrombocytopenic purpura
SOD	superoxidase dismutase		

TTTS	twin-to-twin transfusion syndrome	**VIN**	vulval intraepithelial neoplasia
TV	tidal volume	**VIP**	vasoactive intestinal peptide
		VMA	vanillylmandelic acid
UA	umbilical artery	**VSD**	ventricular septal defect
UHF	ultrahigh frequency	**vWF**	von Willebrand factor
ULGLs	uterine large granulolymphocytes	**VZIg**	varicella zoster immune globulin
UO	urine output	**VZV**	varicella zoster virus
UTI	urinary tract infection		
UV	ultraviolet	**W**	watts
		Wb	weber
V/Q scan	ventilation/perfusion scan	**WBC**	white blood cell
VC	vital capacity		mean
Vd	volume of distribution		
VDRL	Venereal Disease Research Laboratory (test)	**x**	observation
VEGF	vascular endothelial growth factor	$\bar{x}$	mean
		YST	yolk sac tumour

Genetics

Molecular biology

1. Nucleotides
   - Made up of
     i. A sugar molecule
     ii. A nitrogenous base
     iii. A phosphate group
   - Sugar molecule
     i. Composed of 5 carbon atoms in a circular structure forming a pentose ring
        - Deoxyribose in DNA
        - Ribose in RNA
     ii. Base is attached to carbon-1
     iii. Phosphate is attached to carbon-5
   - Nitrogenous base: there are 2 types (*Box 1.1*)
     i. Purines
     ii. Pyrimidines
   - Base pairs
     i. C and G (3 hydrogen bonds)
     ii. A and T/U (2 hydrogen bonds)

Box 1.1 Types of nitrogenous base

Purines	Pyrimidines
• Guanine – G • Adenine – A	• Cytosine – C • Thymine – T (only in DNA) • Uracil – U (only in RNA)

2. Nucleic acids
   - Long polymers of nucleotides
   - Two types – DNA and RNA

- DNA
  - i.   Double-stranded helix held together by hydrogen bond
  - ii. Strands associate into pairs and run in opposite directions (anti-parallel)
  - iii. The sugar is deoxyribose and the pyrimidine is thymine
  - iv. DNA bond = phosphodiesterase ($5' \rightarrow 3'$)
  - v.   Replication involves
    - Unwinding of double-stranded DNA by DNA helicase, resulting in the formation of 2 DNA strands
    - Copying of DNA by DNA polymerase, using one strand as a template
    - Winding back of the DNA strands by DNA ligase, when temperature drops (annealing)
- RNA
  - i.   3 types
    - mRNA = involved in transcription
    - rRNA (ribosomal)
    - tRNA (transfer) = involved in translation
  - ii. The sugar is ribose and the pyrimidine is uracil

3. **Codons**
   - Is genetic code
   - Is made of RNA
   - Consists of 3 sequential nucleotides
   - Is degenerate (i.e. more than 1 codon can specify the same amino acid but no codon specifies more than 1 amino acid)
   - Total possible number of codons is 64 (because DNA contains 4 nucleotides)

4. **Genes**
   - Are a stretch of nucleotides that code for a polypeptide
   - Determine the amino acid sequence and therefore the function of a protein
   - Represent an inherited unit of information
   - Are made up of 2 regions
     - i.   Exons (coding area)
       - They code for the protein that the gene encodes
       - The exon sequence is highly conserved between individuals
     - ii. Introns (non-coding areas)
       - Length outweighs that of exons
       - Not well conserved between individuals
       - Spliced out during processing to mRNA

5. **Chromosomes**
   - Contained in nuclei
   - They are linear strands of DNA that contain genes, regulatory elements, and nucleotide sequences
   - Are 'H' shaped consisting of 2 identical parts called chromatids held together by a centromere (**Fig. 1.1**)
   - There are 22 homologous autosomal pairs and 1 pair of sex chromosomes
   - Size
     - i.   Largest = chromosome 1
     - ii. Smallest = chromosome 22
   - Detected at metaphase
     - i.   Identified by Giemsa staining
     - ii. Colchicine inhibits spindle formation
     - iii. EDTA inhibits deoxyribonuclease

- Structure
  - i. Arms
    - Short = p
    - Long = q
  - ii. Centromeres = the region where the two identical sister chromatids come in contact
- Based on the position of the centromere, the following types of chromosomes have been described
  - i. Metacentric (i.e. the 2 arms of the chromosome are equal in length)
  - ii. Submetacentric
  - iii. Acrocentric
  - iv. Telocentric (do not exist in humans)
  - v. Holocentric (do not exist in humans)
- Can be classified into 7 groups (**Box 1.2**)

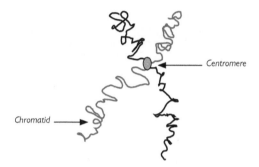

Figure 1.1 Structure of a chromosome

Box 1.2 Human chromosome groups

1–3	4–5	6–12 and X	13–15
• Large • Metacentric	• Large • Submetacentric	• Medium • Submetacentrics	• Medium • Acrocentric

16–18	19–20	21–22 and Y	
• Short • Submetacentric	• Short • Metacentric	• Very short • Acrocentric	

6. **Protein synthesis**
   - DNA is **transcribed** to mRNA (messenger RNA)
     - i. By RNA polymerase
     - ii. DNA strand is read in the $3' \rightarrow 5'$ direction, mRNA is transcribed in the $5' \rightarrow 3'$ direction
   - mRNA is **translated** to amino acids
   - Requires ribosomes

7. **Polymerase chain reaction**
   - PCR amplifies selected areas in a DNA strand
   - Does not work on RNA (would need to be converted to DNA first by the reverse transcriptase enzyme)
   - Needs 3 components
     - i. 2 primers

    ii. 4 deoxynucleotides

    iii. **Taq** polymerase
- Logarithmic amplification

8. **Blotting**
   - Northern = RNA
   - Southern = DNA
   - Western = Protein
     i. Requires protein antibodies

9. **Proteomics**
   - Is the qualitative and quantitative comparison of proteins under different conditions to further unravel biological processes
   - Involves separation using 2-dimensional gel electrophoresis (**Box 1.3**)

Box 1.3 Dimensions of gel electrophoresis

1st Dimension	2nd Dimension
• Based on isoelectric point • Voltage is applied along pH gradient	• Based on size • Voltage is applied perpendicular to the original

Cellular division and replication

1. **Cell cycle**
   - Is a series of events in a cell that lead to its division and replication
   - Has four phases (**Fig. 1.2**)
   - Interphase
     i. Is part of cell cycle consisting of 3 phases (G1, G2, and S)
     ii. Is not a phase in mitosis
   - Chromosome replication occurs only during S phase
     i. Diploid = cells with pairs of homologous chromosomes
     ii. Haploid = contains one member of each homologous pair of chromosomes
   - Proliferation genes
     i. c-Myc
     ii. c-Jun
   - Inhibiting gene
     i. p53

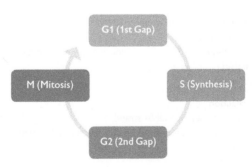

Figure 1.2 Cell cycle phases

2. **Stem cells**
   - Characterized by
     i. Capacity for self-renewal over a prolonged period of time
     ii. Potency
   - Potency is the capacity to differentiate into specialized cell types (**Fig. 1.3**)
   - Totipotent cells can differentiate into extra-embryonic and embryonic cell types

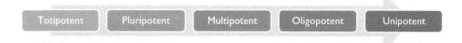

Figure 1.3 Stem cell lineage

3. **Mitosis**
   - Is the process of cell division that results in the production of 2 identical daughter cells from a single parent cell
   - Involves
     i. Nuclear division
     ii. Cytokinesis
   - Occurs exclusively in eukaryotic cells
   - Consists of 4 stages (**Fig. 1.4**)

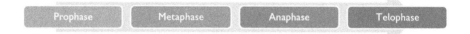

Figure 1.4 Stages of mitosis

   - Prophase
     i. Chromatins condense
     ii. Centrosomes present close to nucleus
     iii. A centrosome consists of a pair of centrioles
   - Metaphase
     i. Nuclei disappear
     ii. Nuclear membrane disintegrate
     iii. Centrioles migrate to both poles
     iv. Mitotic spindles form
     v. Chromosomes align at metaphase plate
   - Anaphase
     i. Kinetochore microtubules shorten separating the chromatids
     ii. Kinetochore is the point on the chromosome where the mitotic spindles attach
   - Telophase
     i. Chromosomes decondense
     ii. Reformation of nuclear membranes
     iii. Mitosis spindles disappear
     iv. Is followed by cytokinesis

4. **Meiosis**
   - Is a type of cell division in which
     i. Germ cells are produced
     ii. 4 haploid daughter cells are produced from a single diploid parent cell

- Involves
  i. Reduction in genetic material
  ii. 2 successive nuclear divisions
- Consist of 2 stages (each stage has 4 phases)
  i. Meiosis 1 – separates homologous chromosomes producing 2 haploid cells
  ii. Meiosis 2 – is similar to **mitosis**
- Meiosis 1 is a reductional division consisting of 4 phases (*Fig. 1.5*)

Prophase 1	Metaphase 1	Anaphase 1	Telophase 1

Figure 1.5 Stages of meiosis 1

- Prophase 1 involves (*Fig. 1.6*)
  i.   Pairing of homologous chromosomes (paired homologous chromosomes are called bivalent)
  ii. Crossing over of chromatids occur at chiasmata
  iii. Migration of centrosome to both poles of the cell
  iv. 3 phases
- Metaphase 1 – Homologous chromosome pairs align at metaphase plate
- Anaphase 1 – Kinetochore microtubules shorten, separating the homologous chromosomes

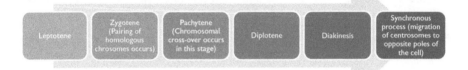

Figure 1.6 Stages of prophase 1

5. **Genetic transfer is based on mendelian inheritance**
   - Derived by Gregor Mendel
   - Mendel's Law has 2 principles
     i. Law of segregation – states that each gamete receives only 1 allele for each gene
     ii. Law of independent assortment – states that alleles of different genes assort independently of one another during gametogenesis
   - 4 models of inheritance
     i.   Autosomal dominant
     ii. Autosomal recessive
     iii. X-linked dominant
     iv. X-linked recessive
     v.   Mitochondrial

Chromosomal abnormalities

Classification of chromosomal abnormalities

1. **There are 2 types of chromosomal abnormalities**

- Aneuploidy = change in number of chromosomes
  i.   Down's syndrome (trisomy 21)
  ii. Edwards' syndrome (trisomy 18)
  iii. Patau's syndrome (trisomy 13)
  iv. Turner's syndrome (monosomy X)
- Structural
  i.   Translocation
  ii. Inversion
  iii. Deletion (forms ring chromosomes)
  iv. Duplication
  v.   Insertion

2. **Mosaics is the presence of 2 or more genetically different cell lines derived from a single zygote**

Examples of aneuploidies

1. **Trisomies – general facts**
   - Due to
     i.   Non-disjunction at meiosis 1 (>70%)
     ii. Non-disjunction at meiosis 2
     iii. Mosaicism (<5%)
   - Increases with maternal age
   - The greater the number of extra chromosomes the greater the probability of learning disabilities if the individual survives

2. **Down's syndrome**
   - Trisomy 21
   - Prevalence is 1 : 700 live births (the incidence is higher at conception; 80% undergo spontaneous pregnancy loss)
   - Due to
     i.   Primary trisomy 21 (accounts for 95% of non-dysjunction at meiosis in maternal (85%) & paternal (15%) cell line)
     ii. Robertsonian translocation of chromosomes 14 : 21 (3%)
     iii. Mosaicism (1%)
   - Features
     i.   Raised nuchal translucency
     ii. Dysmorphic features (small ears, upslanting palpebral fissures, flat facial profile, brachycephaly)
     iii. Hypotonia
     iv. Cardiac abnormalities – arteriovenous (AV) canal defect
     v.   Gastrointestinal tract (GIT) abnormalities
       - Duodenal atresia
       - Imperforate anus
       - Hirschsprung's disease
     vi. Conductive hearing loss
   - Increased risk of
     i.   Alzheimer's disease
     ii. Acute myeloid leukaemia/acute lymphoblastic leukaemia
     iii. Hypothyroidism
   - Maternal age risk for Down's syndrome
     i.   25 years old = 1 : 1500
     ii. 30 years old = 1 : 900
     iii. 35 years old = 1 : 350
     iv. 40 years old = 1 : 100

T. in
Obs
Gyn
Chpt 6.12

   v. 45 years old = 1 : 30

   iii. 50 years old = 1 : 11

   iv. Cut-off for invasive screening = 1 : 250

3. **Edwards' syndrome**
   - Trisomy 18
   - Prevalence is 1 : 3000 live births with a male to female ratio of 1 : 2
   - Features
     i. Increased nuchal translucency
     ii. Musculoskeletal defects
        - Limb defects
        - Rockerbottom feet (convex bottom of foot with projecting heel)
        - Overlapping fingers
     iii. Facial defects
        - Micrognathia
        - Cleft lip
        - Cleft palate
     iv. Cardiac defects
        - Ventricular septal defect (VSD)
        - Atrial septal defect (ASD)
        - Patent ductus arteriosus (PDA)
     v. Abdominal defects
        - Exomphalos
        - Inguinal hernia
        - Diaphragmatic hernia
        - Renal malformations
     vi. Intrauterine growth restriction
   - Mortality rates
     i. By 1 month = 30%
     ii. By 2 months = 50%
     iii. By 1 year = 90%

4. **Patau's syndrome**
   - Trisomy 13
   - Prevalence is 1 : 5000 live births
   - Incidence increases with maternal age
   - Features
     i. Midline defects
        - Hypotelorism (abnormally decreased distance between the eyes)
        - Holoprosencephaly (failure of the prosencephalon to develop into 2 hemispheres)
        - Cleft lip
        - Cleft palate
        - Scalp defects
     ii. Post axial polydactyly
     iii. Congenital heart defects
     iv. Renal abnormalities
     v. Omphalocele
     vi. Intrauterine fetal growth restriction
   - Mortality rates is almost 100% by 1 month of age

5. **Sex chromosome aneuploidies**
   - Incidence in
     i. Males = 1 : 400
     ii. Females = 1 : 600

- Includes
    i. Klinefelter's syndrome (47, XXY)
    ii. Turner's syndrome (45, X0)

6. **Lyon's hypothesis**
    - Barr body
        i. Is inactivated X chromosome
        ii. Present if >2 X chromosomes in a cell
    - Inactivation of 1 X chromosome occurs in females at 15–16 days gestation

T. in
Obs
Gyn

Chpt 2.7

7. **Turner's syndrome**
    - Monosomy 45, X0
    - Prevalence = 1 : 2500 female live births
    - Features
        i. Raised nuchal translucency
        ii. Cystic hygroma
        iii. Lymphoedema
        iv. Neck webbing
        v. Short stature
        vi. Wide carrying angle of arm
        vii. Shield shaped chest with widely spaced nipples
        viii. Coarctation of aorta
        ix. Gonadaldysgenesis
        x. Renal anomalies including horseshoe kidney
    - Intellectually normal
    - Risk of gonadoblastoma

8. **Klinefelter's syndrome**
    - 47, XXY
    - Incidence = 1 : 1000 live births
    - Features
        i. Tall
        ii. Small testes with hypogonadotrophic hypogonadism
        iii. Infertility

Examples of structural chromosome abnormalities

1. **Translocation**
    - Is the exchange of 2 segments of chromosome between non-homologous chromosomes
    - 2 types
        i. Balanced (an even exchange of material with no excess or loss of genetic material)
        ii. Unbalanced (unequal exchange of genetic material resulting in extra or missing genes)
    - Robertsonian translocation results from fusion of the long arms of 2 acrocentric chromosomes

2. **Deletion (Box 1.4)**

Box 1.4 Examples of syndromes due to structural chromosomal abnormalities caused by deletion

Velocardiofacial (DiGeorge) 22q11	Angelman 15q11-13 Maternal deletion	Prader–Willi 15q11-13 Paternal deletion
• Immune deficiency • Parathyroid dysfunction causing hypocalcaemia • Autism • Congenital heart disease • Cleft lip ± palate	• Happy disposition • Macroglossia • Ataxia • Seizures • Learning difficulties	• Obese • Hypogonadism • Hypotonia

Genetic disorders

Types of genetic disorders

1. **Genetic disorders consist of 3 types**
   - Autosomal
     - i.   Autosomal dominant
     - ii. Autosomal recessive
   - Sex linked
   - Mitochondrial

2. **Autosomal dominant**
   - Males and females affected equally
   - Inheritance = 1 : 2
   - New mutations are common
   - Has features of variable expressivity and reduced penetrance
   - Include
     - i.   Myotonic dystrophy
     - ii.   Huntington's chorea
     - iii. Achondroplasia
     - iv.   Neurofibromatosis types 1 and 2
     - v.   Tuberous sclerosis
     - vi.   Familial polyposis coli
     - vii. Marfan's syndrome
     - viii. Osteogenesis imperfecta
     - ix.   Polycystic kidney disease
     - x.   Porphyria
     - xi.   von Willebrand's disease

3. **Autosomal recessive**
   - Both parents must be carriers
   - Inheritance = 1 : 4
   - It is not possible to trace autosomal recessive conditions via the family tree
   - Includes
     - i.   Cystic fibrosis (CF)
     - ii.   Sickle cell disease
     - iii. Thalassaemia
     - iv.   Phenylketonuria
     - v.   Glycogen storage disorders
     - vi.   Congenital adrenal hyperplasia
     - vii. Wilson's disease

4. **X-linked recessive**
   - Inheritance = 1 : 2 sons of carrier females
   - Daughters of all affected males are carriers
   - No male to male transmission
   - Shows a knight's move pattern of transmission (i.e. any male grandchildren of affected male would be at risk)
   - Includes
     - i.   Duchenne muscular dystrophy
     - ii.   Fragile X syndrome
     - iii. Red-green colour blindness
     - iv.   Glucose 6-phosphate dehydrogenase (G6PD) deficiency

     v. Christmas disease (factor XI deficiency)
     vi. Haemophilia A & B (factor VIII & IX deficiency)
     vii. Neurogenic diabetes insipidus
     viii. Lesch–Nyhan syndrome
     ix. Wiskott–Aldrich syndrome
     x. Agammaglobulinaemia

5. **X-linked dominant**
   - Inheritance = 1 : 2 offspring of affected females
   - Often manifest very severely in males, frequently leading to spontaneous loss or neonatal death of affected male pregnancies
   - Includes
     i. Incontinentia pigmenti
     ii. Rett syndrome
     iii. Vitamin D resistance rickets

6. **Mitochondrial**
   - Mitochondrial DNA is inherited through the maternal line because sperm do not contribute to the zygote beyond their nuclear DNA
   - A mitochondrially inherited condition can affect both sexes but is only passed on by affected mothers
   - Includes
     i. Leber's hereditary optic neuropathy
     ii. Leigh's syndrome

Examples of genetic disorders

1. **Tuberous sclerosis**
   - Is a rare multisystem genetic disease that causes tumours to grow in the brain and other vital organs
   - Is caused by mutation of either
     i. *TSC1* gene (encodes for protein hamartin) – located on chromosome 9
     ii. *TSC2* gene (encodes for the protein tuberin) – located on chromosome 16
   - Hamartin and tuberin are suppressors of tumour growth
   - Features
     i. Learning difficulties
     ii. Epilepsy
     iii. Cardiac rhabdomyomas
     iv. Renal angiomyolipomas
     v. Skin manifestations
       - Angiofibromas (rash manifesting in 'butterfly' distribution over nose, nasolabial folds, and cheeks)
       - Hypomelanotic macules ('ash-leaf' spots)
       - Shagreen patches (discoloured leathery patches of skin)
       - Ungual fibromas
     vi. Brain abnormalities
       - Subependymal nodules
       - Cortical tubers

2. **Cystic fibrosis**
   - Is a disease of exocrine secretion
   - Increased chloride in sweat
   - Prevalence is 1 : 2000
   - Carrier rate in Caucasians = 1 : 23

- Is caused by a mutation in the *CFTR* (cystic fibrosis transmembrane conductance regulator) gene
- *CFTR* gene
  i.   Is located on chromosome 7
  ii. Produces a chloride ion protein, which is responsible for anion transport
  iii. There are over 1400 mutations that can affect the *CFTR* gene
  iv. Most common mutation of *CFTR* gene is ΔF508 occurring in 70% of cases
- Chloride ion channel regulates the movement of chloride ions from inside to outside of the cell except in the sweat ducts, where it facilitates chloride movement from sweat to cytoplasm
- Hallmark of CF is viscid (excessive) mucus production, which blocks the ducts of mucus-secreting organs leading to
  i.   Recurrent chest infections
  ii.   Poor alveolar gas exchange
  iii. Infertility
  iv.   Pancreatitis
  v.   Cirrhosis
  vi.   Intestinal obstruction
  vii. Malabsorption (require supplementation with the fat soluble ADEK vitamins)
  viii. Osteoporosis
  ix.   Diabetes
- Infertility is due to
  i.   Congenital absence of vas deferens in males
  ii. Thickened cervical mucus in females

3. **Sickle cell disease (HbS)**

Chpt 7.22

- Is caused by a point mutation in the β-globin chain of haemoglobin
- Is due to a single base change (adenine (GAG) is substituted with thymine (GTG)) causing glutamic acid to be replaced by valine
  i.   Glutamic acid is hydrophilic
  ii. Valine is hydrophobic
- Prevalence in London = 1 : 500
- Two types
  i.   Homozygous = HbSS
  ii. Heterozygous = HbAS
- Causes loss of red blood cell due to loss of (RBC) elasticity and sickling
- Disruption of RBC membrane causes short life span of RBC (10–20 days)
- Anaemia is caused by haemolysis of RBC by spleen (rate of haemolysis > rate of RBC production)
- Complications (**Box 1.5**)
- Types of sickle crisis
  i.   Vaso-occlusive crisis
  ii.   Acute chest syndrome (fever, chest pain, difficulty breathing, and pulmonary infiltrates on chest radiograph (CXR))
  iii. Aplastic crisis (triggered by parvovirus B19)
  iv.   Splenic sequestration crisis
  v.   Haemolytic crisis (common in patients with coexisting G6PD deficiency)
- Blood film shows sickling of RBCs and may show features of hyposplenism (codocytes and Howell–Jolly bodies)
- Treatment
  i.   Cyanate (irreversibly inhibits sickling of RBCs)
  ii.   Hydroxyurea (reactivates fetal haemoglobin production)
  iii. Analgesics

iv. Penicillin

v. Vaccinate for encapsulated organisms (*Haemophilus influenza, Streptococcus pneumoniae, and Neisseria meningitides*)

vi. Blood transfusion and exchange transfusion

vii. Bone marrow transplant

Box 1.5 Complications of sickle cell disease

Infarction	Emboli	Ischaemia	Haemolysis
• Hyposplenism • Autosplenectomy	• Stroke • Pulmonary hypertension	• Avascular necrosis of head of femur • Chronic renal failure	• Jaundice • Cholelithiasis

Infection	In pregnancy
• Osteomyelitis • Overwhelming post-splenectomy infection	• Fetal growth restriction (FGR) • Pre-eclampsia • Miscarriage

Chpt 7.21

4. **Thalassaemia**
   - Results in reduced rate of synthesis of 1 of the globin chains that make haemoglobin (Hb)
   - Types
      i. α – production of α chain affected
      ii. β – production of β chain affected
      iii. δ – production of δ chain affected
      iv. E thalassaemia (similar to β thalassaemia)
      v. S thalassaemia (similar to sickle cell anaemia)
      vi. C thalassaemia
   - Prevalent in
      i. Mediterranean
      ii. Arab
      iii. Maldives – has the highest incidence of thalassaemia in the world
   - Haematological consequences (anaemia) in thalassaemia is due to
      i. Hypochromia (i.e. low intracellular haemoglobin)
      ii. Excess of unimpaired chain – leads to cell membrane damage and reduced RBC survival time
   - RBC morphological abnormalities on blood film include
      i. Anisocytosis
      ii. Poikilocytosis
      iii. Microcytosis
      iv. Hypochromia
      v. Target cells
      vi. Basophilic stippling
      vii. Fragmented RBCs

5. **α-thalassaemia**
   - Severity depends on the number of α-globin gene affected (there are 4)
      i. Silent carrier (1 gene affected)
      ii. Trait (2 genes affected) – associated with mild hypochromic anaemia
      iii. Haemoglobin H disease (3 genes affected) – leads to moderate anaemia with splenomegaly

      iv. Bart's hydrops (4 genes affected) – causes *in utero* death
- Clinical features include
  - i. Tissue hypoxia
  - ii. Hydrops fetalis
- In fetus
  - i. Initial survival is due to haemoglobin Portland
  - ii. Fetal distress is noted after 12 weeks when haemoglobin Portland is replaced by haemoglobin Barts
- Haemoglobin H and Barts have an extreme high affinity for oxygen and thus inhibit delivery of oxygen to tissues

6. **β-thalassaemia**
   - Prevalence in
     - i. UK = 1 : 10 000
     - ii. South Asia = 3 : 100
     - iii. Cyprus = 1 : 7
   - Has 3 classifications
     - i. Major = genetically homozygous for β-thalassaemia gene
     - ii. Minor/trait = genetically heterozygous
     - iii. Intermedia = genetically heterozygous
   - Clinical features include
     - i. Fatigue
     - ii. Anaemia
     - iii. Jaundice
     - iv. Shortness of breath
     - v. Skeletal deformities due to increased erythropoiesis
     - vi. Hepatosplenomegaly due to extramedullary haematopoiesis
     - vii. Haemochromatosis due to excess iron absorption from the gut
     - viii. Delayed physical and sexual development due to haemochromatosis
   - Infants born with β-thalassaemia will usually presents with symptoms from 6 months of age when fetal haemoglobin is replaced by adult haemoglobin
   - Treatment for β-thalassaemia major
     - i. Regular blood transfusion
     - ii. Folic acid supplementation
     - iii. Vitamin D and calcium supplementation
     - iv. Chelation therapy (desferrioxamine) to remove excess iron from the body following repeat transfusions
     - v. Splenectomy
     - vi. Bone marrow transplant
     - vii. Cord blood transfusion

Embryology

Embryogenesis

1. **Definitions**
   - Zygote is a fertilized ovum
   - Embryo = 2–8 weeks following fertilization
   - Fetus = 9 weeks to term

2. **Chronology post fertilization**
   - Fertilization
     - i. Occurs at the ampulla of the fallopian tube
     - ii. Occurs 12 hours post ovulation
   - Second meiotic division is complete following fertilization
   - First mitotic division is complete at 30 hours post fertilization

Chpt 1

3. **Chronology in the 1st week of life (*Fig. 2.1*)**
   - Day 2 – zygote (2 cell) stage
   - Day 3
     - i. Morula (16 cell) stage
     - ii. Reaches uterine cornu
   - Day 4
     - i. Blastocyst stage
     - ii. Enters uterine cavity
   - Day 6 – implantation begins

4. **Blastocyst**
   - Is composed of
     - i. An inner cell mass (known as embryoblast) – which later forms the embryonic tissues
     - ii. An outer layer of cells (known as trophoblast) – which later forms the extra-embryonic tissues, e.g. placenta

- Comprises 70–100 cells
- Has a fluid-filled cavity known as blastocoele
- Prior to gastrulation the trophoblast differentiates into 2 cell lineages
  - i. An outer syncytium (also known as syncytiotrophoblast)
  - ii. An inner layer of cytotrophoblast

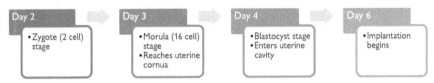

Figure 2.1 Chronology of fetal development in the 1st week of life

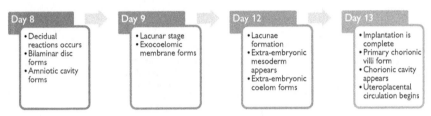

Figure 2.2 Chronology of fetal development in the 2nd week of life

5. **2nd week of development** (*Fig. 2.2*)
   - Day 8
     - i.   Decidual reaction occurs
     - ii. Implantation initiates decidualization of the endometrial stroma
     - iii. Formation of embryonic bilaminar disc
     - iv. Amniotic cavity develops within the epiblast
   - Bilaminar disc is derived from the inner cell mass (embryoblast) and is composed of
     - i. Epiblast (i.e. the dorsal germinal layer)
     - ii. Hypoblast (i.e. the ventral germinal layer)
   - Day 9
     - i. Lacunar stage begins
     - ii. Hypoblast forms the exocoelomic (Heuser's) membrane that lines the yolk sac
   - Day 12
     - i.   Formation of lacunae in syncytiotrophoblast, which communicate with endometrial sinusoids
     - ii. Extra-embryonic mesoderm (derived from yolk sac cells) forms
     - iii. Extra-embryonic coelom forms
       - Also known as chorionic cavity
       - Formed by lacunae which appear within the extra-embryonic mesoderm (between the exocoelomic membrane and cytotrophoblast) that merge
   - Day 13
     - i.   Implantation complete
     - ii. Cytotrophoblast forms primary chorionic villi
     - iii. Yolk sac is called the secondary yolk sac due to the presence of the chorionic cavity
     - iv. Syncytiotrophoblast secretes hCG
     - v.   Uteroplacental circulation begins

- Connecting stalk
  i. Connects embryo to cytotrophoblast
  ii. Derived from extra-embryonic mesoderm
  iii. Is the forerunner of the umbilical cord

6. **3rd week of development (*Fig. 2.3*)**
   - Day 15
     i. Primitive streak appears at the caudal end
     ii. Primitive node appears at the cephalic end of the streak
     iii. Ectodermal cells migrate towards the streak and then detach from it, spreading out laterally and beneath it to form the intra-embryonic mesoderm
   - Intra-embryonic mesoderm lies between the ectoderm and endoderm, except in two locations where the ectoderm meets the endoderm
     i. Prochordal plate (buccopharyngeal membrane)
     ii. Cloacal plate
   - Buccopharyngeal membrane breaks down at 4th week
   - Cloacal membrane breaks down at 7th week
   - Notochord formation
     i. Cells from primitive node migrate cranially towards prochordal plate
     ii. This forms the notochordal plate which becomes the future notochord
   - Day 16
     i. Allantois (allantoenteric diverticulum) appears
     ii. Allantois is the diverticulum that forms from the posterior wall of the yolk sac and extends into the connecting stalk
   - Neurulation
     i. Process of formation of brain and spinal cord
     ii. Neural plate is formed at day 18
   - Primitive heart tube forms at day 20
   - First heart beat is noted at day 21

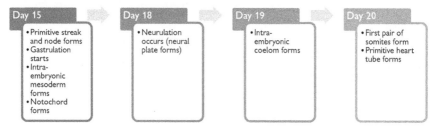

Figure 2.3 Chronology of fetal development in the 3rd week of life

7. **Gastrulation**
   - Is the formation of the 3 germ layers
   - Occurs in the 3rd week of development
   - Ectoderm gives rise to intra-embryonic mesoderm
   - Components derived from the ectoderm, mesoderm, and endoderm are listed in **Box 2.1**

8. **Embryo folding**
   - Occurs in 2 planes
     i. Longitudinal (due to enlargement of cranial end)
     ii. Transverse (due to enlargement of somites)
   - Occurs from day 21–24

Box 2.1 Components derived from the ectoderm, mesoderm, and endoderm

Ectoderm	Mesoderm	Endoderm
• Epidermis • Nervous system	• Muscles • Skeletal system • Connective tissues	• GIT • Respiratory tract • Endocrine glands • Auditory system • Urinary system

9. **Fetal development from week 4 to 7 (*Fig. 2.4*)**

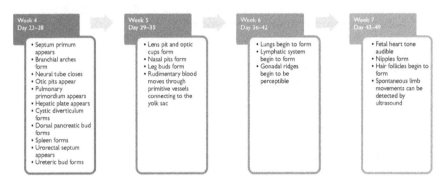

Figure 2.4 Chronology of fetal development from week 4 to 7

10. **Fetal development from week 7 to 20 (*Fig. 2.5*)**

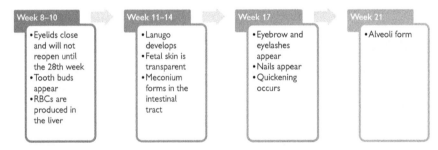

Figure 2.5 Chronology of fetal development from week 7 to 20

11. **Fetal development from week 25 to 37 (*Fig. 2.6*)**

Mesoderm

1. **Mesoderm has 3 parts (*Box 2.2*)**

2. **Somites**
   - Are rounded elevations of paraxial mesoderm which appear on either side of the neural tube under the surface ectoderm on the dorsal aspect of the embryo from base of skull to tail region
   - First pair appears at day 20
   - Develop at a rate of 3 pairs/day

- Maximum number is 42–44 pairs
- Consist of
    i. Dermomyotomes (form connective tissue and muscles)
    ii. Sclerotomes (form bones)

3. **Lateral plate mesoderm**
    - Is continuous with extra-embryonic mesoderm
    - Gives rise to
        i. Somatic mesoderm (lines the amnion)
        ii. Splanchnic mesoderm (lines the yolk sac)

4. **Intra-embryonic coelom**
    - Is formed on day 19
    - Is formed from merging of the clefts within the lateral plate
    - Is continuous with extra-embryonic coelom
    - Is the forerunner of the serous cavities

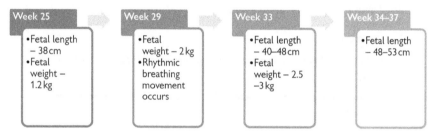

Week 25	Week 29	Week 33	Week 34–37
•Fetal length – 38 cm •Fetal weight – 1.2 kg	•Fetal weight – 2 kg •Rhythmic breathing movement occurs	•Fetal length – 40–48 cm •Fetal weight – 2.5 –3 kg	•Fetal length – 48–53 cm

Figure 2.6 Chronology of fetal development from week 25 to 37

Box 2.2 Parts of the mesoderm

Paraxial mesoderm	Intermediate mesoderm	Lateral plate mesoderm
• Is segmental • Forms somites	• Forms the urogenital system	• Forms the somatic and splanchnic mesoderm

Placenta and fetal membranes

General facts

1. **Embryonic nutrient requirements**
    - During fertilization and initial blastocyte formation nutrients are obtained by diffusion via the zona pellucida from the accumulated fluid in the blastocoele
    - From day 12 to term the embryo obtains nutrients from the maternal blood via the uteroplacental circulation

2. **The endometrial stromal cells become large and accumulate glycogen in response to**
    - Circulating progesterones
    - Blastocyst

3. **Decidual reaction**
    - Are cellular changes at the site of implantation, which include
        i. Syncytiotrophoblast-induced erosion of endometrium
        ii. Congestion and dilation of maternal vessels

      iii. Endometrial tissue oedema

      iv. Endometrial cell shape becoming polyhedral

      v. Increase in endometrial cell glycogen and lipid deposition

      vi. Increase in endometrial vascularization

- Occurs at day 12 of embryonic life

4. **In pregnancy the decidua (endometrium)**
   - Is identifiable as 3 discrete layers
     i. Basalis (i.e. where implantation takes place and the basal plate is formed)
     ii. Capsularis (overlies the chorion)
     iii. Parietalis (covering the rest of the endometrial cavity except the implantation site)
   - Capsularis and parietalis comes into contact with each other and obliterate the uterine cavity at 4 months of gestation

5. **Histology of early pregnancy is characterized by the presence of**
   - Chorionic villi
   - Decidua
   - Trophoblast
   - Fetal membranes
   - Fetal somatic tissue

6. **Presence of decidua on its own in a histological sample is not enough to confirm a diagnosis of pregnancy**

7. **Arias-Stella are changes in the endometrial glands due to the effects of progesterone**

Placenta

1. **The placenta has both maternal and fetal components**
   - Maternal parts are derived from decidua basalis
   - Fetal parts consist of the villi of the chorion frondosum

2. **The placenta is structurally composed of 2 units**
   - Chorionic plate
   - Basal plate (the region of the placenta on the maternal side)

3. **Chorionic plate is of fetal origin and is composed of**
   - Amnion
   - Extra-embryonic mesenchyme
   - Cytotrophoblast
   - Syncytiotrophoblast

4. **The basal plate of the placenta is made up of**
   - Fetal-derived parts from
     i. Cytotrophoblast
     ii. Syncytiotrophoblast
   - Maternal-derived part (from decidua basalis)

5. **Villi**
   - Are chorionic projections suspended in the intervillous space
   - Purpose is to maximize the area of interchange with the maternal blood
   - Each contains a capillary plexus supplied by branches of the umbilical vessels
   - Interchange occurs with maternal blood brought to the intervillous space by branches of the uterine vessels

6. **Development of chorionic villi**
   - Day 9 is the lacunar stage

- Day 12 – formation of primary chorionic villi
  i.   Clefts appear in the syncytiotrophoblast called lacunae, which communicate with maternal endometrial sinusoids
  ii. Cytotrophoblast forms primary chorionic villi
- Day 15 – formation of secondary chorionic villi
  i.   Extra-embryonic mesoderm invades the core of primary chorionic villi converting them into secondary chorionic villi
  ii. Secondary villi line the entire chorion
- Day 21
  i.   Tertiary chorionic villi form
  ii. Tertiary chorionic villi are villi containing blood vessels
- Day 28
  i.   Free villi form
  ii. Cytotrophoblast in the tertiary villi disappears
- Chorion leaf is formed from the chorionic villi located on the anembryonic pole. These become compressed against the decidua capsularis and become avascular
- Chorion frondosum is located at the embryonic pole

7. **Tertiary villi of chorion frondosum**
   - Grow towards the basal plate and attach to the decidual tissue via the cytotrophoblast shell
   - Also known as anchoring villi

8. **Anchoring villi give rise to side branches called intermediate villi, which in turn produce terminal villi**

9. **Terminal villi**
   - Develop as sprouts of syncytiotrophoblast
   - Take over function from intermediate villi in third trimester of pregnancy

10. **Placental villi maturation includes**
    - Capillary enlargement
    - Thinning of syncytiotrophoblast
    - Cytotrophoblast disappearance

11. **Intervillous space**
    - Is blood-filled space between anchoring villi
    - Also known as trophoblastic lacunae

12. **Development of the cytotrophoblast layer**
    - Formed by cytotrophoblast of anchoring villus, which expands into the basal plate until a further layer outside the syncytiotrophoblast arises
    - Penetrates into the decidua and myometrium
    - Colonizes the wall of spiral arteries, leading to destruction of the smooth muscle layer and changes in the elasticity of the spiral arteries
    - This migration is under strict temporal spatial control
    - Insufficient penetration leads to pre-eclampsia
    - Excessive penetration leads to chorion carcinoma

13. **Placental septa**
    - Also known as inter-cotyledon septa
    - Arise from decidua at 4 months of fetal life
    - Divide placenta into 15–20 lobes
    - Do not reach the chorionic plate
    - Do not limit circulation of maternal blood from one cotyledon to the next

14. Placental membrane
- Is the partition between fetal and maternal circulation
- Composed of fetal tissue that is initially 4 layers thick; the layers are
  - i. Fetal capillary endothelium
  - ii. Connective tissue of the villi
  - iii. Cytotrophoblast
  - iv. Syncytiotrophoblast
- From 4 months of fetal life, the placental membrane becomes thinner due to villous maturation

15. Umbilical cord
- Dimensions at term
  - i. Length = 50–60 cm
  - ii. Diameter = 1.5–2 cm
- Contains
  - i. 2 umbilical arteries
  - ii. 1 umbilical vein
  - iii. Wharton's jelly
- 1 : 100 newborns have only 1 umbilical artery and 20% of them will have a coexisting vessel or heart abnormality
- Usually inserts in the placenta near the centre, but other insertions include
  - i. Eccentric – cord insertion is off-centre and up to 2 cm away from the edge
  - ii. Marginal – cord inserts from within 2 cm and up to the edge of the placenta
  - iii. Velamentous – cord inserts into the membranes and then travels within the membranes to the placenta; the exposed vessels are not protected by Wharton's jelly

16. Wharton's jelly
- Is made up of mucopolysaccharides
- Derived from extra-embryonic mesoderm
- Protects umbilical blood vessels
- Contains
  - i. Fibroblasts
  - ii. Macrophages

17. Fibrinoid deposits accumulate in the placenta
- Begins from 4 months of fetal life
- Occurs in 3 regions of the placenta
  - i. Subchorial Langhan's layer within the chorion plate
  - ii. Rohr's layer beneath the stem villi within the basal plate
  - iii. Nitabutch's layer in the deciduas basalis within the basal plate (this is the layer where placenta detaches at birth)
- Can take up a maximum of 30% of placental volume without affecting its function

Fetal membranes

1. Fetal membranes
- Is a term applied to structures derived from the blastocyst that do not contribute to the embryo
- Are made up of 4 components (**Box 2.3**)

2. Amnion
- Amniotic cavity is formed by day 7 of embryonic life
- Has 5 layers
  - i. Cuboidal epithelium

ii. Basement membrane
iii. Compact layer
iv. Fibroblast layer
v. Spongy layer (remnant of extra-embryonic coelom)
- Does not contain blood vessels, lymphatics, or nerves

Box 2.3 Components of the fetal membranes

Amnion	Chorion	Yolk sac	Allantois
• Inner side is formed from ectoderm • Outer side is formed from mesoderm	• Double-layered membrane • Formed by trophoblast and extra-embryonic mesoderm	• Becomes incorporated into the GIT	• Is a diverticulum of the yolk sac • Becomes attached to the urinary bladder

3. **Chorion is composed of 4 layers**
   - Cellular layer
   - Reticular layer
   - Basement membrane
   - Trophoblast

Chpt 6.11

4. **Sharing of placenta and fetal membranes in twins depends on the stage at which a single zygote divides (Box 2.4)**
   - 2 types of twins
     i. Monozygotic
     ii. Dizygotic (constitute 70% of twin pregnancies)
   - Monozygotic twins can be
     i. DCDA: separation occurs at morula stage; by day 3
     ii. MCDA: separation occurs at days 4–8 (accounts for 70% of monozygotic twins)
     iii. MCMA: separation occurs after amnion is formed; between days 9 and 12 (accounts for 1% of monozygotic twins)
     iv. Conjoint: separation occurs after day 12 (incidence is about 1 : 100 000 pregnancies)
   - All dizygotic twins are dichorionic
   - 3% of monochorionic twins have 2 placental masses
   - Chorionicity is better determined by ultrasonography before 14 weeks gestation
     i. λ (lambda) sign indicates dichorionic diamniotic (DCDA)
     ii. 'T' sign indicates monochorionic diamniotic (MCDA)

Box 2.4 Stage of zygote division and resultant type of twining

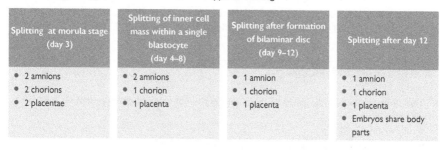

Splitting at morula stage (day 3)	Splitting of inner cell mass within a single blastocyte (day 4–8)	Splitting after formation of bilaminar disc (day 9–12)	Splitting after day 12
• 2 amnions • 2 chorions • 2 placentae	• 2 amnions • 1 chorion • 1 placenta	• 1 amnion • 1 chorion • 1 placenta	• 1 amnion • 1 chorion • 1 placenta • Embryos share body parts

Placental disorders

1. **Molar pregnancy**
   - Is characterized by the presence of hydatidiform mole
   - Prevalence in the UK is 1 : 714 live births
   - Categorized into 2 groups
     - i. Complete moles
     - ii. Partial moles
   - Complete moles
     - i. Characterized by diffuse swelling of villous tissue and diffuse trophoblastic hyperplasia in the absence of embryonic or fetal tissue
     - ii. Occurs when an empty egg is fertilized by one or two normal spermatozoa (dispemic fertilisation is < 20%)
     - iii. Are diploid
     - iv. Genotype is 46, XX or 46, XY
     - v. All nuclear genes are paternal
   - Partial moles
     - i. Characterized by focal swelling of villous tissue and focal trophoblastic hyperplasia in the presence of embryonic tissue
     - ii. Occur when a normal haploid egg is fertilized by two (or three) spermatozoa
     - iii. Are triploid (i.e. contains 3 sets of chromosomes)
     - iv. Genotype is, in decreasing order of frequency: 69, XXY or 69, XXX or 69, XYY
   - Prognosis
     - i. 80% of hydatidiform moles are benign
     - ii. 15% will develop into invasive moles (persistent trophoblastic disease)
     - iii. 2–3% may develop into choriocarcinoma

2. **Placenta accreta**
   - Occurs when the placenta is morbidly adherent to the myometrium
   - Due to deficient deciduas basalis

3. **Placenta increta is the term applied when the placenta invades the myometrium but has not breached the uterine serosa**

4. **Placenta percreta is the term applied when the placenta breaches the serosa of the uterus**

5. **Succenturiate lobe is defined as one or more accessory lobes of the placenta that are attached to the bulk of the placenta by blood vessels running through the fetal membranes**

6. **Twin-to-twin transfusion syndrome (TTTS)**
   - Is due to abnormal connecting blood vessels (arterioarterial or venovenous anastomoses) in the twins' placenta resulting in an imbalanced flow of blood from one twin to another
   - Risk of TTTS
     - i. In monochorionic twins = 15%
     - ii. More common in MCDA than MCMA twins
   - Treatment is fetoscopic laser ablation of interconnecting blood vessels
   - Severity is graded with the Quintero classification system (stages 1–5) (**Box 2.5**)

Body cavities and diaphragm

1. **The embryo takes a 3-dimensional shape during the 4th week of development via folding resulting in**
   - Formation of GIT
   - Conversion of intra-embryonic coelom into a closed cavity

Box 2.5 Quintero classification system of TTTS

Stage 1	Stage 2	Stage 3	Stage 4
• Discrepancy in amniotic fluid volume	• Bladder of donor twin is not visible by ultasonography	• Critically abnormal fetal Doppler studies	• Fetal hydrops present

Stage 5
• Demise of one or both twins

2. **The body cavities**
   - Include
     i. Peritoneal
     ii. Pericardial
     iii. Pleural
   - Arise from coelomic cavity
   - Are lined by 2 serous layers (the somatic and splanchnic mesoderm) (*Box 2.6*)

Box 2.6 Serous layers of body cavities

Somatic mesoderm	Splanchnic mesoderm
• Is in contact with the ectoderm • Gives rise to parietal layer of serous membrane	• Adheres to the endoderm • Forms the visceral layer of the serous membrane

3. **Septum transversum**
   - Is a sheet of mesoderm
   - Appears on day 22
   - Is rostral to (in front of) the developing heart
   - Is cranial to pericardial cavity before folding
   - Forms the central tendon of the diaphragm

4. **Intra-embryonic coelom before folding**
   - Appears as a 'U'-shaped cavity
   - The bend of the 'U' lies anteriorly and represents the pericardial cavity
   - Each arm of the 'U' represents the
     i. Pericardioperitoneal canal
     ii. Peritoneal cavity
   - In the umbilical region the peritoneal cavity opens into the chorionic cavity allowing herniation of midgut into the umbilical cord

5. **After folding**
   - As a result of the head folding, the heart swings ventral to foregut
   - Septum transversum is wedged between heart and yolk sac
   - Pericardial cavity opens into the pericardioperitoneal canal, which opens into the peritoneal cavity
   - At this stage the septum transversum is an incomplete partition between the thorax and abdomen

6. **Division of intra-embryonic coelom forms 4 cavities**
   - 2 pleural
   - 1 peritoneal
   - 1 pericardial

7. **Diaphragm is formed by 5 components**
   - Septum transversum
   - The body wall
     i.   From somatic mesoderm
     ii. The peripheral part of the diaphragm attaches to the ribs – hence receiving its sensory innervation from the lower 6 intercostal nerves
   - Mesentery of the oesophagus (forms the muscular crura of the diaphragm)
   - Pleuroperitoneal membrane
   - Cervical somites
     i.   During the 4th week the septum transversum lies in the cervical region opposite the 3rd, 4th, and 5th cervical somites
     ii. Myoblasts from each somite contribute to the diaphragmatic musculature
     iii. Hence diaphragmatic innervation is via nerves C3–C5
     iv. C3–C5 fuse to form the phrenic nerve

Musculoskeletal system

1. **Mesenchyme**
   - Gives rise to musculoskeletal system
   - Is derived from
     i.   Mesodermal cells of somites
     ii. Somatopleuric layer of lateral plate mesoderm
     iii. Neural crest cells (head region)
   - Has ability to
     i.   Migrate
     ii. Differentiate into many different cell types

2. **Bone formation**
   - Occurs via condensation of mesenchymal cells
   - Consists of 2 types of ossification (*Box 2.7*)
   - Axial skeleton is derived from the paraxial mesoderm which organizes as somites

Box 2.7 Types of ossification

Membranous ossification	Endochondral ossification
• Does not involve cartilage	• Occurs by replacement of hyaline cartilage
• Is responsible for development of flat bones (e.g. skull, clavicle)	• Is responsible for development of long bones

3. **Vertebral column**
   - Development goes through 3 stages
     i.   Mesenchymal condensation around notochord (*Fig. 2.7*)
     ii. Cartilaginous transformation
     iii. Ossification, which starts at 6th week of fetal life and ends at the 25th year of adult life
   - Vertebral arch
     i.   Gives rise to the costal and transverse processes
     ii. Fuses to form the spinous process
   - Formation of vertebral body depends on notochord
   - Formation of vertebral arch depends on sclerotome interaction with the surface ectoderm

- Intervertebral disc has an
  - i.   Outer annulus fibrosus (derived from sclerotomes)
  - ii. Inner nucleus pulposus (derived from notochord)
- The vertebra is intersegmental in origin due to its formation from 2 sclerotomes
- The spinal nerves are segmental

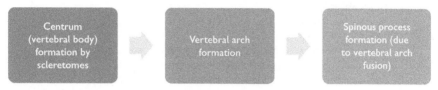

Figure 2.7 Stages of mesenchymal condensation around notochord

4. Sternum
- Develops from a pair of cartilaginous bars that form in the ventral body wall
- These bars fuse in the midline in a craniocaudal sequence

5. Ribs
- Arise from costal process of vertebra
- Grow laterally towards the sternum

6. Skull
- Is composed of
  - i.   Neurocranium (which surrounds the brain)
  - ii. Viscerocranium (which surrounds the mouth, pharynx, and larynx)
- The bones of the cranial base develop
  - i.   From occipital sclerotomes
  - ii. By endochondral ossification
- The skull cap develops
  - i.   From mesenchyme of neural crest
  - ii. By intramembranous ossification

7. Fontanelles
- Are unossified mesenchyme
- There are 6 fontanelles
  - i.   Anterior
  - ii.   Posterior
  - iii. 2 anterior lateral
  - iv.   2 posterior lateral
- Most fontanelles disappear during the 1st year of life
- Anterior fontanelle ossifies at 18 months of life

8. Appendicular skeleton
- In the limbs, bones form initially in the most distal part
- Ossification is via endochondral ossification except for the clavicle
- Ossification centres first appear at 8 weeks of development
- Shaft of limb bones are ossified at 12 weeks of development. However:
  - i.   Carpal bones remain cartilaginous until after birth
  - ii.   Ossification of tarsal bones begin at 16th week of development
  - iii. Smaller tarsal bones do not ossify until 3 years after birth
- At birth
  - i.   The shaft (diaphysis) of long bones are completely ossified

ii. Epiphyses are still cartilaginous

iii. Secondary ossification centres occur in epiphyses few years after birth

9. **Muscles**
    - Skeletal muscles develop from myoblasts derived from somites
    - Head musculature is derived from
        i.   Pharyngeal arches
        ii. Neural crest mesenchyme
    - Each myotome divides into
        i.   Ventral hypomere, which forms muscles of anterior and lateral wall (e.g. rectus abdominis, internal/external oblique, and transversus abdominis)
        ii. Dorsal epimere, which forms muscles of posterior wall (e.g. erector spinae)
    - Dorsal limb muscle mass gives rise to extensor groups
    - Ventral limb muscle mass gives rise to flexor groups

Respiratory system

1. **The epithelial component of the respiratory system develops from the ventral wall of the endodermal lining of the foregut as a diverticulum that grows into the surrounding splanchnopleuric mesoderm.**

2. **Splanchnopleuric mesoderm gives rise to the following components of lower respiratory tract**
    - Visceral pleura
    - Cartilage
    - Smooth muscle
    - Blood vessels

3. **The respiratory diverticulum**
    - Separates from the foregut by development of bilateral longitudinal ridges called the tracheo-oesophageal folds
    - The tracheo-oesophageal folds fuse together to form the tracheo-oesophageal septum
    - Gives rise to
        i.   Trachea (tracheal bifurcation lies at thoracic vertebral level 4 at birth)
        ii. Lung buds

4. **The larynx**
    - Is lined by epithelium from endoderm
    - Laryngeal cartilage and muscles arise from pharyngeal arches

5. **Lung buds**
    - Divide many times to form the bronchial tree
    - This division is known as branching morphogenesis
        i.   Right lung bud divides into 3 secondary lung buds
        ii. Left lung bud divides into 2 secondary lung buds
        iii. Bronchial tree division is not complete until after birth
    - Full lung maturation is reached at 6–7 years of age
    - New alveoli continue to be formed up to 10 years of age

6. **Lung epithelium**
    - Is initially cuboidal and thins with ageing
    - Respiration is not possible until this epithelium thins sufficiently to form squamous epithelium

- This begins at 26 weeks of fetal life
- Consists of 2 types of epithelial cells
    i.   Type 1 (line the alveoli)
    ii. Type 2
        - Produce surfactant
        - Appear at about 24 weeks of fetal life

7. **Pleura is composed of 2 layers**
    - Somatic layer formed by somatopleuric mesoderm
    - Visceral layer formed by splanchnopleuric mesoderm

Cardiovascular system

1. **One of the first systems to develop**

2. **In early embryo nutrients are derived from**
    - Trophoblastic digestion of uterine mucosa
    - Diffusion from the contents of the yolk sac

3. **Initial components of cardiovascular system appear as angiogenic cell clusters in the extra-embryonic mesoderm lining the yolk sac**

4. **The primitive heart begins beating at day 21**

The heart

1. **Heart formation**
    - Angiogenic cell clusters merge in a rostral to prochordal plate direction to form the cardiogenic area
    - Cardiogenic cells form paired heart tubes
    - The dorsal aortae develop on either side of the midline and connect with the heart tubes
    - Heart tubes fuse due to the longitudinal and lateral folding of the embryo
    - The tube is suspended in the pericardial cavity by dorsal mesocardium
    - The dorsal mesocardium breaks down leaving the heart attached merely at the margins of the pericardium
    - The heart tube elongates in the pericardial cavity
    - At day 23 the elongation is more than the volume available in the pericardial cavity
    - Hence the tube bends, forming the cardiac loop
    - Bends occur at
        i.   Bulboventricular groove
        ii. Atrioventricular groove

2. **Heart tube consists of**
    - A single atrium
    - A single ventricle
    - An atrioventricular canal

3. **Atrioventricular valves**
    - Form in the region of the atrioventricular canal
    - Formed by the endocardial cushions

4. **Bulbus cordis**
    - Lies between primitive ventricle and the atrial outflow
    - Proximal third becomes the right ventricle
    - Becomes the conus cordis (eventually becomes the truncus arteriosus)

5. **Atrial septum**
   - Septation begins at about 4 weeks
   - Septum primum
     i.   Develops in the roof of the common atrium
     ii. Grows towards the endocardial cushions
   - Ostium primum
     i.   Is the opening between the septum primum and endocardial cushions
     ii. Closes with further growth
   - Ostium secundum
     i.   Occurs as ostium primum closes
     ii. It is a small hole in the septum primum
   - Septum secundum
     i.   Forms to the right of septum primum
     ii. Grows over septum primum
     iii. Does not completely divide the atria, leaving an opening, the foramen ovale

6. **Foramen ovale**
   - Functional closure occurs after birth due to change in pressure between the two atria (i.e. increased left-sided heart pressure and decreased right-sided pressure caused by air breathing and start of pulmonary circulation)
   - Becomes fossa ovalis after birth

7. **Ventricular septum is composed of 2 components (muscular and membranous parts) (Box 2.8)**

Box 2.8 Components of the ventricular septum

Muscular part	Membranous part
• Develops from floor of ventricle and grows towards endocardial cushions	• Formed by endocardial cushions and aorticopulmonary septum
• This component does not reach the endocardial cushions, leaving a gap	• Accommodates the atrioventricular conducting bundle

8. **Truncus arteriosus gives rise to**
   - Ascending aorta
   - Pulmonary trunk
   - Aortic sac

9. **Aorticopulmonary septum**
   - Forms at week 5
   - Forms from the left and right truncoconal swellings that occur within the conus cordis and truncus arteriosus
   - Develops as a spiralling structure

Venous drainage of the heart

1. **Sinus venosum**
   - Empties into the common atrium via a single opening
   - Consists of
     i.   Left horn (becomes the coronary sinus)
     ii. Right horn
   - Right horn of sinus venosum
     i.   Becomes the dominant horn

ii. Becomes the proximal part of
- Inferior vena cava (IVC)
- Superior vena cava (SVC)
- Drains the following vein pairs
  i. Common cardinal veins
  ii. Vitelline veins
  iii. Umbilical veins

2. **Sinus venarum**
- Consists of the
  i. Right horn of sinus venosum
  ii. Venae cavae
- Lies on the posterior atrial wall

3. **Right auricle is the primitive atrium**

4. **Cristae terminalis**
- A crest that separates the trabeculated right auricle from the smooth sinus venarum
- Corresponds to the sulcus terminalis (is a groove on the exterior of the heart)
- Pectinate muscles project from this crest to the auricle
- Lower part forms the IVC valve in fetal heart
  i. This disappears after birth
  ii. Functions to direct blood to foramen ovale

Arterial system

1. **Arterial system includes**
- Aortic arches
- Paired dorsal aortae (will eventually unite to form the descending aorta)

2. **Aortic arches**
- Aortic sac gives off vessels to the pharyngeal arches (that begin to develop from week 4)
- An artery develops within each pharyngeal arch, each of which meet the aortic sac
- 5 or 6 pair of aortic arches are formed (*Box 2.9*)
- Aortic arch joins the dorsal aorta on each side
- The aortic sac divides to form the right and left dorsal aorta

Box 2.9 Aortic arches and their resultant arteries

1st aortic arch pair	2nd aortic arch pair	3rd aortic arch pair	4th aortic arch pair
• Maxillary artery	• Disappears	• Common carotid • External carotid • Proximal part of internal carotid	• RIGHT – Proximal part of right subclavian artery • LEFT – Arch of aorta

5th aortic arch pair	6th aortic arch pair
• Disappears	• RIGHT – Distal part of right subclavian artery • LEFT PROXIMAL – Pulmonary artery • LEFT DISTAL – Ductus arteriosus

3. Ductus arteriosus
   - Becomes ligamentum arteriosum after birth
   - Closure is stimulated by bradykinin

4. Distal part of internal carotid is formed by dorsal aorta

5. Left subclavian arises from 7th intersegmental artery, which is a branch of the dorsal aorta

6. Right dorsal aorta disappears between the 7th intersegmental artery and the start of the fused dorsal aorta

7. Path of recurrent laryngeal nerve is different on both sides due to the different arrangement of the 6th aortic arch pair
   - Left – the nerve hooks under ductus arteriosus
   - Right – the nerve hooks under right subclavian artery

8. Vitelline artery
   - Supplies the yolk sac
   - Exists as a pair
   - Fuses to form
     i.   Coeliac artery
     ii. Superior mesenteric artery
     iii. Inferior mesenteric artery

9. Umbilical arteries
   - Supply deoxygenated blood from the fetus to the placenta
   - Arise from common iliac artery
   - After birth
     i. The distal portion of the artery obliterates to form the medial umbilical ligaments
     ii. The proximal portions persist as the internal iliac and vesicular arteries

Venous system

1. At week 5 of embryonic life there are 3 major sets of veins
   - Umbilical
   - Vitelline
   - Cardinal (drains head and body)

2. Umbilical veins
   - Initially there are 2 umbilical veins
   - Both proximal portions disappear
   - The right distal portions disappear
   - Left distal umbilical vein
     i. Connects with ductus venosus to bypass the liver
     ii. After birth becomes ligamentum teres and lies in the falciform ligament

3. Ductus venosus
   - Connects to IVC
   - After birth becomes ligamentum venosum

4. Vitelline veins forms
   - Sinus venosus
   - Hepatic vessels

5. Longitudinal venous channels
   - Form by week 5 of embryonic life
   - Are paired

- Include
  i. Azygos veins
  ii. Supracardinal veins
  iii. Subcardinal veins
- Become progressively asymmetrical, resulting in right-sided dominance by week 7, leading to
  i. Formation of the IVC, which includes the supracardinal and subcardinal veins
  ii. The left azygos vein, becoming the hemiazygos vein
  iii. A resultant left to right shunt

Gastrointestinal system

General facts

1. **The endoderm forms the**
   - Foregut
   - Midgut
     i. Is in continuity with the remaining yolk sac
     ii. Vitello-intestinal duct connects the yolk sac and the midgut
   - Hindgut
   - Liver
   - Pancreas

2. **Splanchnopleuric lateral plate mesoderm contributes to**
   - Connective tissue
   - Smooth muscle
   - Serosal layer of gut tube

3. **Dorsal mesentery**
   - Suspends the gut tube in the body of the embryo
   - Formed by serosal membrane
   - Attaches to the posterior wall of the embryo
   - Extends from lower oesophagus to cloaca
   - With further growth the dorsal mesentery is lost for some parts of the gut tube
     i. Duodenum
     ii. Ascending colon
     iii. Descending colon

4. **Dorsal mesogastrium**
   - Is the dorsal mesentery of the stomach
   - Becomes the greater omentum

5. **Ventral mesentery**
   - Forms at the caudal part of foregut
   - Is derived from the septum transversum
   - Covers the
     i. Stomach
     ii. Terminal oesophagus
     iii. Initial portion of duodenum
   - The liver develops within the ventral mesentery and divides it into 2 parts
     i. Falciform ligament (connects liver to ventral wall of embryo)
     ii. Lesser omentum (lies between stomach and liver)
   - Mesenteries are double layered, allowing structures (such as nerves and blood vessels) to lie within them

6. A structure is intraperitoneal when it is completely invested in splanchnopleuric mesoderm all around

7. A structure is retroperitoneal when it is not suspended by dorsal mesentery

Foregut

1. **Foregut consists of**
   - Oesophagus
   - Stomach
   - Duodenum
   - Pancreas
   - Liver

2. **The foregut is divided into the**
   - Cranial portion
     i. Forms the pharynx
     ii. Associated with pharyngeal arches
   - Caudal portion

3. **Oesophagus**
   - Is the part of the caudal foregut
   - Lies in the posterior mediastinum
   - Gives rise to the respiratory diverticulum
   - Lengthens due to the growth of thoracic organs

4. **Stomach**
   - Undergoes a clockwise 90° rotation (i.e. rotates to the right)
   - This pulls the dorsal mesentery over to the left side
   - Consequently a small gap is formed between the stomach and the dorsal wall, called the lesser sac

5. **Spleen develops in the dorsal mesogastrium**

6. **Gastrosplenic ligament is the portion of the dorsal mesogastrium that lies between the stomach and the spleen**

7. **Lienorenal ligament is the portion of the dorsal mesogastrium that lies between the spleen and the dorsal wall of the embryo**

8. **Pancreas**
   - Lies in the dorsal wall of the embryo
   - Develops from endodermal lining of the duodenum
   - At 4 weeks of embryonic development 2 pancreatic buds arise
     i. Dorsal
        - Lies within the dorsal mesentery
        - Is the larger of the 2 buds
        - Its duct is the main pancreatic duct
     ii. Ventral (lies within the ventral mesentery)
   - As the duodenum rotates right
     i. The ventral bud moves dorsally to lie superior to the dorsal bud
     ii. Entrapping the superior mesenteric blood vessel between the dorsal and ventral buds
     iii. Both the buds fuse
   - Both pancreatic ducts fuse
     i. Entering the medial wall of the duodenum

ii.   To form the major duodenal papilla
- Tail of pancreas lies within the double layer of the lienorenal ligament

9. Lesser sac
- Is limited in its extend by the greater omentum (as the double layer of the greater omentum fuse laterally)
- Communicates with the greater sac via the aditus

10. Duodenum
- Arises from
  i.   Foregut
  ii. Midgut
- The bile duct lies in the junction between foregut and midgut
- Lumen of duodenum
  i.   Initially is hollow
  ii. At 2 months of fetal development it is solid
- Lies in the posterior abdominal wall
- Gives rise to the pancreas which lies within the mesoduodenum
- Is 'C' shaped
- Has a dual arterial supply

11. Mesoduodenum is lost with further development
- Consequently the duodenum is covered with peritoneum only on its anterior surface, known as the parietal peritoneum
- The posterior leaf of the mesoduodenum regresses
  i.   Thus the posterior surface of duodenum is attached to the dorsal wall of embryo
  ii. This seals off the lower extent of the aditus to the lesser sac

12. Liver
- Hepatic diverticulum
  i.   Arises on the ventral wall of duodenum and just above the ventral pancreatic duct
  ii. Pushes into the septum transversum
- Gall bladder
  i.   Arises from a ventral outpouching of the hepatic diverticulum
  ii. Its duct initially is solid (failure to recanalize the duct results in extrahepatic biliary atresia)
- The peritoneum covers all of the liver except the bare area (this is the area in contact with the diaphragm)
- Kupffer cells
  i.   Are bone marrow derived
  ii. Line liver sinusoids
- At 10 weeks of embryonic life liver produces blood cells

Midgut

1. Starts at the midpoint of the duodenum

2. Terminates approximately 2/3 of the way along the transverse colon

3. Its artery is the superior mesenteric artery

4. The midgut rapidly elongates but as the peritoneal cavity is small it
- Herniates out of the abdominal cavity into the umbilical cord
- Herniation occurs at 6 weeks and returns at 10 weeks. This is a physiological umbilical hernia

- As the gut enters the umbilical cord it rotates 90° anticlockwise
- On return to the abdomen it rotates a further 180° anticlockwise resulting in the caecum moving from its subhepatic position to the right iliac fossa
- The rotation is about the axis of the vitello-intestinal duct
- Abnormal herniation of midgut is of 2 types (*Box 2.10*)

Box 2.10 Types of abnormal midgut herniation

Omphalocoele	Gastroschisis
• Indirect herniation • Herniates via the umbilicus • Covered with a layer of amnion • Associated with other structural and chromosomal abnormalities (e.g. Trisomy 18 – Edwards' syndrome)	• Direct herniation via abdominal wall • Lies in the amniotic sac and hence is not covered by amnion • Not associated with chromosomal abnormalities

5. **The midgut forms**
   - The second half of the duodenum
   - Ileum
   - Jejunum
   - Ascending colon
   - Proximal 2/3 of the transverse colon

6. **The mesentery of the following organs are reabsorbed**
   - Duodenum
   - Ascending colon
   - Descending colon

7. **The transverse mesocolon**
   - Is the dorsal mesentery of the transverse colon
   - It fuses with the anterior 2 layers of the greater omentum, thus appearing that the transverse colon is attached to the posterior surface of the greater omentum

8. **Meckel's diverticulum**
   - Is a remnant of the vitello-intestinal duct
   - Rules of 2
     i.   2 inches (5 cm) long
     ii. 2 ft (61 cm) from ileocaecal valve
     iii. 2% of population has it
   - Contains
     i. Gastric mucosa
     ii. Pancreatic mucosa
   - Inflammation of it is often mistaken for appendicitis

Hindgut

1. **Forms the**
   - Distal 1/3 of the transverse colon
   - Descending colon
   - Rectum
   - Upper half of anal canal

2. **Forms epithelial layer of**
   - Urinary bladder
   - Urethra

3. Initially opens into the primitive cloaca, which communicates with the allantois

4. Urorectal septum
   - A band of mesenchymal tissue
   - Divides the primitive cloaca into
     i.   Urogenital sinus anteriorly
     ii. Rectum posteriorly
   - Becomes the perineal body when it reaches the cloacal membrane
   - Perineal body divides the perineum into
     i.   Urogenital triangle
     ii. Anal triangle
   - Cloacal membrane breaks down at 7 weeks of embryonic development

5. Allantois
   - Non-functional
   - Connects primitive cloaca to umbilicus
   - Becomes the urachus, which eventually becomes the median umbilical ligament
   - In some species the allantois contributes to the formation of the placenta

6. Anal canal
   - Mucosa of anal canal derived from
     i.   Upper half – endoderm
     ii. Lower half – ectoderm (proctodeum)
   - Pectinate line
     i.   Demarcates the two embryological parts of the anal canal
     ii. Located at base of anal columns
     iii. Marks a change in
       - Blood supply
       - Nerve supply
       - Epithelial lining
   - Anal canal lumen
     i.   Occluded at 7 weeks by the ectoderm
     ii. At 9 weeks this is recanalized

Urinary system

1. Origins of the urinary system
   - Bulk of the urogenital system is derived from intermediate intra-embryonic mesoderm (forms the nephrogenic cord that underlies the urogenital ridge)
   - Develops in the trunk
   - Craniocaudal development (*Box 2.11*)

Box 2.11 Development of the urinary system

Pronephros	Mesonephros	Metanephros
• Non-functional • Temporary	• Produces urine	• Produces urine • Becomes the definitive human kidney

2. The initial structures that develop in the urogenital system have excretory functions

3. **Two components are necessary for development of an excretory system**
   - Capillary bed
   - Tubules (glomeruli)

4. **Mesonephros**
   - Develops in the lower thoracic and lumbar region
   - Cavities appear in the mesonephros
     i. Which become the tubules (Bowman's capsules)
     ii. Join laterally to form the mesonephric duct
   - Mesonephric duct
     i. Drains into the urogenital sinus
     ii. Forms the bladder trigone
     iii. In males – produces ductus deferens and efferent ductules of testes
     iv. In females – produces Gardner's ducts

5. **Metanephros**
   - Consists of
     i. Ureteric bud
     ii. Metanephric blastema
   - Ureteric bud
     i. Outgrowth of mesonephric duct and eventually grows into the metanephric duct
     ii. Forms the
       - Definitive ureter
       - Renal pelvis
       - Calyces
       - Collecting ducts
   - Metanephric blastema
     i. Condensation of nephrogenic cord tissue around ureteric bud
     ii. Forms the nephrons (formation continues until 32 weeks of intrauterine life)
   - Functional from 10 weeks (urine produced passes into the amniotic fluid as the cloacal membrane disappears at week 7)

6. **Bladder arises from the urogenital sinus after the cloaca has been divided**

Chpt 2.1

Reproductive system

1. **Indifferent gonad**
   - Develops from intermediate mesoderm
   - Situated on the gonadal ridge (which is the medial portion of the urogenital ridge)
   - Primordial germ cell migration
     i. Starts at week 6 of embryonic life
     ii. Originates from the wall of the yolk sac
     iii. Cells migrate to the genital ridge
     iv. Path is via dorsal mesentery of the hindgut
     v. Induced formation of primitive sex cord
   - Primitive sex cord is derived from mesonephros and overlying coelomic epithelium

2. **Testis**
   - The default is for the gonad to develop into an ovary
   - Sex determining region of Y chromosome (known as the *SRY* gene)
     i. Produces testis-determining factor
     ii. Promotes testicular development
     iii. Induces differentiation of gonad mesenchymal cells into interstitial Leydig cells

- Primitive sex cords
  i. Penetrate the medulla and form the testicular cords, which anastomose to form the rete testis
  ii. Differentiate into Sertoli cells
  iii. Become seminiferous tubules (which are solid cylinders until after puberty, when they are canalized)
- Rete testis is continuous with mesonephric duct
- Leydig cells produce testosterone from week 8
- Sertoli cells produce anti-Mullerian hormone from week 8

3. **Ovary**
   - Absence of testis-determining factor causes
     i. Sex cords in the medulla to degenerate
     ii. Formation of vascular medullary stroma
   - Surface epithelium gives rise to second-generation cortical cords
   - At 4 months of fetal life primordial germ cells invest in the secondary cords

4. **The development of a female internal genitalia occurs in the absence of testosterone and anti-Mullerian hormone**

5. **Initially 2 pairs of genital ducts arise**
   - Mesonephric (also known as Wolffian or Leydig's ducts)
   - Paramesonephric (also known as Mullerian ducts)

6. **Mesonephric duct**
   - Loses its urinary function once the metanephros supersedes the mesonephros
   - Persists in males and regresses in females
   - Forms
     i. Ductus deferens
     ii. Epididymis
     iii. Seminal vesicles
     iv. Prostatic utricle
     v. Trigone
   - Opens into the urogenital sinus
   - Differentiation is due to testosterone being produced from week 8 of embryonic life

7. **Paramesonephric duct**
   - Persists in females and regresses in males
   - Regression is due to anti-Mullerian hormone
   - Lies lateral to mesonephric duct
   - Is a longitudinal invagination of the coelomic epithelium overlying the urogenital ridge
   - The cranial end of the duct
     i. Opens into the peritoneal cavity
     ii. Becomes the fimbriae of the uterine tubes
   - Caudal ends of the duct
     i. Fuse in the midline bringing together the 2 peritoneal folds forming the broad ligament
     ii. Form the uterovaginal canal

8. **Uterovaginal canal**
   - Forms the
     i. Uterus
     ii. Upper half of vagina
   - Fuses with the sinovaginal bulb (swelling on the urogenital sinus)

9. **Sinovaginal bulb**
   - Gives rise to the lower half of the vagina

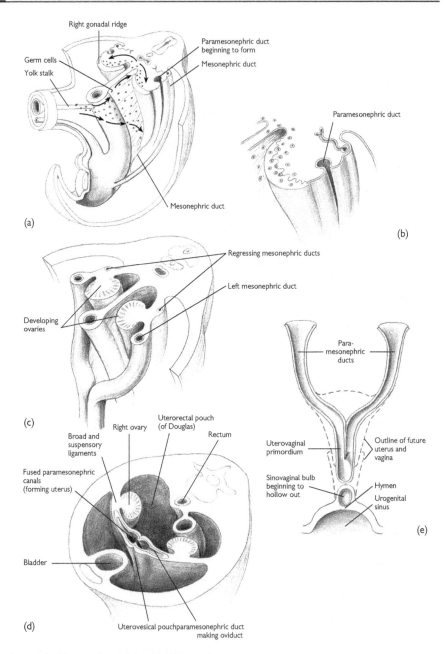

Figure 2.8 Development of the internal genitalia

Reproduced from the *Oxford Textbook of Functional Anatomy*, Vol. 2, by Patricia MacKinnon and John Morris © Oxford University Press 2005.

- Forms the vaginal plate
- Initially is solid and is later canalized

10. Urogenital sinus
- Forms
    - i.   Bartholin's glands

    ii. Skene's gland (paraurethral/ lesser vestibular) – is analogous to the male prostate
- Has 3 portions
    i. Vesico-ureteric (gives rise to bladder)
    ii. Pelvic (gives rise to prostate)
    iii. Phallic

11. Testicular descent
- Mediated through guidance of the gubernaculums
- Is towards the labioscrotal swelling
- Gubernaculum in females becomes
    i. Ovarian ligament
    ii. Round ligament
- Processus vaginalis
    i. An outpouching of peritoneum from the coelomic cavity protruding into the labioscrotal swelling, into the space created by the gubernaculum
    ii. Precedes the testis into the scrotum
    iii. Forms the inguinal canal as it pushes through the 3 layers of abdominal wall
    iv. Becomes the tunica vaginalis
- Has 2 phases
    i. Independent phase (testis reaches deep inguinal ring at 7 months of fetal life)
    ii. Hormone dependent (from 7–9 months of fetal life)
- Factors determining testicular descent
    i. Elongation of fetal trunk
    ii. Increase in intra-abdominal pressure
    iii. Regression of gubernaculum

12. External genitalia (*Fig. 2.9*)
- Are undifferentiated until 9 weeks of fetal life
- The default development is towards a female phenotype
- Dihydrotestosterone (DHT) stimulates external genitalia virilization in the male embryo
- At 5 weeks a cloacal fold forms
    i. On either side of the cloacal membrane
    ii. Fuses anteriorly to give rise to the genital tubercle
    iii. Forms the
        ■ Labia minora
        ■ Penile urethra (at the end of 3 months of development the cloacal folds fuse anteriorly)
- Lateral to the cloacal fold are the genital swellings
    i. In the female they form the labia majora
    ii. In the male they fuse to form the scrotum
- Genital tubercle elongates under hormonal influence to form
    i. Clitoris in female
    ii. Penis in male

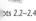

Reproductive development disorders

1. Ambiguous genitalia at birth
- Incidence is 1 : 4000
- Aetiology is either virilization of a genetically female infant or under-masculinization of a genetically male infant (*Box 2.12*)
- Severity of the ambiguity is classified according to the Prader stages 1–5 (*Box 2.13*)

2. Partial or complete androgen insensitivity
- X-linked inheritance disorder in 2/3 of cases

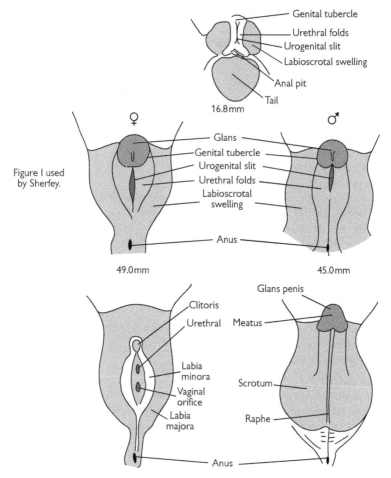

Figure 2.9 Development of the external genitalia

Reproduced from the *Oxford Textbook of Functional Anatomy*, Vol. 2, by Patricia MacKinnon and John Morris © Oxford University Press 2005.

Box 2.12 Aetiology of ambiguous genitalia at birth

46, XY under-masculinization	46, XX virilization	Ovotesticular disorder of sexual development
• Partial androgen insensitivity (PAIS) • Complete androgen insensitivity (CAIS) • 5α-reductase deficiency (unable to convert testosterone to DHT) • Gonadal dysgenesis (e.g. Swyer's syndrome)	• Congenital adrenal hyperplasia • Placental aromatase deficiency • *In-utero* exposure to maternal androgens	• True hermaphroditism

Box 2.13 Prader stages

Typical girl	Stage 1	Stage 2	Stage 3
	• Isolated clitoromegaly • The rest of the genital area and internal organs resemble those of a typical girl	• Clitoromegaly • Partially fused labia • The vagina and urethra open into a funnel-shaped area	• Clitoromegaly • Completely fused labia • The vagina and urethra share a single opening (the urogenital sinus)

Stage 4	Stage 5	Typical boy
• Micropenis • The labia are completely joined like a scrotum • The vagina and urethra share a single opening near the base of the phallus	• Isolated crypto-orchidism • The external genitalia look like a typical boy's • The vagina and urethra share a single opening at the tip of the phallus	

- Characterized by
    i. Normal testicular production of androgens
    ii. Abnormal androgen receptors
- Leads to incomplete virilization of external genitalia
- The testes are usually positioned in the inguinal canal bilaterally

T. in Obs Gyn

Chpt 2.4

3. **Mayer–Rokitansky–Kuster–Hauser syndrome is a congenital malformation of the female internal genitalia due to Mullerian duct failure that leads to an absent or rudimentary uterus but with normal ovarian function**

Nervous system

1. **Forms mainly from ectoderm**

2. **Formation starts at 3 weeks of intrauterine life**

3. **Neurulation is formation of**
    - Neural plate (day 18)
    - Neural fold (day 20)
    - Neural tube (day 22)

4. **Neural plate**
    - Is an ectodermal thickening
    - Widest at cranial end

5. **Neural folds**
    - Are lateral to the neural plates on each side
    - Form the neural groove
    - Ultimately fuse to form the neural tube
    - Give rise to neural crest

6. **Neural crest**
    - Lies beneath surface ectoderm
    - Migrates laterally
    - Gives rise to a wide range of structures (see **Box 2.14**)

7. **Neural tube**
   - Cranially forms the brain
   - Caudally forms the spinal cord
   - An opening at each end of the tube, called the neuropore
     i.   Anterior neuropore closes at day 24
     ii. Posterior neuropore closes at day 26
   - Lined with neuroepithelium
   - Neural tube lumen becomes the ventricular system

Box 2.14 Neural crest derivatives

Brain	Nerves	Cells	Other
• Arachnoid and pia matter • Glial cells • Schwann cells	• Dorsal root ganglia • Cranial nerve ganglia • Paravertebral sympathetic ganglia • Parasympathetic ganglia in GIT	• Melanocytes • Odontoblasts • C cells (thyroid parafollicular cells) – also derived from the 5th pharyngeal pouch	• Adrenal medulla • Dermis of face • Skull cap bones

8. **Nerve cells arise from**
   - Neuroepithelium (neuro-ectoderm), giving rise to
     i.   Neuroblasts
     ii. Glioblasts
          - Astrocytes
          - Oligodendrocytes
     iii. Ependyma
   - Bone marrow (mesoderm), giving rise to microglial cells

9. **There are 4 types of neural tube defect (NTD)**
   - Spina bifida occulta (unfused vertebral arch)
   - Spina bifida cystica (2 subtypes)
     i.   Neural tube and its coverings protrude through the vertebral arch
     ii. Meningocoele
          - Neural tube lies in its normal position
          - Cyst formed by protruding subarachnoid membrane and space
     iii. Meningomyelocoele – neural tube lies ectopically in the cystic space
     iv. Associated with hydrocephalus
   - Rachischisis
     i.   No neural tube
     ii. Neural tissue is fused with skin

Spinal cord

1. **Consists of 3 zones**
   - Neuroepithelial (ventricular) layer
   - Mantle zone – becomes the grey matter
   - Marginal zone
     i.   Contains axons entering and leaving the mantle zone
     ii. After myelination this area looks white

2. **Has 2 plates divided by the sulcus limitans**
   - Alar
     i.   Dorsal plate

    ii. Sensory region
- Basal
  - i. Ventral plate
  - ii. Motor region

3. Extends the entire length of the vertebral column until the 3rd month of intrauterine life after which it ends at lumbar vertebral level 2 (L2) due to overgrowth of the vertebral column

Brain

1. 3 dilatations occur at the cranial end of the neural tube
   - Prosencephalon (forebrain)
   - Mesencephalon (midbrain)
   - Rhombencephalon (hindbrain)

2. Due to limited space the tube bends at 2 places
   - Cervical – lies between rhombencephalon and spinal cord
   - Cephalic – lies in mesencephalon

3. The 3 primary vesicles develop into 5 secondary vesicles
   - Prosencephalon develops in to
     - i. Telencephalon
       - Bilateral portions
       - Become the cerebral hemispheres
     - ii. Diencephalon – becomes thalamus and hypothalamus
   - Mesencephalon
   - Rhombencephalon develops into
     - i. Metencephalon – becomes pons and cerebellum
     - ii. Myelencephalon – becomes medulla

4. Ventricular system
   - The neural tube lumen becomes the ventricular system
   - 4th ventricle lies in the rhombencephalon
   - 3rd ventricle lies in the diencephalons
   - Lateral ventricles lie in the telencephalon
   - Cerebral aqueduct connects the 3rd and 4th ventricles
   - Intraventricular foramen connects the lateral and 3rd ventricles

5. Meninges
   - Dural sac ends at sacral vertebral level 2 (S2)
   - Spinal cord meninges arise from the paraxial mesoderm
   - Cephalic meninges arise from
     - i. Neural crest
     - ii. Mesoderm
       - Choroid plexus
       - Dura

6. Pituitary gland develops from 2 sources
   - Downgrowth from the floor of the diencephalons forming the posterior pituitary (neurohypophysis)
   - Upgrowth from the stomodaeum (ectodermal portion of oral cavity)
     - i. Known as Rathke's pouch
     - ii. Appears at 3rd week of intrauterine life
     - iii. Loses its connection with oral cavity at the 8th week of intrauterine life
     - iv. Forms the anterior pituitary (adenohypophysis)

Face and neck development

1. **The face and neck are derived from a series of branchial arches that lie on either side of the stomodaeum**

2. **Pharyngeal arches (Table 2.1)**
   - Develop in the 4th week of embryonic life
   - Arise from neural crests
   - Five pairs of arches (1, 2, 3, 4, and 6)
   - 5th pharyngeal arch
     - i. Is rudimentary
     - ii. Disappears
   - Each arch consists of
     - i. A core of mesenchyme, which differentiates into
       - Cartilage
       - Muscle
       - Aortic arch artery
     - ii. An inner endoderm (gives rise to pharyngeal pouches)
     - iii. An outer ectoderm (gives rise to pharyngeal clefts)
   - Each pharyngeal arch is supplied by a cranial nerve

Table 2.1 Pharyngeal arches

Arch	Nerve	Muscles	Bones and cartilages
1st	Trigeminal	Of mastication 1. Mylohyoid 2. Anterior belly of digastric 3. Tensor veli palatine 4. Tensor tympani	Malleus Incus Sphenoid
2nd	Facial	Of facial expression 1. Buccinator 2. Stapedius 3. Stylohyoid 4. Posterior belly of digastric	Stapes Styloid process Lesser horn of hyoid bone
3rd	Glossopharyngeal	Stylopharyngeus	Greater horn (lower part) of hyoid bone
4th	Vagus	Pharyngeal Cricothyroid	Thyroid cartilage Cricoid cartilage
6th	Vagus	Muscles of 1. Larynx 2. Oesophagus	Arytenoid cartilages

3. **Pharyngeal clefts**
   - Only the first pair contributes (forms the external acoustic meatus)
   - 2nd pharyngeal arch enlarges and grows as a flap covering the remaining clefts and forms the platysma muscle
   - Remnants of lower cleft may form a cervical sinus

4. **Pharyngeal pouches (Box 2.15)**
   - Derived from endoderm of the foregut growing laterally as pockets on each side of the pharynx

- 3rd and 4th pharyngeal pouches have dorsal and ventral portions
- Tympanic membrane is formed by
  - i.   Ectoderm of 1st pharyngeal arch
  - ii. Intermediate layer
  - iii. Endoderm layer of 1st pharyngeal pouch

Box 2.15 Pharyngeal pouches and their derivatives

1st	2nd	3rd	4th
• Tubotympanic recess • Middle ear • Auditory tube • Tubal tonsil	• Palantine tonsil	• DORSAL – Inferior parathyroid glands • VENTRAL – Thymus gland	• DORSAL – Superior parathyroid glands • VENTRAL – Ultimobranchial body

5th
• Ultimobranchial body (fuses with lateral lobe of thyroid gland) • Parafollicular cells (produce calcitonin)

5. **Thyroid gland**
   - Grows from the thyroid diverticulum
     - i.   Divides into the left and right thyroid lobes
   - Thyroglossal duct
     - i.   Connects the foramen caecum to the thyroid gland
     - ii. Detaches from the pharyngeal floor
     - iii. Gives rise to the pyramidal lobe of the thyroid

Tongue

1. **Develops from**
   - Epithelium of the floor of the pharynx
   - Muscles invade the tongue in 2nd month from occipital myotomes bringing hypoglossal nerve innervation with it

2. **Anterior 2/3 of the tongue is formed by 3 swellings from the 1st pharyngeal arch**
   - 2 lateral lingual swellings
   - Tuberculum impar

3. **Posterior 1/3 of the tongue is formed by the hypobranchial eminence derived from**
   - 3rd pharyngeal arch
   - 4th pharyngeal arch

4. **Sulcus terminalis**
   - V shaped groove
   - Represents line of fusion between 1st and 3rd pharyngeal arches

5. **Foramen caecum**
   - Is a midline depression in the sulcus terminalis
   - Appears as an invagination of the endoderm at the floor of the pharynx between the 1st and 2nd pharyngeal pouches
   - Marks the origin of the thyroid diverticulum

6. **Nerve innervation**
   - Anterior 2/3
     i. Lingual branch of mandibular nerve (trigeminal nerve)
     ii. Chorda tympani nerve (facial nerve)
   - Posterior 1/3
     i. Vagus
     ii. Glossopharyngeal
   - Vallate papillae (lies anterior to sulcus terminalis)
     i. Glossopharyngeal nerve (due to forward migration of posterior 1/3 of the tongue mucosa across the sulcus terminalis)

Face

1. **Develops from neural crest as 5 swellings**
   - Frontonasal prominence forms
     i. Forehead
     ii. Nose
     iii. Philtrum
     iv. Primary palate
   - Paired maxillary prominences form
     i. Cheek
     ii. Maxilla
     iii. Zygoma
     iv. Lateral portions of upper lip
     v. Secondary palate
   - Paired mandibular prominences form
     i. Cheek
     ii. Lower lip
     iii. Mandible

2. **Events that shape the facial appearance**
   - Nasal placodes
     i. Appear on frontonasal prominence
     ii. Medial nasal processes fuse to form intermaxillary segment
   - Maxillary prominences
     i. Fuse with the lateral and medial nasal processes to form the upper lip
   - Nasolacrimal groove
     i. Separates the lateral nasal process from the maxillary prominence
     ii. Ectoderm floor forms the nasolacrimal duct
     iii. Upper end forms the nasolacrimal sac
   - Mandibular prominences
     i. Fuse laterally with the maxillary prominences to form the mouth and cheek
     ii. Fuse in the midline to form the lower jaw

3. **Nasal cavity**
   - Nasal placodes invaginate to form the nasal pit
   - Nasal pit
     i. Becomes the nasal sac
     ii. Also known as anterior nares
   - Nasal sac
     i. Grows upwards
     ii. Separated from oral cavity by oronasal membrane
     iii. Oronasal membrane breaks down at 7th week of intrauterine life

- Posterior nares open into the pharynx
- Nasal septum
  i.   Develops at the 9th week of intrauterine life
  ii. Develops from the medial nasal processes
  iii. Grows towards the palate
- Maxillary sinus
  i.   Grows from lateral nasal cavity
  ii. Grows into maxillary bones
- The remainder of the paranasal sinuses develop after birth

4. **Palate develops from fusion of**
   - Primary palate (derived from the intermaxillary segment)
   - Secondary palate (formed by a pair of palatine process from the maxillary prominence)

Eye development

1. **Placodes**
   - Are thickened areas of ectoderm in the head region of the embryo
   - Form as a result of interaction between the neural tube and the overlying ectoderm
   - Become columnar
   - Invaginate
   - Migrate deep to the surface ectoderm

2. **Optic vesicles**
   - Are the earliest indication of the eye
   - Develop at 4th week of intrauterine life
   - Are an outgrowth from the lateral wall of the forebrain
   - Induce development of the lens placode
   - Become the optic cup

3. **Optic stalk is the connection between the optic vesicle and the forebrain**

4. **Lens vesicle**
   - Formed by lens placode
   - Detaches from surface ectoderm
   - Sinks into optic vesicle

5. **Hyaloid artery**
   - Branch of ophthalmic artery
   - Supplies
     i.   Lens (the branch of which eventually regresses)
     ii. Retina
   - Runs along the choroidal fissure

6. **Retina**
   - Formed by 2 layers of the optic cup
     i.   Outer layer forms the pigmented layer
     ii. Inner layer forms the rods and cones
   - At the rim of the optic cup the retina gives rise to
     i.   Ciliary body
     ii. Iris

7. **The mesenchyme around the optic cup condenses to form**
   - Inner choroids
   - Outer sclera

8. **Cornea**
   - Anterior part of the sclera
   - Transparent

9. **Eyelids**
   - Develop as folds of ectoderm
   - Grow over the cornea
   - Both the eyelids fuse initially (they separate at 5–7 months of intrauterine life)
   - The inner layer of the eyelid (ectoderm) becomes the conjunctiva

Ear development

1. **The ear develops from 3 different regions**
   - External ear – 1st pharyngeal cleft
   - Middle ear – 1st pharyngeal pouch
   - Inner ear – otic placode

2. **Otic placode**
   - Close to hindbrain
   - First part of ear to develop at 22 days of embryonic life
   - Invaginates as the otic vesicle

3. **Otic vesicle**
   - Forms
     i.   Dorsal vestibular portion
     ii. Ventral cochlear portion
   - Gives rise to the endolymphatic sac
   - Vestibular portion has 2 parts
     i.   Larger – utricle
     ii. Smaller – saccule
   - Utricle gives rise to 3 semicircular ducts
   - Structures within the otic vesicle form the membranous labyrinth

Anatomy

CONTENTS

Trunk surface anatomy

1. **Vertebral levels**
   - T2 – Suprasternal notch
   - T5 – Angle of Louis
   - T9 – Xiphoid
   - L1 – Transpyloric plane of Addison
     i. Halfway between suprasternal notch and pubis
     ii. One hand width below xiphoid
     iii. Crosses
        - Pancreatic neck
        - Duodenojejunal flexure
        - Fundus of gall bladder
        - Tip of 9th costal cartilage
        - Renal hilum
     iv. Termination of spinal cord
   - L3 – Subcostal plane (line that joins the inferior margins of 10th rib)
   - L4 – Iliac crest plane
     i. Bifurcation of aorta
   - S2 – Posterior superior iliac spines
     i. Termination of dural sheath

2. **Position of umbilicus is variable, but is usually at vertebral level L3–L5**

3. **Costal margin is the medial margins formed by the false ribs (7–10)**

4. **Linea semilunaris is the lateral border of the rectus abdominis**

5. **McBurney's point is 2/3 of the way laterally along the line from the umbilicus to the anterior superior iliac spine on the right side**

6. Palmer's point is 2/3 of the way laterally along the line from the umbilicus to the point of intersection between the midclavicular line and the costal margins of the 9th rib

7. **Arcuate line of Douglas is**
    - Where inferior epigastric vessels enter the rectus sheath
    - Point of termination of posterior rectus sheath
    - Halfway between the umbilicus and the pubis

8. **Linea alba**
    - Is a fusion of abdominal muscle aponeuroses
    - Stretches from xiphoid to pubic symphysis

9. **Organs palpable in a normal adult**
    - Liver – lower border
    - Right kidney – lower pole
    - Caecum
    - Sigmoid
    - Aorta

10. **Paracentesis is done at**
    - Midline (linea alba)
    - Lateral to McBurney's point (to avoid inferior epigastric vessels)

Abdomen

Abdominal wall

1. **Abdominal fasciae**
    - Trunk has **only** superficial fascia composed of
      i.   Fatty layer of Camper
      ii. Deep fibrous layer of Scarpa
    - Scarpa's fascia
      i.   Blends in with deep fascia of upper thigh
      ii. In the perineum it continues as Colles' fascia

2. **Abdominal wall muscles (*Table 3.1*)**
    - Anterior wall muscles
      i.   Rectus abdominis
    - Lateral wall muscles
      i.   External oblique
      ii. Internal oblique
      iii. Transversus abdominis
    - Posterior wall muscles
      i.   Diaphragm
      ii. Quadrates lumborum
      iii. Psoas major
      iv. Iliacus

3. **Rectus sheath aponeurosis**
    - Is made up of
      i.   Anterior leaf
      ii. Posterior leaf
    - Posterior leaf is present only from below the costal margins to the arcuate line
    - Composition (*Table 3.2*)

Table 3.1 Abdominal wall muscles

	Muscle	Origin	Insertion	Innervation/notes
Anterior abdominal wall	Rectus abdominis	5–7th costal cartilages	Pubic crest	Tendinous insertions 1. 3 between xiphoid and umbilicus 2. 1 below umbilicus 3. Only on anterior rectus 4. Superior epigastric vessels pierce the rectus at this sites
	External oblique	Outer surface of the lower 8 ribs	1. Xiphoid 2. Linea alba 3. Pubic crest 4. Pubic tubercle 5. Anterior half of iliac crest	Innervated by anterior primary rami of T7–T12
	Internal oblique	1. Lumbar fasciae 2. Anterior 2/3 of Iliac crest 3. Lateral 2/3 of Inguinal ligament	1. Lower 6 costal cartilages 2. Linea alba 3. Pubic crest	Innervated by anterior primary rami of T7–T12
	Transversus abdominis	1. Lower 6 costal cartilages 2. Lumbar fascia 3. Anterior 2/3 of Iliac crest 4. Lateral 1/3 of Inguinal ligament	1. Linea alba 2. Pubic crest	Innervated by anterior primary rami of T7–T12
Posterior abdominal wall	Psoas major	Transverse process of lumbar vertebrae	Lesser trochanter of femur	Innervated by anterior primary rami of L1 and L2 Acts as hip flexor
	Psoas minor	Bodies of T12 and L1	Iliopectineal eminence	Lies on psoas major Absent in 40% of people
	Iliacus	Upper 2/3 of inner aspect of Iliac crest	Lateral side of psoas major tendon	Innervation is via the femoral nerve Acts as hip flexor

Table 3.2 Rectus sheath composition

	Above the costal margins	Costal margins to arcuate line of Douglas	Below the arcuate line of Douglas
Anterior leave	External oblique	External oblique Internal oblique	External oblique Internal oblique Transversus abdominis
Posterior leave	None	Internal oblique Transversus abdominis	None

Ligaments, canals, and fossae

1. **Inguinal ligament**
   - Also known as ligament of Poupart
   - Runs from anterior superior iliac spine (ASIS) to pubic tubercle
   - Aponeurosis formed by external oblique

2. **Inguinal canal**
   - 3.8 cm long
   - Lies parallel and above inguinal ligament
   - Runs from internal to external ring
   - Internal ring
     - i.   Lies on the transversalis fascia
     - ii. Midpoint of inguinal ligament
     - iii. Medially demarcated by inferior epigastric vessels
     - iv. 1.26 cm above femoral artery
   - External ring
     - i.   V shaped
     - ii. Defect in external oblique aponeurosis
     - iii. Lies above and medial to pubic tubercle
   - Canal relations (*Fig. 3.1*)

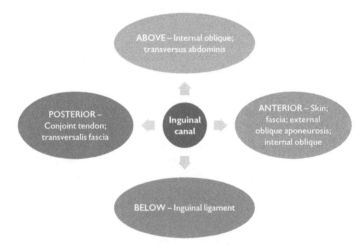

Figure 3.1 Inguinal canal relations

3. **Conjoint tendon**
   - Fusion of
     - i.   Internal oblique
     - ii. Transversus abdominis
   - Inserts into
     - i.   Pectineal line
     - ii. Pubic crest

4. **Spermatic cord comprises of**
   - 3 fascial layers
     - i.   External spermatic (formed by external oblique aponeurosis)
     - ii. Cremasteric (formed by internal oblique)
     - iii. Internal spermatic (formed by transversalis fascia)

- 3 arteries
  i. Testicular (branch of aorta)
  ii. Vas (branch of inferior vesicle)
  iii. Cremasteric (branch of inferior epigastric)
- 3 nerves
  i. Ilioinguinal (on top of cord)
  ii. Cremasteric (branch of genitofemoral nerve)
  iii. Sympathetic
- 3 other structures
  i. Vas deferens
  ii. Pampiniform plexus of veins
  iii. Lymphatics

5. **Femoral triangle**
   - Content
     i. Femoral nerve
     ii. Femoral artery
     iii. Femoral vein
     iv. Deep inguinal nodes
   - Boundaries (*Fig. 3.2*)

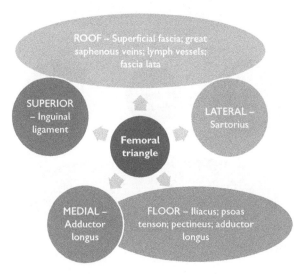

Figure 3.2 Femoral triangle boundaries

6. **Femoral sheath (*Fig. 3.3*)**
   - Is derived from extraperitoneal intra-abdominal fascia
     i. Anterior = Transversalis fascia
     ii. Posterior = Iliacus fascia
   - Contains the
     i. Femoral canal
     ii. Femoral artery
     iii. Femoral vein
   - Does **not** contain the femoral nerve

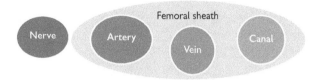

Figure 3.3 Femoral sheath content (from lateral to medial)

7. **Femoral ring**
   - Entrance to femoral canal
   - Is oval
   - Larger in females
   - Diameter = 1.25 cm
   - Contains
     i. Fat
     ii. Lymph node (Cloquet's)
   - Boundaries (*Fig. 3.4*)

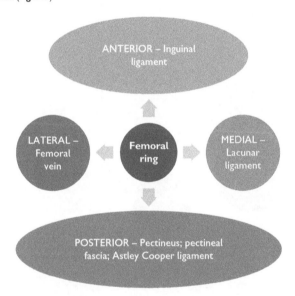

Figure 3.4 Femoral ring boundaries

8. **Lacunar ligament**
   - Also known as Gimbernat's ligament
   - Is part of aponeurosis of external oblique that is reflected backwards and lateralwards and is attached to the pectineal line of pubis
   - Larger in males
   - Posterior margin is attached to pectineal ligament
   - Anterior margin is attached to inguinal ligament

9. **Adductor canal**
   - Also known as
     i. Subsartorial
     ii. Hunter's

- Aponeurotic tunnel in the middle third of the thigh
- Extends from apex of femoral triangle to the adductor hiatus
- Boundaries
  i.   Anterior and lateral = vastus medialis
  ii. Posteriorly = adductor longus and magnus
- Lying on the aponeurosis is the sartorius muscle
- The canal contains
  i.   Femoral vessels
  ii. Saphenous nerve

10. Hasselbach's triangle
- Is a space bounded by
  i.   Laterally – inferior epigastric artery
  ii. Medially – rectus abdominus
  iii. Inferiorly – inguinal ligament
- Also known as the inguinal triangle
- Site of direct inguinal hernia

Peritoneal cavity

1. Peritoneal cavity is
- Formed by primitive coelomic cavity of the embryo
- Serous lined
- Closed in the male
- Consist of the (*Fig. 3.5*)
  i.   Greater sac
  ii. Lesser sac

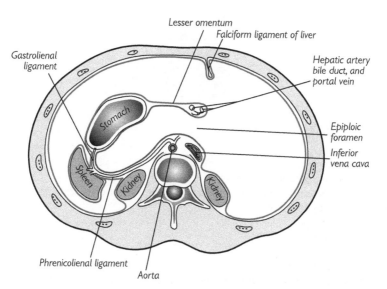

Figure 3.5 Relations of the lesser (marked in dark grey) and greater (marked in purple) sac
Reproduced from *Gray's Anatomy*, 20 US ed., http://www.bartleby.com/107/246.html, with permission from Bartleby.com, Inc.

2. Lesser sac
- Is the cavity formed by the lesser and greater omentum

- Also known as omental bursa
- Projects downwards between the layers of greater omentum (usually obliterated)
- Boundaries
  - i. Left = spleen
  - ii. Right = epiploic foramen
  - iii. Superior = liver
  - iv. Anterior = stomach
  - v. Posterior = pancreas

3. **Epiploic foramen**
   - Is also known as foramen of Winslow
   - Is the entrance to the lesser sac
   - Borders (*Fig. 3.6*)

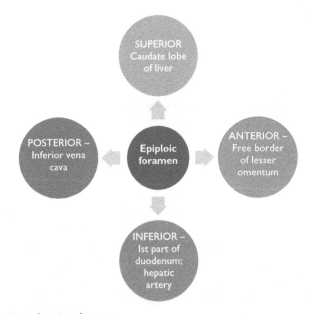

Figure 3.6 Borders of epiploic foramen

4. **Lesser omentum**
   - Also known as gastrohepatic omentum
   - Is a double layer of peritoneum extending from liver to lesser curvature of the stomach
   - Is divided into 4 ligaments
     - i. Hepatogastric
     - ii. Hepatoduodenal
     - iii. Hepatophrenic
     - iv. Hepato-oesophageal
   - Free border of lesser omentum contains portal vein, common bile duct, and hepatic artery enclosed in Glisson's capsule (*Fig. 3.7*)

5. **Greater omentum**
   - Also known as gastrocolic omentum
   - It is a large fold of peritoneum that extends from the stomach to the posterior abdominal wall after encasing the transverse colon

- Is continuous with
  - i.   Duodenum on the right
  - ii. Gastrolienal ligament on the left
  - iii. Blood supply = right and left gastroepiploic vessels
- Is divided into 4 ligaments
  - i.   Gastrocolic
  - ii. Gastrosplenic
  - iii. Gastrophrenic
  - iv. Splenorenal

6. **Ligaments within the peritoneal cavity**
   - Umbilical ligaments
     - i.   Median (also known as urachus, an embryological remnant of the allantois)
     - ii. Medial (an embryological remnant of the umbilical artery)
     - iii. Lateral (overlies the inferior epigastric artery)
   - Falciform ligament (runs from umbilicus to liver)
   - Ligamentum teres
     - i.   Remnants of umbilical vein
     - ii. Passes between quadrate and left liver lobes
     - iii. Attaches to the free border of falciform ligament

7. **Intraperitoneal fossae – there are 4**
   - The lesser sac
   - Intersigmoid
   - Paraduodenal (between duodenojejunal junction and inferior mesenteric vessels)
   - Retrocaecal

8. **Subphrenic spaces – there are 5**
   - Subphrenic
     - i. Right and left
     - ii. Divided by falciform ligament
   - Right subhepatic (Morison's)
   - Left subhepatic (lesser sac)
   - Right extraperitoneal (between bare area of liver and diaphragm)

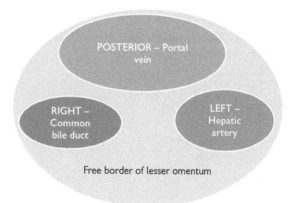

Figure 3.7 Content of the free border of the lesser omentum

Pelvis

Bones and ligaments

1. **Pelvis is made up of**
   - Innominate bones
   - Sacrum
   - Coccyx

2. **Innominate bones consist of 3 bones**
   - Ilium
   - Ischium
   - Pubis

3. **Iliopectineal eminence**
   - Is the point of fusion between the pubis and ilium
   - Lateral to it, 2 muscles pass in a groove
     i.   Iliacus
     ii. Psoas major

4. **Obturator foramen is bounded by the pubis and ischium**

5. **Acetabulum is the fusion point of all 3 innominate bones**

6. **Sacrum**
   - Is made up of 5 fused vertebrae
   - Is triangular
   - Sacral promontory represents the anterior border of the upper part of sacrum
   - Consists anteriorly of
     i.   Central mass
     ii. 2 x row of 4 anterior sacral foramina
     iii. 2 × lateral mass
     iv. 2 × ala (superior aspect of lateral mass)
   - Consists posteriorly of
     i.   Sacral canal
     ii. 2 × row of 4 posterior sacral foramina
     iii. Sacral hiatus (transmits the 5th sacral nerve)
     iv. Sacral cornua
     v.   Superior articular facet
   - Dural sheath terminates at S2, beyond which the sacral canal contains
     i.   Fatty tissue of extradural space
     ii. Cauda equina
     iii. Filum terminale

7. **Coccyx is made up of 3–5 fused vertebrae**

8. **Pelvic joints**
   - Symphysis pubis is **not** a synovial joint
   - Sacroiliac joint is a synovial joint

9. **Pelvic brim is bounded by**
   - Pectineal line
   - Arcuate line

- Sacral promontory
- Upper margins of symphysis pubis

10. Linea terminalis consists of
- Arcuate line
- Pectineal line
- Pubic crest

11. Pelvic outlet
- Is bounded by
  - i.   Pubic arch (ischiopubic rami)
  - ii. 2 × sciatic notch
  - iii. Coccyx
- Diamond in shape

12. Dimple just above the buttocks defines
- S2
- Sacroiliac joint
- Termination of dural sheath
- Posterior superior iliac spines

13. Sacrospinous ligament runs from the ischial spine to the sacrum/coccyx

14. Sacrotuberous ligament runs from sacrum to ischial tuberosity

15. Boundaries of greater sciatic foramen (*Fig. 3.8*)

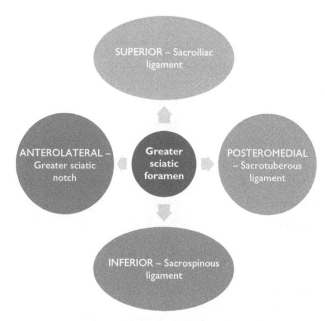

Figure 3.8 Boundaries of the greater sciatic foramen

16. Boundaries of lesser sciatic foramen (*Fig. 3.9*)

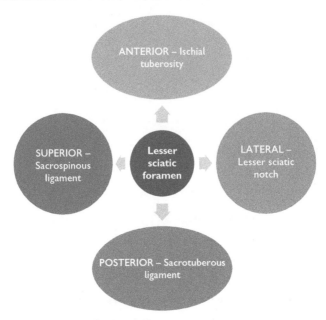

Figure 3.9 Boundaries of the lesser sciatic foramen

17. Female versus male pelvis (*Table 3.3*)

Table 3.3 Female versus male pelvis

	Male	Female
Acetabulum	Large	Small
Obturator foramen	Round	Oval
Ischial tuberosity	Inturned	Everted
Pelvic inlet	Heart shaped	Oval
Pelvic canal	Long	Short
Pelvic outlet	Small	Large
Inferior pubic rami angle	Acute	Wide (90°)
Ischial tuberosity angle	–	Admits 4 knuckles
Sacrum	Long and narrow	Short and wide

18. Pelvis measurements (*Table 3.4*)
- Plane of inlet = 60° to the horizontal
- Diagonal conjugate = 12.7 cm (promontory of sacrum to lower border of pubic symphysis)
- Anteroposterior outlet is from midpoint of pubic symphysis to apex of coccyx
- Transverse outlet is the distance between the ischial tuberosities
- Oblique outlet is from midpoint of sacrotuberous ligament to junction of opposite ischial and pubic rami

Table 3.4 Pelvic measurements in centimetres

	Transverse	**Oblique**	**Anteroposterior**
Inlet	12.7	11.5 Iliopectineal eminence – opposite sacroiliac joint	10 Sacral promontory – symphysis pubis
Mid	11.5	11.5 Lower sacroiliac joint – midpoint of obturator membrane	11.5 S3 – Midpoint of pubic symphysis
Outlet	10 Distance between ischial tuberosities	11.5	12.7 Pubis to sacrococcygeal joint

Pelvic muscles (Table 3.5)

Table 3.5 Pelvic muscles

Muscle	Origin	Insertion	Notes

Piriformis	1. Anterior part of sacrum
	2. Greater sciatic foramen
	3. Anterior surface of
	   sacrotuberous ligament
		Greater trochanter
		of femur
			1. Exits pelvis via greater
			   sciatic foramen
			2. Is pierced by the common
			   peroneal nerve

Obturator internus	1. Medial surface of obturator membrane 2. Ischium 3. Pubis	Greater trochanter of femur	Exits pelvis via lesser sciatic foramen
Obturator externus	1. Obturator membrane 2. Obturator foramen	Greater trochanter of femur	

Fasciae

1. **Pelvic fascia**
   - Is the term applied to the connective tissue of the covering of the pelvis
   - Includes the fascial coverings of
     i. Levator ani
     ii. Obturator internus

2. **Endopelvic fascia**
   - Is the extraperitoneal tissue of the
     i. Uterus (parametrium)
     ii. Vagina
     iii. Bladder
     iv. Rectum
   - Gives rise to 3 sets of ligaments
     i. Cardinal ligaments
     ii. Uterosacral ligaments
     iii. Pubocervical ligaments (extend from cardinal ligaments to pubis)

- These 3 ligaments
  i.   Support the cervix and vaginal vault
  ii. Are lengthened in pelvic floor prolapse

3. **Cardinal ligaments**
   - Also known as
     i.   Transverse ligaments
     ii. Mackenrodt's ligaments
   - Pass laterally from the cervix and upper vagina
   - Attach to pelvic side walls along the line of insertion of the levator ani
   - Pierced by ureters

4. **Uterosacral ligaments**
   - Originate
     i.   From posterolateral aspect of cervix
     ii. At the level of isthmus
   - Attached to
     i.   Periosteum of sacroiliac joints
     ii. Lateral part of S3
   - Encircle the pouch of Douglas

5. **Round ligament**
   - Together with the ovarian ligament is equivalent to the male gubernaculum
   - Blood supply is via uterine artery

Pelvic floor

1. **The pelvic floor is made up of 2 components**
   - Pelvic diaphragm (**Table 3.6**)
     i.   Levator ani
     ii. Coccygeus muscle
   - Superficial muscles of the perineum forming
     i.   Anterior (urogenital) triangle
     ii. Posterior (anal) triangle

Table 3.6 Pelvic diaphragm

Pelvic floor muscle	Origin	Insertion	Notes
Levator ani	1. Posterior aspect of pubic bone 2. Fascia of side wall of pelvis (covering obturator internus) 3. Ischial spine	1. Perineal body 2. Anal sphincter 3. Coccyx 4. Median fibrous raphe	Forms 1. Levator prostate 2. Sphincter vaginae 3. Puborectalis 4. Pubococcygeus 5. Iliococcygeus
Coccygeus	1. Sacrospinous ligament 2. Ischial spine	Coccyx	

2. **Anterior (urogenital) triangle is bound by**
   - Line across ischial tuberosities
   - Ischiopubic inferior rami

3. **Perineal membrane**
   - Is attached to the urogenital triangle
   - Is pierced by
     i. Urethra
     ii. Vagina
   - Forms 2 spaces
     i. Deep perineal pouch
     ii. Superficial perineal pouch

4. **Deep perineal pouch**
   - Is bound by perineal membrane and levator ani fascia
   - Contains
     i. External urethral sphincter
     ii. Deep transverse perineal muscle
     iii. Bulbourethral glands (Cowper's)

5. **Superficial perineal pouch**
   - Boundaries
     i. Superiorly = perineal membrane
     ii. Inferiorly = perineal fascia (Colles' fascia)
   - Contains
     i. Superficial perineal muscles
     ii. Bulbospongiosus
     iii. Ischiocavernosus
     iv. Bartholin's glands (greater vestibular glands)
     v. Crura of clitoris

6. **Perineal body**
   - Is a fibromuscular node
   - Lies in the midline at the junction of the anterior and posterior perineum
   - Is the point of attachment for
     i. External anal sphincter
     ii. Bulbospongiosus
     iii. Transverse perineal muscles
     iv. Levator ani

7. **Posterior (anal) triangle**
   - Is the space between the ischial tuberosities and coccyx
   - Contains
     i. Ischiorectal fossa
     ii. Levator ani
     iii. Anus

8. **Ischiorectal fossa**
   - Contains
     i. Lobulated fat
     ii. Anus
     iii. External anal sphincter
     iv. Alcock's canal
   - Fossae on either side communicate with each other behind the anus
   - Boundaries (*Fig. 3.10*)

9. **External anal sphincter attaches to**
   - Perineal body

- Coccyx
- Puborectalis

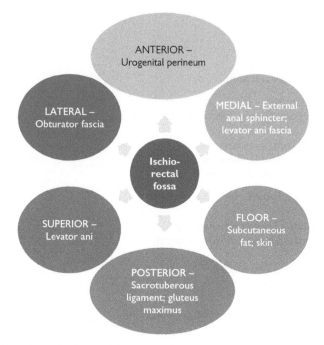

Figure 3.10 Boundaries of ischiorectal fossa

Gastrointestinal tract

Stomach

1. **Is J shaped**

2. **Consists of**
   - Fundus
   - Body
   - Pyloric antrum

3. **Body secretes**
   - Pepsin
   - HCl (oxyntic cells)

4. **Pyloric antrum secretes**
   - Alkaline juices
   - Gastrin

5. **Incisura angularis marks the junction between the body and pyloric antrum**

6. **Vein of Mayo marks the junction between the pylorus and duodenum**

7. **Sphincters**
   - Cardia
   - Pylorus

8. Borders (*Fig. 3.11*)

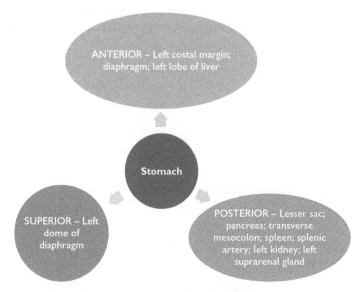

Figure 3.11 Relationship of stomach to other abdominal organs

9. **Blood supply is via branches of the coeliac axis** (*Fig. 3.12*)
   - Left gastric artery
   - Splenic artery
   - Hepatic artery

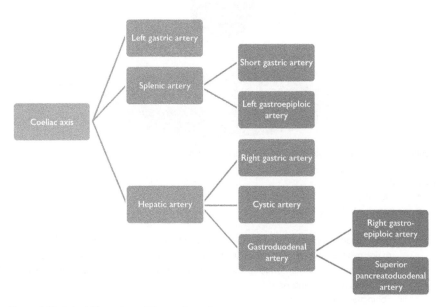

Figure 3.12 Arterial branches of the coeliac axis

10. Lymphatics
- Area 1 (superior 2/3 of stomach) drains directly to aortic nodes
- Area 2 (right 2/3 of inferior 1/3 of stomach) drains via subpyloric node to aortic nodes
- Area 3 (left 1/3 of inferior 1/3 of stomach) drains via suprapancreatic node to aortic nodes

11. Nerve supply
- Vagus nerve
- Posterior nerve of Latarjet

Duodenum

1. C shaped

2. Contains Brunner's glands

3. 25.5 cm long

4. Covered by peritoneum for 2.5 cm then becomes retroperitoneal

5. Divided into 4 parts

6. **1st part**
   - 5 cm long
   - Relations (*Fig. 3.13*)

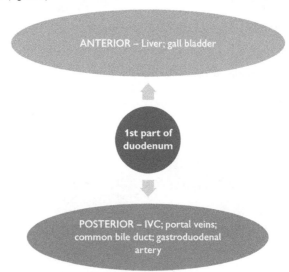

Figure 3.13 1st part of duodenum and its spatial relations

7. **2nd part**
   - 7.5 cm long
   - Curves around head of pancreas
   - Contains
     i. Major duodenal papilla (also known as ampulla of Vater) – which is the opening of the major pancreatic duct (also known as duct of Wirsung) and the common bile duct
     ii. Minor duodenal papilla – which is the opening of the accessory pancreatic duct (also known as duct of Santorini)
     iii. Sphincter of Oddi
   - Relations (*Fig. 3.14*)

8. **3rd part**
   - 10 cm long
   - Runs transversely towards the left
   - Relations (*Fig. 3.15*)

9. **4th part is 2.5 cm long**

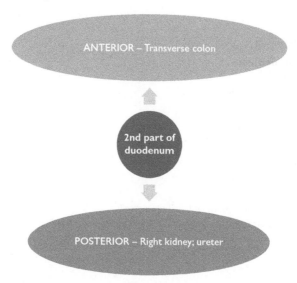

Figure 3.14 2nd part of duodenum and its spatial relations

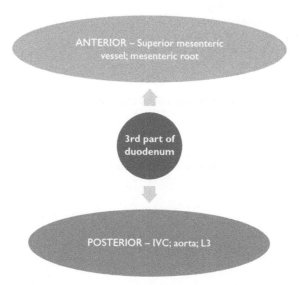

Figure 3.15 3rd part of the duodenum and its spatial relations

10. **Duodenojejunal junction is identified by**
   - Ligament of Treitz (a peritoneal fold from the right crus of the diaphragm containing some smooth and skeletal muscle fibres)

• Inferior mesenteric vessels descend from behind the pancreas immediately to the left of the junction

11. Blood supply
• Superior pancreatoduodenal artery
• Inferior pancreatoduodenal artery (branch of superior mesenteric artery)

Small intestines

1. Measure 3–10 m long

2. Small intestine mesentery
• Is 15 cm long
• Starts at duodenojejunal junction (L2)
• Ends at right sacroiliac joint

3. Have valvulae conniventes

4. Jejunum versus ileum
• Jejunum has a thicker wall
• Jejunum has a larger diameter
• Jejunum lies in the umbilical region
• Ileum has a thicker and more fat laden mesentery
• Mesenteric vessels form 1–2 arcades at the jejunum while at the ileum they form 3–5 arcades

Large intestine

1. Comprises 7 portions
• Caecum (along with the appendix)
• Ascending colon (20 cm long)
• Transverse colon (45.5 cm long)
• Descending colon (25.4 cm long)
• Sigmoid (12.7–76 cm long)
• Rectum (12.7 cm long)
• Anal canal (3.8 cm long)

2. Has appendices epiploicae (fat-filled peritoneal tags) except for
• Appendix
• Caecum
• Rectum

3. Has taenia coli (3 flattened bands running from base of appendix to retrosigmoid junction) except for
• Appendix
• Rectum

4. Has sacculations

5. Peritoneal coverings (Box 3.1)

6. Mucosa has
• Goblet cells
• No villi

7. Nerve plexus
• Meissner's (in submucosa layer)
• Auerbach's (between muscular layers)

Box 3.1 Peritoneal coverings of the large intestine

Peritonized	Non-peritonized	Inconsistent
• Transverse colon	• Ascending colon	• Caecum
• Sigmoid	• Descending colon	• Appendix

Rectum

1. **Has no peritoneal covering in its**
   - Upper 1/3 posteriorly
   - Middle 1/3 posteriorly and laterally
   - Entire lower 1/3

2. **Commences at S3**

3. **Ends at level of**
   - Lower 1/4 of vagina in women
   - Apex of prostate in men

4. **Has**
   - 3 lateral inflexions (left, right, left)
   - Valves of Houston

5. **Denonvilliers' fascia separates the rectum from anterior structures**

6. **Relations (*Fig. 3.16*)**

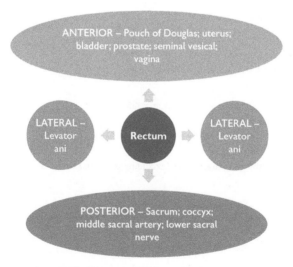

Figure 3.16 Rectum and its spatial relations

Anal canal

1. **Epithelium**
   - Lower half = squamous
   - Upper half = columnar (columns of Morgagni)
   - This junction is separated by valves of Ball

2. **Blood supply**
   - Upper 1/2 = superior rectal vessel
   - Lower 1/2 = inferior rectal vessel

3. **Lymphatics**
   - Upper 1/2 = lumbar nodes
   - Lower 1/2 = inguinal nodes

4. **Relations**
   - Anterior = perineal body
   - Posterior = coccyx
   - Lateral = ischiorectal fossa

5. **Haemorrhoids = dilatation of superior rectal veins**

Appendix

1. **Also known as vermiform appendix**

2. **Connects to the caecum**

3. **Base is 2.5 cm below the ileocaecal valve**

4. **Lies posteromedial to caecum**

5. **Length = 2.5–23 cm**

6. **Blood supply = ileocolic artery**

7. **Has 2 folds of peritoneal attachment**
   - Ileocaecal fold
   - Appendix mesentery

8. **Ileocaecal fold**
   - Passes from the front of the ileum to the appendix
   - Is also known as bloodless fold of Treves

9. **Appendix mesentery**
   - Descends from behind the ileum to the appendix
   - Contains the ileocolic artery

Portal vein system

1. **Drains blood from the alimentary tract (excluding the anus) to the liver**

2. **Formation**
   - Inferior mesenteric vein joins the splenic vein above L3
   - Superior mesenteric vein joins the splenic vein behind neck of pancreas at L1, giving rise to the portal vein
   - Portal vein divides into right and left branches

3. **Collateral pathways between portal and systemic venous systems**
   - Oesophageal branch of left gastric vein and oesophageal vein of Azygos system
   - Superior rectal and inferior rectal veins
   - Portal branches of liver and
     - i. Veins of diaphragm (bare area)
     - ii. Veins of abdominal wall (via falciform ligament)

- Portal tributaries in mesocolon, mesentery, and retroperitoneal veins to
  i.   Renal veins
  ii. Lumbar veins
  iii. Phrenic veins

Meckel's diverticulum

1. **Remnant of vitello-intestinal duct (communication between midgut and yolk sac)**

2. **Always on anti-mesenteric border**

3. **Rules of 2**
   - Prevalence = 2%
   - Male : female = 2 : 1
   - 2 inches (5 cm) long
   - Situated 2 ft (61 cm) from ileocaecal junction

Accessory gastrointestinal and other organs

Liver

1. **Largest organ in the body**

2. **Has 4 lobes**
   - Right
   - Left
   - Anterior quadrate
   - Posterior caudate

3. **Contains**
   - Falciform ligament
   - Ligamentum teres (remnant of left umbilical vein)
   - Ligamentum venosum (remnant of ductus venosum)

4. **Lesser omentum arises from**
   - Porta hepatis
   - Ligamentum venosum

5. **Porta hepatis**
   - 5 cm long
   - Contains (*Fig. 3.17*)

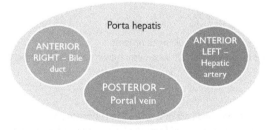

Figure 3.17 Content of porta hepatis

6. **Venous drainage – 3 in total**
   - Left
   - Right
   - Central

7. **Blood supply**
   - Left hepatic artery
   - Right hepatic artery
   - Cystic artery

Biliary system

1. **Common hepatic duct**
   - Formed from fusion of right and left hepatic ducts
   - 3.8 cm long

2. **Cystic duct = 3.8 cm long**

3. **Common bile duct**
   - Formed from fusion of common hepatic duct and cystic duct
   - 10 cm long

4. **Gall bladder**
   - Holds 50 mL of bile
   - Separates the right and quadrate lobes of the liver
   - Epithelium = columnar

Pancreas

1. **Weighs 80 g**

2. **Contains islets of Langerhans which secrete**
   - Glucagon (from α cells)
   - Insulin (from β cells)
   - Somatostatin (from δ cells)
   - Pancreatic polypeptide (from F cells)

3. **Is retroperitoneal**

4. **Is both an endocrine and exocrine organ**

5. **Relations (*Fig. 3.18*)**

6. **Blood supply**
   - Splenic artery
   - Pancreatoduodenal artery

7. **Development**
   - Ventral bud
     - i. It is smaller
     - ii. Forms part of the head and uncinate process
     - iii. It is drained by the duct of Wirsung (also known as the major pancreatic duct)
   - Dorsal bud
     - i. It is larger
     - ii. Forms the body, tail, and part of the head and uncinate process
     - iii. Contains the accessory duct of Santorini (also known as the accessory pancreatic duct) which is non-functional

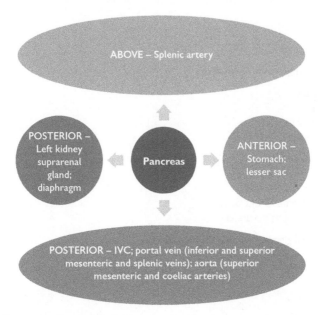

Figure 3.18 Pancreas and its spatial relations

Spleen

1. Size = a cupped hand

2. Ligaments
   - Gastrosplenic
     i. Runs to greater curve of stomach
     ii. Carries short gastric and left gastroepiploic artery
   - Lienorenal
     i. Runs to posterior abdominal wall
     ii. Contains splenic artery and tail of pancreas

3. Accessory spleen tissue can occur in
   - Ovary
   - Testes
   - Omentum
   - Small bowel mesentery
   - Tail of pancreas

Urinary system

Kidney

1. Is retroperitoneal

2. Right kidney is 1.26 cm lower than the left

3. Relations (*Fig. 3.19*)

4. Vessel order at the hilum (front to back)

- Vein
- Artery
- Pelvis of ureter

5. **Supplied by sympathetic nerve fibres**

6. **Has 3 capsules**
   - Renal fascia
   - Perinephric fat
   - True capsule

7. **Renal fascia blends with**
   - Above = diaphragm
   - Medially = IVC and aorta
   - Laterally = transversalis fascia
   - Inferiorly = tracts the ureter

8. **The suprarenal glands are not in the renal fascia**

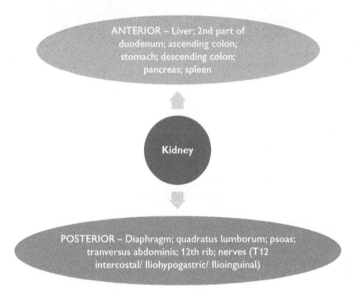

Figure 3.19 Kidney and its spatial relations

Ureters

1. **Are 25.4 cm long**

2. **Are valveless**

3. **Route**
   - Pass anterior to the medial edge of psoas major
   - Separated from tip of transverse process (L2–L5) by psoas major
   - Cross into pelvis at the bifurcation of common iliac artery in front of sacroiliac joint
   - Run on lateral wall of pelvis
   - Run in front of internal iliac artery
   - Pass under uterine artery

- Pass 1.5 cm lateral to supravaginal cervix
- Cross into bladder at ischial spine
- Pierce cardinal and broad ligaments

4. **Relations (Fig. 3.20)**

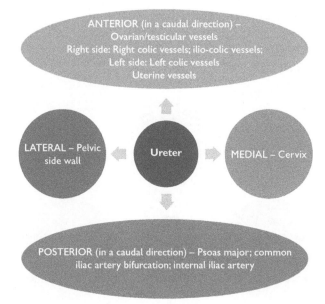

Figure 3.20 The ureter and its relationship to other organs

5. **Crossed by (in a caudal direction)**
   - Ovarian/testicular vessels
   - Right colic vessels and ileocolic vessels on the right side
   - Left colic vessels on the left side
   - Uterine vessels

6. **Blood supply (in a caudal direction) is from branches of the**
   - Aorta
   - Renal artery
   - Ovarian/testicular artery
   - Internal iliac artery
   - Inferior vesical artery

7. **Narrowing occurs at 3 sites**
   - Junction with the renal pelvis
   - Pelvic brim
   - Ureteric orifice

8. **Common sites of ureteral injury during surgery are**
   - Lateral to the uterine vessel
   - In the tunnel of the cardinal ligament
   - Base of the infundibulopelvic ligament (as the ureters cross the pelvic brim at the ovarian fossa)
   - The lateral pelvic wall (just above the uterosacral ligament)

Bladder

1. **Is extraperitoneal**

2. **Is intra-abdominal in children <3 years old**

3. **Ureteric orifices are 2.5 cm apart**

4. **Trigone is the triangular area bounded by**
    - Ureteric orifices
    - Internal meatus

5. **Relations** (*Fig. 3.21*)

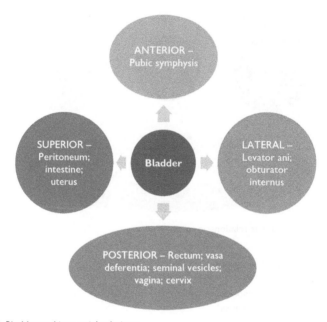

Figure 3.21 Bladder and its spatial relations

Urethra

1. **In females**
    - Is 3.8 cm long
    - Lies 2.5 cm behind the clitoris

2. **In males**
    - Is 25.4 cm long
    - Is divided into 3 portions (*Box 3.2*)
    - Prostatic utricle
        i.   Opens into the colliculus seminalis (verumontanum)
        ii. Is a blind tract
        iii. Is the remnant of paramesonephric duct
        iv. Is the equivalent of the vagina

3. **Has spiral grooves on the inside**

Chpt 2

Box 3.2 Portions of the male urethra

Prostatic	Membranous	Spongy
• Posterior wall bears the urethral crest and prostatic sinus	• Located in deep perineal pouch • Contains external urethral sphincter • Narrowest part of urethra • Bulbourethral glands enter here	• Also known as cavernous or penile portion

4. **Epithelium changes between**
   - Transitional (near the bladder)
   - Stratified columnar
   - Stratified squamous (near the external urethral orifice)

5. **Contains mucus-secreting urethral glands**

6. **Urethral sphincter**
   - Has two parts
   - i. Internal
     - Located at the junction of the urethra and bladder
     - Composed of smooth muscle (as a continuation of the bladder's detrusor muscle)
     - Under autonomic sympathetic control from the inferior hypogastric plexus
     - In males it prevents retrograde flow of semen in the bladder during ejaculation
     - In females it is not anatomically distinct, although smooth muscle fibres are still present
   - ii. External
     - Located at the junction of the urethra and bladder in females and after the prostate in males
     - Composed of skeletal muscle
     - Under voluntary control via the perineal branch of the pudendal nerve (but not exclusively)

Male genital tract

1. **External genitalia consist of**
   - Scrotum
   - Testes
   - Epididymides
   - Vasa deferentia
   - Penis, consisting of
     - i. A pair of corpus cavernosa
     - ii. Corpus spongiosum

2. **Internal genitalia consist of**
   - Seminal vesicles
   - Ejaculatory ducts
   - Prostate gland
   - Bulbourethral glands (Cowper's)

3. **Scrotum**
   - Is pigmented and rugose

- Contains
  - i.   Median longitudinal raphe
  - ii. Sebaceous glands
  - iii. Dartos muscle
- Divided into 2 sacs
- Temperature is 2.5 °C lower than body temperature

4. **Epididymides**
   - Consist of
     - i.   Head
     - ii. Body
     - iii. Tail
   - Measure 6 m long
   - Lined by ciliated epithelium
   - Passage of sperm through them takes 8–14 days

5. **Vasa deferentia**
   - Measure 45 cm long
   - Join the spermatic cord
   - Connect to the epididymides
   - Similar length to
     - i.   Femur
     - ii. Thoracic duct
     - iii. Spinal cord
     - iv. Distance from incisor to cardiac end of stomach

6. **Seminal vesicles**
   - Irregular-shaped sacs
   - Lie between base of bladder and rectum
   - Measure 5 cm long
   - Functions
     - i. Reservoir for spermatozoa
     - ii. Secrete nourishing fluid for sperm

7. **Ejaculatory ducts**
   - Measure 2.5 cm long
   - Eject sperm into urethra
   - Connect vas deferens to urethra

8. **Bulbourethral (Cowper's) glands**
   - Situated at root of penis
   - Pea sized

Testes

1. **The left testis lies lower than the right**

2. **Oval shaped**

3. **Measurements**
   - Dimensions = 55 × 30 mm
   - Weight = 10–15 g
   - Volume = 15–30 mL

4. **Have 3 layers**
   - Tunica vaginalis

- Tunica albuginea
- Tunica vasculosa

5. **Functions**
   - Produce spermatozoa
   - Produce testosterone

6. **Consist of 2 types of cell**
   - Sertoli cells
   - Leydig cells

7. **Structure**
   - Divided in to 300 lobules
   - Each lobule has 1–3 seminiferous tubules
   - Each tubule = 61 cm (2 ft) long
   - Seminiferous tubules anastomose at rete testes

8. **Seminiferous tubules**
   - Lined with germinal epithelium
   - Make up 90% of testes
   - Have a basement membrane that acts as a blood barrier

9. **Testicular artery anastomoses with vas artery (the vas artery is a branch of the inferior vesical artery)**

10. **Lymph drainage**
    - Para-aortic lymph nodes
    - Cervical nodes

11. **Nerve supply is via T10**

12. **Development (fetal life)**
    - 3 months – reach iliac fossa
    - 7 months – traverse inguinal canal
    - 8 months – situated at external ring
    - 9 months – descend in scrotum

13. **Embryological remnants**
    - Appendix testes is the remnant of the paramesonephric duct
    - Appendix epididymis is the remnant of the mesonephros

14. **Sertoli cells**
    - Situated within seminiferous tubules
    - Nourish spermatozoa
    - Produce inhibin and oestrogen
    - Contain follicle-stimulating hormone (FSH) receptors

15. **Leydig cells**
    - Situated between seminiferous tubules
    - Produce testosterone
    - Contain luteinizing hormone (LH) receptors

Prostate

1. **Measures 4 × 3 cm**

2. **Pyramidal in shape**

3. **Relations (*Fig. 3.22*)**

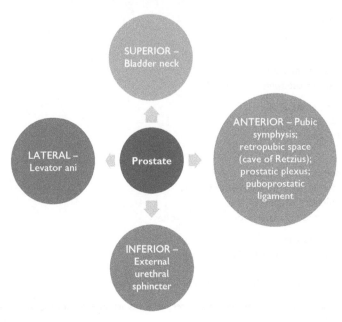

Figure 3.22 Prostate and its spatial relations

4. **Has 2 capsules**
   - True capsule
   - False capsule, which is the extraperitoneal fascia (continues with bladder and Denonvilliers' fascia)

5. **Blood supply = inferior vesical artery**

6. **Prostatic plexus**
   - Lies between the 2 capsules of the prostate
   - Receives the dorsal vein of the penis
   - Drains into
     i.   Internal iliac vein
     ii. Valveless vertebral veins of Batson

Female genital tract

1. **External genitalia**
   - Collectively known as the vulva
   - Extend from
     i.   Anteriorly – mons pubis
     ii. Posteriorly – perineum
     iii. Laterally – labium majora
   - Consist of
     i.   Mons pubis
     ii. Labia majora
     iii. Labia minora
     iv. Vestibule
     v.   Clitoris

2. **Mons pubis is the pad of fatty tissue that lies above the symphysis pubis**

3. **Labia majora**
   - Extend from mons pubis to perineum
   - Analogous to the scrotum
   - Contain
     i.   Hair-bearing skin
     ii. Sebaceous glands
     iii. Smooth muscle (tunica Dartos)
     iv. Nerve endings (free and corpuscles = Ruffini/Pacini/Merkel/Meissner)
   - Insertion point of round ligament
   - Nerve supply
     i.   Iliohypogastric nerve
     ii. Ilioinguinal nerve
     iii. Genitofemoral nerve
     iv. Posterior femoral cutaneous nerve
     v.   Pudendal nerve

4. **Labia minora**
   - Hairless skin folds
   - Give rise to
     i.   Prepuce
     ii. Frenulum
     iii. Fourchette
   - Contain sweat and sebaceous glands

5. **Vestibule**
   - Is the area enclosed by labia minora
   - Contains
     i.   Urethral orifice
     ii. Vaginal orifice
   - Blood supply
     i.   Azygos artery of vagina
     ii. Pudendal artery

6. **Clitoris**
   - Contains erectile tissues
   - Consists of
     i.   A glans
     ii. A shaft that is attached to the pubis
     iii. Paired crura that are attached to the inferior pubic rami
   - Ischiocavernosus muscles
     i.   Overlie the crura of the clitoris
     ii. Originate from ischial tuberosity
   - Bulbospongiosus (also known as bulbocavernosus) muscle
     i.   Originates from perineal body
     ii. Inserts into clitoral shaft
     iii. Overlies vestibular bulb and Bartholin's glands

7. **Bartholin's glands**
   - A pair of glands that lie
     i.   Between the perineal membrane and bulbospongiosus muscle
     ii. At the tail end of the vestibular bulb
     iii. Deep to posterior labia majora

- Pea sized
- Duct = 2.5 cm long
- Drains at 5 'clock and 7 'clock positions between the hymen and labium minus

8. **Introitus**
   - Is the vaginal orifice
   - Situated in the vestibule
   - Covered with hymen
   - Remnants of hymen are called carunculae myrtiformes

9. **Vagina**
   - Vaginal orifice is demarcated by the hymen (carunculae myrtiformes)
   - Length
     i. Anterior wall = 7.5 cm
     ii. Posterior wall = 10 cm
     iii. Length is proportional to height of the individual
   - Cervix projects into anterior part of vaginal vault
   - Has no glands
   - Is kept moist by
     i. Cervical glands
     ii. Seepage of fluid from blood capillaries
   - Relations (*Fig. 3.23*)

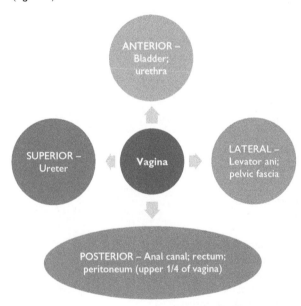

Figure 3.23 Borders of the vagina

- Peritoneum covers only the posterior upper 1/4 of the vagina
- Ureters lie above and lateral to the fornix, 1.5 cm away from the cervix
- Blood supply
  i. Uterine artery
  ii. Vaginal artery
  iii. Internal pudendal artery
  iv. Middle rectal artery

- Lymphatic drainage (*Box 3.3*)

Box 3.3 Lymphatic drainage of the vagina

Upper 1/3 of vagina	Middle 1/3 of vagina	Lower 1/3 of vagina
• External iliac nodes • Internal iliac nodes	• Internal iliac nodes	• Inguinal nodes

- Gartner's duct cyst is a mesonephric remnant in the vagina
- Vaginal fluid
  - i. pH = 4
  - ii. High K^+ content
  - iii. Low Na^+ content
  - iv. Remains alkaline 6 h post coitus
- Vaginal wall is composed of 4 layers
  - i. Inner squamous epithelium
  - ii. Connective tissue
  - iii. Muscular layer (inner circular and outer longitudinal)
  - iv. Connective tissue
- Epithelium is arranged in folds (arbour vitae)
- Vagina contains Doderlein's bacilli (converts glycogen to lactic acid)
- Nerve supply is via the sacral plexus

T. in
Obs
Gyn

*Chpts 2.4
& 12.2*

10. Uterus
- Pear-shaped organ
- Weighs
  - i. Nulliparous = 50 g
  - ii. Multiparous = 70 g
  - iii. Term = 1 kg
- Measures 7.5 × 5 × 2.5 cm
- Consists of
  - i. Fundus
  - ii. Body
  - iii. Isthmus
  - iv. Cervix
- Ante-flexed or retroflexed
  - i. Flexion of uterus at the level of the internal os
  - ii. Is usually 170°
- Anteversion or retroversion
  - i. Axis of cervix on vagina
  - ii. Is usually 90°
- Relations (*Fig. 3.24*)
- Lymphatic drainage (*Box 3.4*)
- Uterus is made up of 3 layers of tissue
  - i. Endometrium
  - ii. Myometrium
  - iii. Perimetrium
- Endometrium consist of 2 layers
  - i. Functional layer
  - ii. Basal layer
- Cervical endometrium is not shed during menstrual cycle

- Myometrium is composed of 3 layers of muscle
    i.   Inner circular
    ii. Middle oblique
    iii. Outer longitudinal
- Perimetrium is made up of peritoneum
- Nerve supply is via sacral plexus
- Blood supply
    i.   Basal layer – straight arterioles
    ii. Functional layer – spiral arterioles

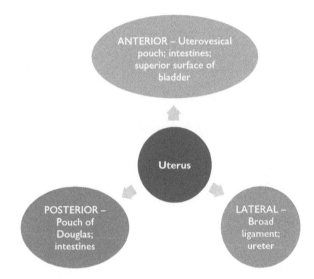

Figure 3.24 Uterus and its and its spatial relations

Box 3.4 Lymphatic drainage of the uterus

Fundus	Body
• Via round ligament to inguinal node • Via ovarian vessel to para-aortic node	• Via broad ligament to external iliac node

11. Cervix
- Epithelium consists of
    i.   Supravaginal portion = columnar cells
    ii. Vaginal portion = stratified squamous cells
- Cervical mucosa displays
    i.   Arbour vitae
    ii. Spinnbarkeit
- Lymphatic drainage (*Box 3.5*)

12. In pregnancy
- Lower segment of uterus is composed of
    i.   Isthmus = 70%
    ii. Cervix = 30%
- Internal os lies in the cervix
- Shortening of the upper segment is called retraction

Box 3.5 Lymphatic drainage of the cervix

Lateral aspect	Posterolateral aspect	Posterior aspect
• Via broad ligament to external Iliac node	• Via uterine vessels to internal iliac node	• Sacral node

- Decidua
  - i. Is endometrium under the influence of progesterone
  - ii. Has high glycogen content
  - iii. Produces prolactin and insulin-like growth factor (IGF)
- Braxton Hicks
  - i. Can occur as early as 8 weeks
  - ii. 25 mmHg of pressure is sufficient to cause cervical dilatation

13. Fallopian tubes
- 10 cm long
- Composed of
  - i. Isthmus – 2.5 cm
  - ii. Ampulla – 5 cm
  - iii. Infundibulum – 2.5 cm
  - iv. Fimbriae
- Have 4 layers
  - i. Lined by ciliated columnar epithelium
  - ii. Inner circular muscle
  - iii. Outer longitudinal muscle
  - iv. Peritoneum
- Nerve supply is via ovarian plexus

14. Uterine ligaments consist of
- Broad ligaments (is a double fold of perimetrium)
- Round ligaments (run from cornua to labia majora)
- Cardinal ligaments (run from cervix to lateral wall of pelvic cavity)
- Uterosacral ligaments (run from cervix to periosteum of sacrum)
- Pubocervical ligaments (run from cervix to pubic bone)

15. Infundibulopelvic ligaments
- Are folds of broad ligament
- Extend from infundibulum to lateral wall of the pelvis
- Contain ovarian vessels

16. Ovaries
- Measure 3 cm × 2 cm × 1 cm
- Weight 5–8 g
- Irregular surface
- Almond shaped
- Have 4 layers
  - i. Germinal epithelium
  - ii. Tunica albuginea
  - iii. Cortex (contains ovarian follicles)
  - iv. Medulla (contains vessels)
- Ovarian support ligaments
  - i. Infundibulopelvic ligament

    ii. Broad ligament

    iii. Ovarian ligament

- Attached to back of broad ligament by mesovarium
- Lie in the ovarian fossae
- Nerve supply is via T10
- Ovarian epithelium is cuboidal

17. Ovarian fossa (Waldeyer's fossa)
- Shallow depression on the lateral wall of the pelvis
- Contains the obturator nerve
- Boundaries (*Fig. 3.25*)

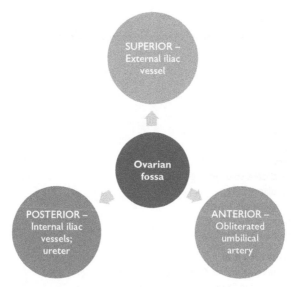

Figure 3.25 Boundaries of the ovarian fossa

18. Breasts
- Are modified sudoriferous glands which produce milk
- Overlie
  - i. 2nd–6th rib
  - ii. Serratus anterior
  - iii. Pectoralis major
  - iv. Rectus sheath
- Structure
  - i. Have 20 lobules
  - ii. The lobules are drained to the nipple via lactiferous ducts
- Ligaments of Cooper
  - i. Separate the lobules
  - ii. Run from subcutaneous tissue to fascia of chest wall
- Glands of Montgomery
  - i. Lubricates areola
  - ii. Are modified sebaceous glands
- Tail of Spence is the superior lateral quadrant of the breast that extends towards the axilla

- Blood supply
  - i. Axillary artery via
    - Lateral thoracic artery
    - Acromiothoracic artery
  - ii. Internal thoracic artery
  - iii. Intercostal arteries
- Nerve supply of the breast is from T4–T6
- Nerve supply to the nipple is from T4
- Lymphatic drainage
  - i. Axillary
  - ii. Parasternal
  - iii. Abdominal
- Develops from ectoderm

19. Homologous male structures
- Skene's gland = prostate
- Bulbourethral gland (Cowper's) = Bartholin's
- Prostatic utricle = vagina
- Labia majora = scrotum
- Clitoris = penis

Vascular tree – arteries

1. Aorta
- Branches
  - i. Inferior phrenic arteries
  - ii. Coeliac trunk
  - iii. Suprarenal arteries
  - iv. Superior mesenteric artery
  - v. Renal arteries
  - vi. Gonadal arteries
  - vii. Lumbar (4 paired lateral arteries)
  - viii. Inferior mesenteric artery
  - ix. Median (also known as middle) sacral artery
- Bifurcates at L4 into the 2 common iliac arteries
- Enters abdomen at the level of T12

2. Common iliac arteries
- Commence at the level of L4
- End at L5/S1
- Bifurcate at sacroiliac joints
- Relations (*Fig. 3.26*)

3. External iliac arteries
- Branches
  - i. Inferior epigastric arteries
  - ii. Deep circumflex iliac arteries
- Relations (*Fig. 3.27*)

4. Internal iliac arteries
- Also known as hypogastric arteries
- Arise at bifurcation of common iliac arteries (level of L5/S1)

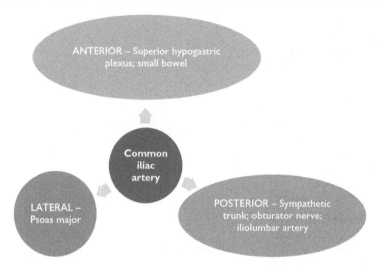

Figure 3.26 Common iliac artery and its spatial relations

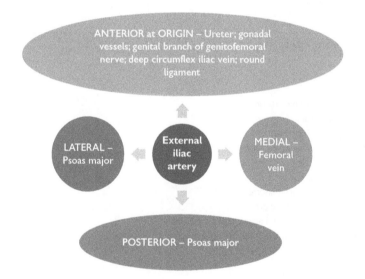

Figure 3.27 External iliac artery and its spatial relations

- Are the main arteries of the pelvis
- Supply
  i.   Pelvic organs
  ii. Buttocks
  iii. Medial compartment of thighs
- Relations (*Fig. 3.28*)
- Divide into 2 branches at the margin of the greater sciatic foramen (*Box 3.6*)
- Collateral circulations – anastomoses
  i.   Uterine and ovarian arteries
  ii. Middle rectal and superior rectal arteries

iii. Obturator and inferior epigastric/medial circumflex femoral arteries
iv. Superior and inferior vesical arteries
v. Profunda femoris and inferior gluteal arteries
vi. Superior gluteal and lateral sacral arteries
vii. Lateral sacral and median sacral arteries
viii. Iliolumbar and lumbar arteries
ix. Iliolumbar + superior gluteal and superficial iliac circumflex arteries

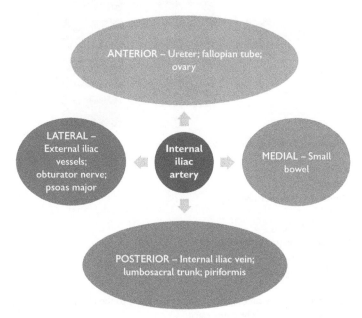

Figure 3.28 Internal iliac artery and its spatial relations

Box 3.6 Branches of the internal iliac artery

Brances of anterior branch	Branches of posterior branch
• Uterine	• Ilio lumbar
• Vaginal	• Lateral sacral
• Vesical (inferior and superior)	• Superior gluteal
• Umbilical	
• Obturator	
• Gluteal	
• Rectal	
• Internal pudendal	

5. **Femoral arteries**
   - Branches of external iliac
   - Route
     i. Run medial to femur
     ii. Cross via the adductor hiatus (a hole in the tendon of adductor magnus)
     iii. Enter into popliteal fossa
     iv. Become the popliteal arteries
   - Pass under inguinal ligament

- Lie
    i.   In the femoral triangle
    ii. On the tendon of psoas major
- Branches (*Fig. 3.29*)

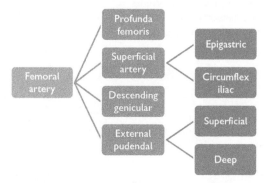

Figure 3.29 Branches of the femoral artery

6. **Obturator arteries**
    - Arise from
        i.   Internal iliac (anterior division)
        ii. Rarely
            ▪ External iliac
            ▪ Internal iliac (posterior division)
            ▪ Superior gluteal
            ▪ Inferior epigastric
    - Route
        i.   Pass anteroinferiorly on the lateral wall of the pelvis to the obturator foramen
        ii. Leave pelvic cavity via obturator canal
        iii. Rarely
            ▪ Pass lateral to femoral ring
            ▪ Curve on the free margin of the lacunar ligament
    - Branches (*Fig. 3.30*)

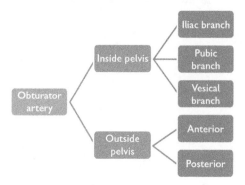

Figure 3.30 Branches of the obturator artery

    - Communicate with
        i.   Iliolumbar
        ii. Inferior epigastric
    - Relations (*Fig. 3.31*)

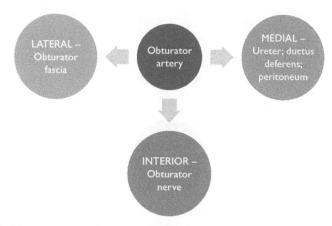

Figure 3.31 Obturator artery and its spatial relations

7. **Internal pudendal arteries**
   - Supply the external genitalia
   - Are the terminal branches of the anterior division of the internal Iliac arteries
   - Smaller in females compared with males
   - Route
     i.   Exit pelvis via greater sciatic foramen
     ii. Curve around sacrospinatous ligament
     iii. Enter ischio-anal fossa via lesser sciatic foramen
     iv. Travel in the pudendal (Alcock's) canal
   - Branches (*Fig. 3.32*)

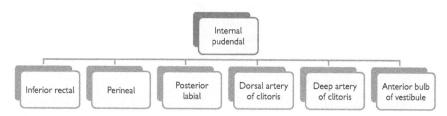

Figure 3.32 Branches of the internal pudendal artery

8. **Homologous male and females structures**
   - Vaginal artery = inferior vesical artery in male
   - Uterine artery = middle rectal artery in male

Vascular tree – veins

1. **IVC**
   - Commences at level of L5
   - Terminates at level of T8
   - Relations (*Fig. 3.33*)

2. **Gonadal veins**
   - Right drains directly in to IVC
   - Left drains to left renal vein

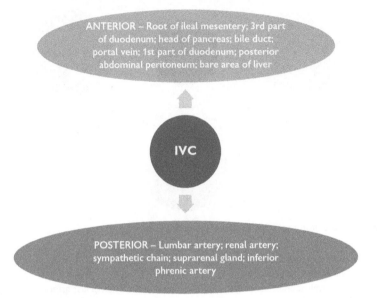

Figure 3.33 IVC and its spatial relations

3. **Greater saphenous veins**
   - Large superficial veins
   - Originate from dorsal vein of big toe
   - Route
     i. Pass anterior to the medial malleolus
     ii. Run over posterior border of medial epicondyle of femur
     iii. Enters fascia lata via saphenous opening on the anterior aspect of the thigh
     iv. Join femoral vein in femoral triangle
   - Receive
     i. Tibial veins
     ii. Femoral vein branches

4. **Thoracoepigastric veins**
   - Connect femoral and axillary veins
   - Run lateral to the superficial epigastric veins

Lymphatic system

Chpt 4

1. **Thoracic duct**
   - Originates from cisterna chyli at the level of T12
   - Drains into the left subclavian vein
   - Measures 45 cm

2. **Right lymphatic duct**
   - Arises anterior to scalenus anterior
   - Drains into the right subclavian vein
   - Measures 10 mm

3. **Drainage of abdominal lymph glands** (*Fig. 3.34*)

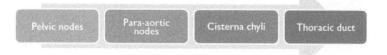

Figure 3.34 Abdominal lymph gland drainage

Neuroanatomy

Chpt 4   *Brain*

1. **Brain consists of 4 principal parts**
   - Brain stem consisting of
     i.   Midbrain
     ii. Pons
     iii. Medulla oblongata
   - Cerebellum
   - Diencephalon consisting of
     i.   Thalamus
     ii. Hypothalamus
     iii. Pineal gland
   - Cerebrum

2. **Cerebrum**
   - The superficial layer is the grey matter and is called cerebral cortex
   - Consists of
     i. Gyri
     ii. Sulci
   - Corpus callosum is white matter that connects the cerebral hemispheres
   - Each hemisphere is divided into 4 lobes
     i.   Frontal
     ii. Parietal
     iii. Temporal
     iv. Occipital
   - Precentral gyrus
     i. Located anterior to the central sulcus
     ii. Is the primary motor area
   - Postcentral gyrus
     i. Located posterior to the central sulcus
     ii. Is the primary somatosensory area

3. **Basal ganglia**
   - Are several groups of nuclei in each cerebral hemisphere
   - Consist of
     i.   Corpus striatum
     ii. Substantia nigra
     iii. Red nuclei
     iv. Subthalamic nuclei

- Corpus striatum is made up of
  - i. Caudate nucleus
  - ii. Lenticular nucleus
- Lenticular nucleus is made up of
  - i. Putamen
  - ii. Globus pallidus

4. **Cerebrospinal fluid (CSF)**
   - Circulates in the subarachnoid space
   - There are 4 CSF-filled cavities within the brain
     - i. 2 lateral ventricles
     - ii. Third ventricle
     - iii. Fourth ventricle
   - Measurements
     - i. Total CSF volume in body = 80–150 mL
     - ii. Rate of production = rate of absorption = 20 mL/h
   - Produced
     - i. By choroid plexus
     - ii. Via filtration of blood plasma
   - Flow of CSF (*Fig. 3.35*)

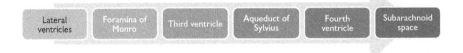

Lateral ventricles → Foramina of Monro → Third ventricle → Aqueduct of Sylvius → Fourth ventricle → Subarachnoid space

Figure 3.35 CSF flow

- Reabsorption occurs via
  - i. Arachnoid villi in the superior sagittal sinus
  - ii Choroid plexus

Cranial nerves

1. **Cranial nerves – there are 12 pairs (*Table 3.7*)**

Somatic pathways

1. **Somatic motor and sensory pathways (*Fig. 3.36*)**
   - Motor
     - i. Pyramidal tract
     - ii. Extrapyramidal pathway
   - Sensory
     - i. Posterior column
     - ii. Spinothalamic column

2. **Spinothalamic tract**
   - Formed by 3 neurone sets
     - i. Pseudounipolar neurones in the dorsal root ganglion
     - ii. Tract cells (i.e. secondary neurones in the substantia gelatinosa or the nucleus proprius)
     - iii. Several nuclei in the thalamus (i.e. third order neurones)
   - The pathway decussates at the level of the spinal cord in the anterior white commissure

Table 3.7 Cranial nerves

Cranial nerve	Origin	Runs via	Exits via
Olfactory			Olfactory foramina
Optic			Optic canal
Oculomotor	Midbrain	Lateral wall of cavernous sinus	Superior orbital fissure
Trochlear	Midbrain	Cavernous sinus	Superior orbital fissure
Trigeminal	Pons	Cavernous sinus	Ophthalmic nerve – Superior orbital fissure
			Maxillary nerve – Foramen rotundum
			Mandibular nerve – Foramen ovale
Abducens	Pons	Cavernous sinus	Superior orbital fissure
Facial	Cerebellopontine angle	Internal acoustic canal and facial canal	Stylomastoid foramen
Vestibulocochlear	Cerebellopontine angle		Internal acoustic canal
Glossopharyngeal	Medulla		Jugular foramen
Vagus	Medulla	Carotid sheath	Jugular foramen
Accessory		Foramen magnum	Jugular foramen
Hypoglossal	Medulla	Lies on carotid sheath	Hypoglossal canal

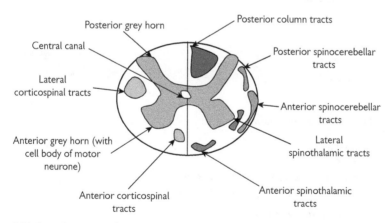

Figure 3.36 Somatic motor and sensory pathways in the spinal cord

- Consists of two tracts
  i.   Lateral spinothalamic tract (transmits pain and temperature)
  ii. Anterior spinothalamic tract (transmits touch)
- Type of impulse modality conducted
  i.   Pain

ii.   Temperature

iii. Touch

iv. Pressure

- Pathway (*Fig. 3.37*)

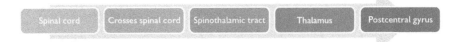

Figure 3.37 Spinothalamic pathway

3. Posterior column

- Also known as dorsal column-medial lemniscus pathway
- Formed by 3 neurone sets

  i.   First set = Meissner's corpuscles

  ii. Second set = gracile and cuneate nucleus (forms the medial lemniscus)

  iii. Third set = ventral posteromedial nucleus of the thalamus

- Types of impulse modality conducted

  i.   Proprioception

  ii. Discriminative touch

  iii. 2-point tactile discrimination

  iv. Pressure

  v.   Vibration

- Composed of

  i.   Fasciculus gracilis

  ii. Fasciculus cuneatus

- This pathway is tested with Romberg's test
- Pathway (*Fig. 3.38*)

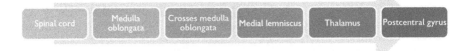

Figure 3.38 Posterior column pathway

4. Corticospinal tracts

- Consist of

  i.   Lateral corticospinal tract – 90% (*Fig. 3.39*)

  ii. Anterior corticospinal tract – 10% (*Fig. 3.40*)

5. Extrapyramidal pathway consists of

- Rubrospinal tract
- Tectospinal tract
- Vestibulospinal tract

Spinal nerves

1. Meninges

- Are connective tissue covering the brain and spinal cord

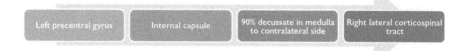

Figure 3.39 Lateral corticospinal pathway

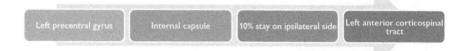

Figure 3.40 Anterior corticospinal pathway

- Composed of 3 layers
  i.   Dura matter (runs from brain to 2nd sacral vertebrae)
  ii. Arachnoid
  iii. Pia matter

2. **Spinal cord**
   - Extends from medulla oblongata to vertebral level
     i. In adults – L1
     ii. In infants – L3/L4
   - Conus medullaris
     i.   Is the conical portion of the spinal cord
     ii. Ends at L1
     iii. Gives rise to filum terminale
   - Filum terminale
     i. Is the extension of the pia matter
     ii. Ends at the coccyx
   - Cauda equina are nerve roots that arise inferior to the conus medullaris
   - Potential spaces
     i.   Epidural space – between wall of vertebral canal and dura
     ii. Subdural space – between dura and arachnoid
     iii. Subarachnoid space – between arachnoid and pia matter

3. **Spinal nerves**
   - There are 31 pairs
     i.   Cervical – 8
     ii. Thoracic – 12
     iii. Lumbar – 5
     iv. Sacral – 5
     v.   Coccygeal – 1
   - Have 2 roots
     i. Posterior (dorsal) root – contains sensory fibres
     ii. Anterior (ventral) root – contains motor fibres
   - Posterior root has a ganglion

Peripheral nerves

1. **Nerve plexuses**
   - Cervical (C1–C5)
   - Brachial (C5–T1)
   - Lumbar (T12–L5)
   - Sacral (L4–S5)

2. **Lumbar plexus**
   - Gives rise to
     i. Iliohypogastric nerve (L1)
     ii. Ilioinguinal nerve (L1)
     iii. Genitofemoral nerve (L1–L2)
     iv. Lateral femoral cutaneous nerve (L2–L3)
     v. Obturator nerve (L2–L4)
     vi. Femoral nerve (L2–L4)
   - Originates from the anterior primary rami of L1–L4
   - Traverses the psoas major and emerges from its lateral borders except for the
     i. Obturator nerve (emerges from the medial border)
     ii. Genitofemoral nerve (emerges from the anterior aspects of the muscle)

3. **Iliohypogastric nerve**
   - Originates from the anterior ramus of L1 (which also contains some fibres from T12)
   - Emerges on the lateral border of psoas major
   - Perforates the transversus abdominis muscle
   - Branches
     i. Lateral cutaneous
     ii. Anterior cutaneous
   - Communicates with the ilioinguinal nerve (which also originates from the anterior ramus of L1)

4. **Genitofemoral nerve**
   - Emerges from the anterior surface of psoas major
   - Branches
     i. Femoral branch (lumboinguinal)
     ii. Genital branch
   - Femoral branch travels
     i. Lateral to external iliac artery
     ii. Beneath inguinal ligament
   - Genital branch innervates (via the deep inguinal ring)
     i. Cremaster muscle
     ii. Scrotum
     iii. Mons pubis
     iv. Labia majora

5. **Obturator nerve**
   - Arises from L2–L4
   - Emerges from the medial border of psoas major
   - Route
     i. Passes behind common iliac vessels
     ii. Lateral to internal iliac vessels and ureter
     iii. Runs along lateral wall of lesser pelvis
     iv. Runs above and in front of the obturator vessels
     v. Enters the thigh via the obturator canal and divides into anterior and posterior divisions

- Branches
  i. Anterior
  ii. Posterior
- Both anterior and posterior branches are divided by
  i. Obturator externus muscle
  ii. Adductor brevis muscle
- Innervations
  i. Medial aspect of thigh
  ii. Knee joint
  iii. Adductor muscles of lower limb
- Adductor muscles of lower limb innervated by the obturator nerve include
  i. External obturator
  ii. Pectineus
  iii. Adductor longus
  iv. Adductor brevis
  v. Adductor magnus
  vi. Gracilis

6. **Femoral nerve**
   - Largest branch of lumbar plexus
   - Arises from L2–L4
   - Emerges from lateral border of psoas major
   - Route
     i. Passes between psoas major and iliacus muscles
     ii. Runs behind the iliac fascia
     iii. Divides into 2 divisions beneath the inguinal ligament which straddle the lateral circumflex femoral artery
   - Branches
     i. Anterior
     ii. Posterior
   - Anterior femoral branch consists of
     i. Intermediate anterior cutaneous nerve
     ii. Medial anterior cutaneous nerve
   - Posterior femoral branch consists of
     i. Saphenous nerve
     ii. Vastus lateralis
     iii. Vastus medialis
     iv. Vastus intermedius
   - Innervates
     i. Hip joint
     ii. Knee joint
     iii. Anterior compartment of thigh
   - Anterior compartment of thigh muscles innervated by the femoral nerve include
     i. Quadriceps
     ii. Sartorius
     iii. Pectineus

7. **Saphenous nerve**
   - Branch of femoral nerve
   - Route
     i. Descends in the femoral triangle
     ii. Enters adductor canal

    iii. Continues with long saphenous vein

    iv. Crosses anterior to the medial malleolus (where it is palpable)

8. **Sacral plexus**
   - S1–S4
   - Lies between the piriformis muscle and the pelvic fascia
   - In front of it are
     i. Internal iliac vessels
     ii. Ureter
     iii. Sigmoid colon
   - Gives rise to
     i. Superior gluteal nerve (L4–S1)
     ii. Sciatic nerve (L4–S3)
     iii. Inferior gluteal nerve (L5–S2)
     iv. Posterior cutaneous nerve (S1–S3)
     v. Pudendal nerve (S2–S4)

9. **Posterior cutaneous nerve**
   - Innervates
     i. Perineum
     ii. Skin of posterior thigh and leg
   - Route
     i. Exits pelvis via the greater sciatic foramen
     ii. Descends beneath gluteus maximus with inferior gluteal artery
     iii. Runs down the back of the thigh beneath the fascia lata
     iv. Pierces the deep fascia at the knee and accompanies the small saphenous vein

10. **Superior gluteal nerve**
    - Innervates
      i. Gluteus medius
      ii. Gluteus minimus
      iii. Tensor fascia lata
    - Route
      i. Leaves the pelvis via the greater sciatic foramen above piriformis
      ii. Accompanies the superior gluteal vessels

11. **Inferior gluteal nerve**
    - Innervates the gluteus maximus
    - Leaves the pelvis via the greater sciatic foramen below piriformis

12. **Sciatic nerve**
    - L4–S3
    - Longest single nerve in the body
    - Innervates
      i. Nearly the entire skin of the leg
      ii. Obturator internus
      iii. Biceps femoris
      iv. Semitendinosus
      v. Semimembranosus
      vi. Adductor magnus
      vii. Hip joint
    - Route
      i. Exits the pelvis via the greater sciatic foramen below piriformis

   ii. Descends between greater trochanter of femur and tuberosity of ischium
   iii. Divides at lower 1/3 of posterior thigh into 2 branches
- Branches
  i. Tibial
     - Passes through the popliteal fossa
     - Innervates
        - All muscles of the foot except extensor digitorum brevis
        - Knee joint
        - Ankle joint
        - Skin over lateral aspect of foot
     - Branches
        - Sural nerve (provides the cutaneous innervation)
        - Plantar nerve
  ii. Fibular (or common peroneal) divides into 2 branches
     - Deep (innervates extensor digitorum brevis)
     - Superficial
- The division can take place from any point between the sacral plexus to the lower 1/3 of the thigh
- Accompanied by
  i. Posterior femoral cutaneous nerve
  ii. Inferior gluteal artery
- Crossed by long head of biceps femoris
- Covered by gluteus maximus

13. Pudendal nerve
- Arises from S2–S4
- Route
  i.   Passes between piriformis and coccygeus muscles
  ii. Leaves the pelvis via the greater sciatic foramen
  iii. Crosses the ischial spines
  iv. Re-enters pelvis via lesser sciatic foramen
  v.   Runs along the pudendal vessels in the ischiorectal fossa
  vi. Contained in the obturator internus fascia called pudendal (Alcock's) canal
- Branches
  i.   Inferior anal nerve (arises at greater sciatic foramen)
  ii. Perineal (superficial)
  iii. Dorsal nerve of penis/clitoris (traverses the deep perineal pouch)
- Innervates
  i.   Penis
  ii. Scrotum
  iii. Clitoris
  iv. Bulbospongiosus
  v.   Ischiocavernosus
  vi. Anus

Autonomic nerves

1. Autonomic plexuses
- Coeliac
  i. Formed by coeliac ganglia
  ii. Supplied by greater splanchnic nerve and vagus nerve
- Superior mesenteric

- Aortic
- Inferior mesenteric
- Superior hypogastric – lies at the bifurcation of the aorta
- Inferior hypogastric
  i.   Two plexuses, each located on either pelvic side wall
  ii. Together form the pelvic hypogastric plexus

2. **Splanchnic nerve**
   - Preganglionic sympathetic fibres form
     i.   Greater splanchnic nerve (T5–T9)
     ii. Lesser splanchnic nerve (T10–T11)
     iii. Least splanchnic nerve (T12)
     iv. Lumbar splanchnic nerve (S1–S4) – joins superior hypogastric plexus
     v.   Sacral splanchnic nerve (L1–L4) – joins inferior hypogastric plexus
   - Preganglionic parasympathetic fibres form
     i.   Pelvic splanchnic nerve (S2–S4) – joins inferior hypogastric plexus

3. **Pelvic splanchnic nerve**
   - Also known as nervi erigentes
   - Located on the side of the rectum
   - Provides motor innervation to
     i.   Beyond the left 1/3 of the transverse colon
     ii. Uterus
     iii. Bladder
   - Provided sensory innervation to
     i.   Bladder
     ii.   Urethra
     iii. Rectum
     iv.   Anal canal
     v.   Cervix
     vi.   Upper vagina
     vii. Prostate

4. **Inferior hypogastric plexus postganglionic sympathetic innervations**
   - Motor
     i.   Seminal vesicles
     ii. Prostate
     iii. Anal sphincter
     iv. Urethral sphincter
   - Sensory
     i.   Upper rectum
     ii   Body of uterus

Endocrine anatomy

1. **Hypothalamus**
   - Located
     i.   Below the thalamus
     ii. Above the brain stem
   - Forms the floor of the 3rd ventricle
   - Includes

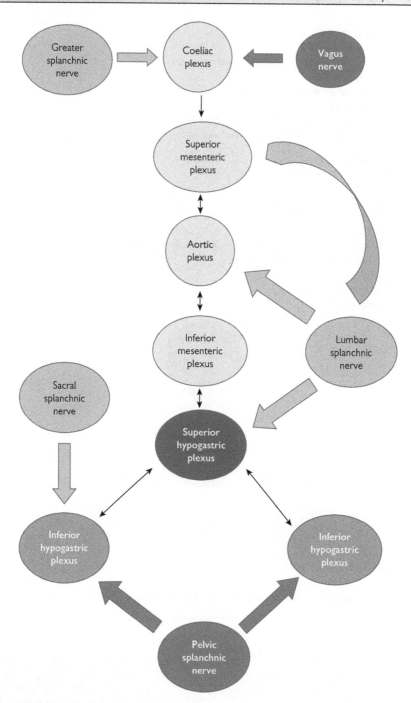

Figure 3.41 Nervous plexus pathways

    i.   Optic chiasm
    ii. Tuber cinereum
    iii. Infundibular stalk (connects to posterior pituitary)
    iv. Mamillary bodies
    v.   Posterior perforated substance
- Has 2 portions
    i. Posteromedial (has sympathetic innervation)
    ii. Anterolateral (has parasympathetic innervation)

2. **Pituitary gland**
   - Also known as hypophysis
   - Pea sized
   - Sits on sella turcica (pituitary fossa) in the sphenoid bone
   - Covered by a dural fold (sella diaphragm)
   - Has 3 parts
     i.   Anterior lobe (adenohypophysis) – develops from Rathke's pouch
     ii. Posterior lobe (neurohypophysis)
     iii. Pars intermedia
   - Develops from ectoderm
   - Borders (*Fig. 3.42*)

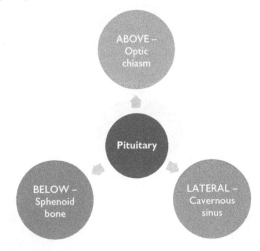

Figure 3.42 Boundaries of the pituitary

   - Blood supply to anterior pituitary lobe is via the infundibulum (*Fig. 3.43*)

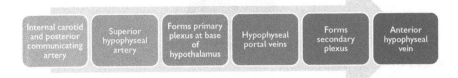

Figure 3.43 Vascular network of the anterior pituitary

- Blood supply to posterior pituitary lobe (*Fig. 3.44*)

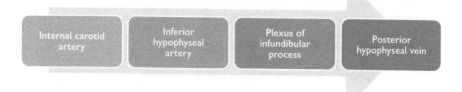

Figure 3.44 Vascular network of the posterior pituitary

- Anterior lobe composed of 3 cell types
  i. Chromophobe
  ii. Eosinophilic
  iii. Basophilic
- Adenohypophysis secretes 6 hormones
  i. Gonadotrophins (FSH and LH)
  ii. Prolactin
  iii. Growth hormone
  iv. Thyroid-stimulating hormone (TSH)
  v. Adrenocorticotrophic hormone (ACTH)
  vi. Melanocyte-stimulating hormone
- Neurohypophysis stores and secretes 2 hormones, which are produced by the hypothalamus
  i. Oxytocin
  ii. Antidiuretic hormone (ADH)

3. **Pineal gland**
   - Secrets melatonin
   - Often calcified
   - Attached to roof of 3rd ventricle
   - Covered by a capsule formed by pia matter

4. **Thyroid gland**
   - 1st endocrine organ to appear at day 24 of embryonic development
   - Weights 30 g
   - Blood supply = 120 mL/min
   - Arterial supply
     i. Superior thyroid (branch of external carotid artery)
     ii. Inferior thyroid (branch of subclavian artery)
     iii. Thyroid ima (branch of aortic arch/ brachiocephalic artery)
   - Venous drainage
     i. Superior thyroid (drains to internal jugular vein)
     ii. Middle thyroid (drains to internal jugular vein)
     iii. Inferior thyroid (drains to left brachiocephalic)
   - Is made up of
     i. Isthmus (overlying 2nd and 3rd tracheal ring)
     ii. Lateral lobes (extends to 6th tracheal ring)
     iii. Pyramidal lobe (also known as the Lalouette's pyramid)
   - Is enclosed in pretracheal fascia

- Thyroid follicles contain 2 cell types
  i. Follicular
  ii. Parafollicular (C cells)
- 3 principal hormones are secreted
  i.   Thyroxine (T_4)
  ii. Triiodothyronine (T_3)
  iii. Calcitonin (from C cells)
- Relations (**Fig. 3.45**)

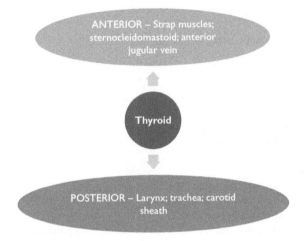

Figure 3.45 Thyroid gland and its spatial relations

5. **Parathyroid glands**
   - There are usually 4 (10 g each)
   - Pea sized
   - Yellowish-brown in colour
   - Contain 2 cell types
     i. Chief
     ii. Oxyphilic

6. **Carotid sheath**
   - Extends from base of skull to 1st rib and sternum
   - Contains
     i.   Internal carotid artery (medial)
     ii. Internal jugular vein (lateral)
     iii. Vagus nerve
     iv. Deep cervical lymph node
   - Nerves that pierce the sheath
     i.   Glossopharyngeal
     ii. Accessory
     iii. Hypoglossal

7. **Suprarenal (adrenal) glands**
   - Lie above the kidneys
   - Measure 3 cm × 5 cm
   - Weigh 5 g

- Have 2 regions
  - i. Cortex
    - Derived from mesoderm
    - Subdivided into 3 zones
  - ii. Medulla
    - Derived from ectoderm
    - Contain chromaffin cells
- Adrenal cortex zones
  - i. Zona glomerulosa (secretes mineralocorticoids)
  - ii. Zona fasciculata (secretes glucocorticoids)
  - iii. Zona reticularis (secretes androgens)
- Chromaffin cells
  - i. Are sympathetic postganglionic cells
  - ii. Secrete catecholamines (adrenaline (epinephrine) and noradrenaline (norepinephrine))
- Blood supply
  - i. Renal artery
  - ii. Phrenic artery
  - iii. Aorta
- Venous drainage
  - i. Right suprarenal drains into the IVC
  - ii. Left suprarenal drains into the left renal vein
- Fetal adrenals produce surfactant
- Nervous supply
  - i. Receives preganglionic sympathetic fibres
  - ii. No parasympathetic supply

Fetal skull

1. **Fetal skull bones (9 in total)**
   - 2 × frontal
   - 2 × parietal
   - 2 × temporal
   - 2 × sphenoidal
   - 1 × occipital

2. **Fetal skull sutures (8 in total)**
   - 1 × frontal
   - 1 × sagittal
   - 2 × coronal
   - 2 × lambdoidal
   - 2 × squamous (lie between parietal and temporal bones)

3. **Fetal skull fontanelles (6 in total) (Box 3.7)**
   - 1 × anterior
   - 1 × posterior
   - 2 × sphenoidal
   - 2 × mastoid

4. **Designations**
   - Vertex is the area encompassed by the anterior fontanelle, posterior fontanelle and the 2 parietal eminences

- Occiput is behind the posterior fontanelle
- Sinciput is the area in front of the anterior fontanelle, divided into
  i. Brow (area above root of nose)
  ii. Face (area below root of nose)

5. Dimensions

Chpt 9.10

- Diameter
  i. Biparietal = 9.5cm
  ii. Bitemporal = 8.5cm
  iii. Suboccipitobregmatic (presenting in an occipital position) = 9.5cm
  iv. Occipitofrontal (presenting in a vertex position) = 11.5cm
  v. Mentovertical (presenting in a brow position) = 14cm
  vi. Submentobregmatic (presenting in a face position) = 9.5cm
- Circumferences
  i. Subocipitobregmatic x biparietal (presenting in a vertex position) = 28cm
  ii. Occipitofrontal x biparietal (presenting in a occiput posterior position) = 33cm
  iii. Mentovertical x biparietal (presenting in a brow position) = 35.5cm

Box 3.7 Fetal skull fontanelles

Anterior (Bregma)	Posterior	Sphenoidal (anterolateral)	Mastoid (posterolateral)
• Bordered by frontal and parietal bones • Diamond shaped • Closes at 18 months of life	• Bordered by parietal and occipital bones • Closes at 2 months of life	• Bordered by frontal, parietal, temporal and sphenoidal bones • One on each side	• Bordered by parietal, temporal and occipital bones • One on each side

Physiology

CONTENTS

Acid–base balance

Fluids

1. **H_2O balance**
   - Total body volume = 42 L (60% total body weight) (*Fig. 4.1*)
   - Total blood volume = 5.6 L (plasma + RBC)
   - Fluid losses occur by 4 routes (exact amount depends on ambient temperature, humidity, and intake)
     i.   Lungs – 400 mL/day of water is lost in expired air
     ii. Skin – 1 L/day
     iii. Faeces – 100 mL/day
     iv. Urine – 1.5 L/day (minimum UO/day = 400 mL)
   - Maintenance fluid requirement = 30 mL/kg/day

2. **Hormones that regulate extracellular fluid (ECF) volume**
   - Directly
     i.   ADH
   - Indirectly
     i.   Atrial natriuretic peptide (ANP)
     ii. Renin–angiotensin system – this primarily regulates plasma osmolarity and indirectly blood volume via aldosterone
   - Minor regulators with some effect
     i.   Glucocorticoids
     ii. Catecholamines

3. **Osmosis**
   - Movement of water from low solute concentration to a higher one via a semi-permeable membrane

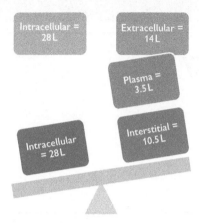

Figure 4.1 Distribution of total body fluid volume

- Opposed by hydrostatic power
- 1 osmol/L depresses freezing point by 1.86 °C
- Osmolarity
  i.   Defined as number of osmoles of solution per litre of solution (Osm/L)
  ii. Is a measure of solute concentration
- Osmolality is a measure of osmoles of solutes per kilogram of solvent (Osm/kg)

4. **Plasma osmolarity**
   - Total plasma osmolarity = 300 mOsm/L
   - Consist of
     i. Na^+ = 140 mOsm/L (Na^+ is the main contributor to plasma osmolarity)
     ii. Cl^- = 140 mOsm/L
     iii. K^+ = 4 mOsm/L
     iv. Anion = 4 mOsm/L
     v.   Glucose = 5 mOsm/L
     vi. Urea = 5 mOsm/L

5. **Starling's law of the capillaries**
   - Refers to fluid movement across capillary membrane as a result of filtration
   - Starling's forces shows the relationship between hydrostatic and oncotic pressures (**Box 4.1**)

Box 4.1 Starling's forces

Oncotic pressures (mmHg)	Hydrostatic pressures (mmHg)
• Blood (BOP) = 26 • Interstitial (IOP) = 1	• Arterial (B_AHP) = 35 • Venous (B_VHP) = 16 • Interstitial (IHP) = 0

- Net filtration pressure (NFP) = pressure promoting filtration (BHP + IOP) – pressure promoting reabsorption (BOP + IHP)
  i.   NFP arterial end = (35 + 1) – (26 + 0) = 10 mmHg
  ii. NFP venous end = (16 + 1) – (26 + 0) = –9 mmHg

6. **Oedema (Box 4.2)**
   - Signifies increased fluid in interstitial space
   - Anasarca is generalized oedema with subcutaneous tissue swelling

- Pathophysiology of oedema
  i. Increased hydrostatic pressure
  ii. Reduced plasma oncotic pressure
  iii. Lymphatic obstruction
  iv. Sodium retention
  v. Inflammation

Box 4.2 Causes of oedema

Lymphatic obstruction	Sodium retention
• Inflammatory	• Increased renin–angiotensin secretion
• Neoplastic	
• Post-surgical	
• Post-irradiation	

Acid–base balance

1. **Main organs involved in regulating acid–base balance**
   - Respiratory system
   - Kidney
   - Blood
   - Bone
   - Liver (generates HCO_3^- and NH_4^+ by glutamine metabolism)

2. **Anion gap (Box 4.3)**
   - Is the difference between the concentrations of the body's cations and anions
   - Normal values range between 8 and 16 mEq/L

Box 4.3 Causes of altered anion gap

↑ Anion gap	↓ Anion gap
• Lactic acidosis (methanol; salicylate; paraldehyde)	• Bromide
• Ketoacidosis	• Myeloma
• Hypoalbuminaemia	

3. **Henderson–Hasselbach equation**
   - $CO_2 \Leftrightarrow HCO_3^- + H^+$
   - If H^+ is generated reaction shifts to the **left**
     i. Generates CO_2
     ii. Consumes HCO_3^-
   - If HCO_3^- is lost reaction shifts to the **right**
     i. Generates H^+
     ii. Consumes CO_2
   - A net gain in H^+ is the same as a net loss in HCO_3^-

4. **pH**
   - Is a logarithmic relationship
   - Is the negative logarithm (with base 10) of hydrogen ion concentration ($- \log_{10} [H+]$)
   - $pH = pK + \log_{10} [HCO_3^-]/[CO_2]$

5. **Normal maternal arterial values (Box 4.4)**

6. **Normal fetal values (Box 4.5)**

Box 4.4 Normal maternal arterial blood values

Oxygen sats	pO$_2$	pCO$_2$	Base excess
• > 97%	• 100 mmHg	• 40 mmHg • 4 kPa	• −2 to 2

HCO$_3^-$	pH	Haemoglobin
• 24 mEq/L	• 7.34–7.44	• 12 gm/dL

Box 4.5 Normal fetal blood values

Oxygen sats	pO$_2$ (mmHg)	pCO$_2$	Base excess
• Venous = 75% • Arterial = 25%	• Venous = 35 • Artery = 25	• 8–10 kPa	• Vein = −1 to 9 • Artery = −2.5 to 10

pH	Haemoglobin
• Vein = 7.17–7.48 • Artery = 7.05–7.38	• 18 gm/dL

7. **Respiratory compensation**
   - Occurs **only** in metabolic disorders
   - Is instantaneous
   - Cannot compensate for primary respiratory disorders

8. **Metabolic compensation**
   - Is via kidneys
   - Compensates for
     i. Respiratory disorders
     ii. Metabolic disorders not originating from the kidneys
   - Slow process

9. **HCO$_3^-$**
   - Is alkaline
   - Is manufactured in
     i. Distal convoluted tubule (DCT)
     ii. Collecting duct
   - Proximal convoluted tubule (PCT) is not involved with acid–base balance
   - DCT cells
     i. Have carbonic anhydrase
     ii. Produce CO$_2$ (CO$_2$ reacts with water to form carbonic acid [H$_2$CO$_3$], a reaction catalysed by carbonic anhydrase. H$_2$CO$_3$ is an unstable organic acid, which rapidly dissociates into H$^+$ and HCO$_3^-$)

$$CO_2 + H_2O \rightarrow H_2CO_3 \rightarrow H^+ + HCO_3^-$$

   - iii. HCO$_3^-$ enters general circulation
     iv. H$^+$ enters urine and is buffered with
       - NH$_4^+$
       - HPO$_4^{2-}$
     v. NH$_4^+$ is produced by the kidneys and increases in acidosis

10. In long-term acidosis
- H^+ enters cell (due to high extracellular fluid concentration of H^+)
- K^+ is driven out of the cell to maintain electrical neutrality
- Hyperkalaemia occurs

11. Base deficit/excess
- Is the amount of acid or alkali required to restore 1 L of blood to a normal pH at a
  - i. pCO_2 of 5.3 kPa
  - ii. Temperature of 37 °C
- Is calculated using the serum bicarbonate concentration and pH values
- Base excess = $0.93 \times [HCO_3^- - 24.4 + 14.8 (pH - 7.4)]$
- Normal range is −2 to +2 mEq/L
- A negative base excess indicates metabolic acidosis
- A positive base excess indicates metabolic alkalosis
- Actual base excess
  - i. Is the base excess value of blood
  - ii. Is not a true representation of the base excess of the total ECF
- Standard base excess
  - i. Is the base excess value calculated when the haemoglobin is at 5 g/dL
  - ii. Gives a better representation of the base excess of the total ECF
- Total body bicarbonate deficit = $0.3 \times$ base deficit $\times$ body weight (in kg)

Acid–base changes in pregnancy

1. In the fetus
- Cord compression leads to respiratory acidosis
- Placental insufficiency leads to metabolic acidosis
- Anaerobic metabolism leads to increased lactate
- Shift to anaerobic metabolism occurs when O_2 saturation <25%

2. Electrolyte changes in pregnancy
- Osmolarity decreases by 10 mOsm/L (in response to progesterone)
- Decreased HCO_3^- (in response to decreased CO_2)
- Decreased Na^+ (in response to fall in HCO_3^- and resetting of the plasma osmolarity)

Calcium homeostasis

Calcium

1. Ca^{2+} functions
- Bone formation
- Muscle contraction
- Enzyme co-factor
- Blood clotting (necessary for the function of some of the coagulation cascade complexes)
- Secondary messenger
- Stabilization of membrane potentials

Chpt 7

2. Distribution of Ca^{2+}
- Total body calcium is 1 kg of which 99% is located in the skeleton
- Extracellular (plasma) Ca^{2+}
  - i. Ionized (45%)
  - ii. Bound (55%)

- Ca^{2+} is bound to
  i.   Plasma proteins
  ii. PO_4^{3-}
  iii. HCO_3^-
- Acidosis causes increased ionized calcium
- Daily requirement
  i.   Adult = 1 g/day
  ii. Pregnant = 1.5 g/day

3. **There are 3 major pools of Ca^{2+} in the body**
   - Extracellular compartment (plasma)
     i.   The concentration of ionized calcium in ECF is 12 000 times the Ca^{2+} concentration within the intracellular compartment
   - Intracellular compartment
     i. Ca^{2+} is sequestrated almost exclusively out of the cytosol and within the endoplasmic reticulum and mitochondria. It can only be released by certain stimuli or cell damage
     ii. Intracellular free Ca^{2+} concentrations fluctuates from 100 nM to 1 µM
   - Bone

4. **Ca^{2+} modulation is via**
   - Parathyroid hormone (PTH)
   - Parathyroid hormone-related peptide (PTHrP)
   - Calcitonin

5. **Ca^{2+} absorption from GIT via**
   - Active uptake – Na^+/Ca^{2+} ATPase
   - Transcellular transport – Calbindin
   - Endocytosis – Ca^{2+}–calbindin complex via TRPV6 membrane Ca^{2+} channel

6. **Phosphate functions**
   - Important in intracellular metabolism (ATP synthesis)
   - Phosphorylation of enzymes
   - Forms phospholipids in membranes

Calcium regulatory hormones

1. **PTH**
   - Peptide hormone (consist of 84 amino acids and has many isoforms)
   - Acts on G-protein receptors
   - Secreted by parathyroid gland
   - Half life = minutes
   - Store supplies last for 90 min
   - Functions
     i.   Increases Ca^{2+}
     ii. Decreases PO_4^{3-}
     iii. Calcitonin antagonist
   - Does not cross placenta
   - Acts on 3 body components (**Box 4.6**)

2. **PTHrP**
   - Made by
     i.   Most tissues
     ii. Cancer cells
   - Functions
     i.   Similar to PTH

    ii. Does not increase vitamin D levels

    iii. Regulates chondrocyte proliferation

    iv. Important for placental Ca^{2+} transport

Box 4.6 Action of PTH

Bone	Kidney	Intestines
• Increases bone resorption	• Increases Ca^{2+} absorption from DCT • Decreases PO_4^{3-} re-absorption from PCT • Increases vitamin D production via increasing 1α-hydroxylase • Promotes calcitriol formation	• Increases Ca^{2+} and PO_4^{3-} absorption

3. **Calcitonin**
   - Is a polypeptide (consists of 32 amino acids)
   - Secreted in response to high levels of PO_4^{3-} and Ca^{2+}
   - Produced by C cells (parafollicular cells) in the thyroid gland
   - Decreases circulating Ca^{2+} levels in 3 ways
     i. Prevents osteoclast action
     ii. Decreases reabsorption of PO_4^{3-} and Ca^{2+} in PCT
     iii. Decrease Ca^{2+} absorption in GIT

4. **Phosphaturic hormone**
   - Functions
     i. Increases PO_4^{3-} in urine
     ii. Decreases PO_4^{3-} in blood
   - Counteracts actions of vitamin D
   - Predominantly made by osteoblasts

5. **Vitamin D**
   - Is a pro-hormone
   - 2 major forms
     i. Vitamin D_2 (ergocalciferol)
     ii. Vitamin D_3 (cholecalciferol)
   - Made in
     i. Skin
     ii. Placenta
     iii. Decidua

6. **Calcitriol = $1,25(OH)_2D_3$**
   - Is the active form of vitamin D found in the body
   - Controls
     i. Osteoblast and osteoclast differentiation
     ii. Increases Ca^{2+} uptake from GIT
     iii. Increases Ca^{2+} and PO_4^{3-} reabsorption from kidneys
   - Functions
     i. Has anti-tumour activity
     ii. Inhibits release of calcitonin
   - Synthesis
     i. 7-dehydro-cholesterol (skin) → UV light → vitamin D_3
     ii. Vitamin D_3 (liver) → 25-hydroxylase → $25(OH)D_3$
     iii. $25(OH)D3$ (kidney) → 1α-hydroxylase → $1,25(OH)_2D_3$

- $25(OH)D_3$
  - i.   Half life = 1.5 months
  - ii. Is a form of stored vitamin D
- $1,25(OH)_2D_3$ half life = 0.25 days
- Deficiencies cause
  - i.   2° hyperparathyroidism (renal osteodystrophy)
  - ii. Rickets
  - iii. Osteomalacia
  - iv. X-linked rickets

Calcium disorders

1. **Hyperparathyroidism**
   - There are 3 types (*Box 4.7*)

Box 4.7 Types of hyperparathyroidism

1° hyper-PTH	2° hyper-PTH	3° hyper-PTH
• Causes hypercalcaemia • Due to benign tumours	• Response to decreasing Ca^{2+} levels	• Secondary to 2° hyper-PTH • Chronic process

- 1° hyperparathyroidism is due to
  - i.   Parathyroid adenoma (80%)
  - ii. Primary parathyroid hyperplasia (15%)
  - iii. Parathyroid carcinoma (2%) – can occur as part of familial endocrinopathies; all of which are autosomal dominant traits
    - Multiple endocrine neoplasia (MEN) 1
    - MEN 2A
    - Isolated familial hyperparathyroidism
- 2° hyperparathyroidism is due to
  - i.   Kidney disease
  - ii. Decreased vitamin D
  - iii. Decreased serum Ca^{2+}
- 2° hyperparathyroidism results in renal osteodystrophy by
  - i.   Increased Ca^{2+} resorption from bones
  - ii. Reduced glomerular filtration rate (GFR) by 50%

2. **Pathological calcification**
   - Is the abnormal tissue deposition of Ca^{2+} salts with smaller amount of other mineral salts
   - It is a common process
   - 2 forms
     - i. Dystrophic calcification
       - Deposition occurs locally in dying tissue or areas of necrosis
       - Occurs despite normal serum levels
       - Occurs despite normal calcium metabolism
     - ii. Metastatic calcification
       - Deposition in normal tissues
       - Due to hypercalcaemia

3. **Hypercalcaemia**
   - Causes of hypercalcaemia
     - i. Hyperparathyroidism
     - ii. Renal failure

- Leads to accumulation of PO_4^{3-} and
- Secondary hyperparathyroidism

iii. Vitamin D-related disorders
  - Sarcoidosis (causes dysregulation of vitamin D production with an increase in its extrarenal production)
  - Vitamin D excess
  - Williams' syndrome (idiopathic hypercalcaemia of infancy)

iv. Destruction of bone tissue
  - Primary bone tumours
  - Skeletal metastasis (breast cancer)
  - Immobilization
  - Accelerated bone turnover (Paget's disease)

v. Drug induced
  - Vitamin A intoxication
  - Thiazide diuretics
  - Lithium
  - Oestrogens

vi. Endocrinopathies
  - Thyrotoxicosis
  - Phaeochromocytoma

- Classic clinical features (**Box 4.8**)

Box 4.8 Clinical features of hypercalcaemia

Stones	Bones	Abdominal groans	Psychic moans
• Renal calculi	• Osteitis fibrosa	• Constipation	• Depression
• Nephrocalcinosis	• Osteoporosis	• Vomiting	• Memory loss
	• Osteomalacia	• Peptic ulcer	• Psychoses, paranoia
	• Rickets	• Pancreatitis	• Coma

Others
• Proximal muscle weakness
• Keratitis
• Conjunctivitis

- Treatment includes
  i. Rehydration
  ii. Pamidronate disodium (is a bisphosphonate drug that inhibits osteoclastic bone resorption)
  iii. Calcitonin
  iv. Plicamycin

4. **Hypocalcaemia**
  - Is defined as the presence of low serum calcium in blood
    i. Ionized Ca^{2+} < 1.1 mmol/L
    ii. Total Ca^{2+} < 2.1 mmol/L
  - Aetiology
    i. Hypoparathyroidism
    ii. Vitamin D deficiency
    iii. Hypomagnesaemia
    iv. Acute pancreatitis
    v. Citrated blood transfusion

- Clinical features include
  i. Perioral tingling
  ii. Paraesthesia
  iii. Tetany
     - Carpopedal spasm
     - Trousseau's sign
     - Chvostek's sign
  iv. Cardiac arrhythmias
  v. ECG changes
     - Prolonged QT interval
     - Prolonged ST interval
  vi. Subcapsular cataract
- Causes of hypoparathyroidism
  i. Surgical or post-radiation
  ii. Idiopathic
  iii. Neonatal
  iv. Familial
  v. Autoimmune (DiGeorge's syndrome)
  vi. Deposition of metals (iron, copper, aluminium)
  vii. Hypomagnesaemia

Bone and osteoporosis

1. **Bone**
   - Remodelling cycle takes 90–200 days
   - Turnover occurs at bone surfaces
     i. Periosteal
     ii. Endosteal
   - Total surface area = 1000–5000 m^2
   - Osteoblast modulators
     i. PTH
     ii. Oestrogen
     iii. Glucocorticoids
     iv. Thyroid hormone
   - Osteoclast modulators
     i. TNF
     ii. IL-1/IL-6
     iii. GM-CSF
   - Peak bone mass density occurs at the age of 25

2. **Osteoclast**
   - Has no PTH receptors
   - Osteoclast is a product of osteoblast
   - Osteoblast has PTH receptors

3. **Biochemical markers of bone turnover**
   - AlPO$_4$
   - Type 1 collagen (urine)
   - Hydroxyproline (urine)
   - Pyridinolines (urine)
   - TRAP

4. **Osteoporosis**
   - Is a bone disease characterized by

   i.   Reduced bone mineral density
   ii. Disruption of bone microarchitecture
- Prevalence in age >50 years old
   i.   Male = 20%
   ii. Female = 50%
- Diagnosis based on T-scores
   i.   BMD <1 SD = normal
   ii. BMD 1–2.5 SD = osteopenia
   iii. BMD >2.5 SD = osteoporosis
- Aetiology (*Box 4.9*)

Box 4.9 Causes of osteoporosis

Environmental	Autoimmune disorders	Drugs	Endocrine
- Smoking - Alcohol - Malnutrition - Immobilization	- Diabetes mellitus - Coeliac disease	- Immunosuppresive drugs - Steroids - Proton pump inhibitor	- Hyperthyroidism - Hyperparathy roidism - Hypogonadal states - Cushing's - Pregnancy - Lactation - ↓ Oestrogen - Hyperprolactinaemia

Haematological	Metabolic
- Lymphoma - Myeloma - Sickle cell	- Haemochromatosis - Glycogen storage disease - Homocystienuria - Porphyria

- Risk factors
   i.   BMI <19 kg/m^2
   ii. Family history of maternal fractures before the age of 75
   iii. Untreated premature menopause
   iv. Chronic medical disorders
   v.   Prolonged immobility

5. **Treatment of osteoporosis includes prescription of**
- Calcium (1 g)
- Vitamin D (800 IU)
- Bisphosphonates
   i.   If >75 years it can be given without a dual energy X-ray absorptiometry (DEXA) scan
   ii. If 65–75 years give if osteoporosis confirmed on DEXA
   iii. If <65 years give if low bone mineral density (BMD) or high risk factors
- Hormone replacement therapy (HRT) or raloxifene (SERM)
- Teriparatide (a form of PTH) – used in women aged >65 years with low BMD
- Strontium (promotes osteoblasts and inhibits osteoclasts)
- Calcitonin
- Calcitriol
- Testosterone

Calcium and pregnancy

1. **Pregnancy**
   - Is a hypocalcaemic (although the free ionized calcium levels remain the same) state caused by
     i.   Active transplacental transport of Ca^{2+} to the fetus
     ii. Increased renal loss of Ca^{2+} (due to increased renal GFR)
     iii. Decreased serum albumin
   - Is associated with an
     i.   Increased calcitriol
     ii. Increased PTH
     iii. Increased calcitonin

2. **Fetus**
   - Contains 21–33 g calcium
   - Is hypercalcaemic compared to the mother (ratio 1.4 : 1)
   - Ca^{2+} and PO_4^{3-} is actively transported
   - Ossification occurs in 3rd trimester
   - Produces PTH from 12 weeks

Cardiovascular system

Cardiac

1. **The cardiovascular system consists of**
   - The heart
   - Blood vessels
   - Blood

2. **Cardiac anatomy**
   - Heart weighs ≈ 250 g
   - Approximately same size as the person's fist
   - Composed of 3 layers
     i.   Epicardium – is part of the pericardium
     ii. Myocardium
     iii. Endocardium
   - Has 4 valves
     i.   Mitral (bicuspid valve)
     ii. Tricuspid (composed of 3 cusps)
     iii. Aortic (semilunar valve)
     iv. Pulmonary (semilunar valve)

3. **Cardiac cycle**
   - Electrical impulse travels via (**Fig. 4.2**)

SAN   AVN   Bundle of His   Purkinje fibres

Figure 4.2 Cardiac electrical impulse pathway

   - Divided into 3 phases
     i.   Relaxation (0.4 s)
     ii. Ventricular filling (0.1 s)
     iii. Ventricular contraction (0.3 s)

- Last for 0.8 s
- Isovolumetric contraction phase
  i.   Both atrioventricular and semilunar valves are closed
  ii. Volume in ventricular chamber is constant

4. **Central venous pressure**
   - Wave forms
     i.   A wave = atrial systole
     ii. X wave = occurs at the end of atrial systole
     iii. C wave = ventricular systole
     iv. V wave = atrial filling against closed tricuspid valve
     v.   Y descent occurs following tricuspid valve opening
   - Normal value = 0–10 mmHg

5. **Heart sounds (*Fig. 4.3*)**
   - 1st = Atrioventricular valve closure (occurs at the beginning of ventricular systole)

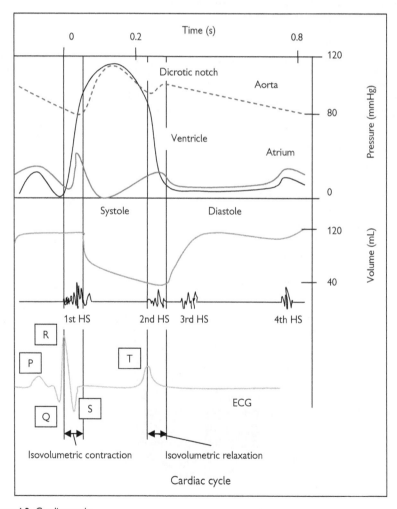

Figure 4.3 Cardiac cycle

- 2nd = Semilunar valve closure
  - i.   Occurs at the end of ventricular systole
  - ii. Usually split
- 3rd
  - i.   Occurs at beginning of ventricular diastole
  - ii. Due to rapid ventricular filling
  - iii. Common in pregnancy and young adults
- 4th
  - i.   Atrial systole
  - ii. Absent in atrial fibrillation (AF)

6. **ECG**
   - PR interval
     - i.   Is 0.1–0.2 s
     - ii. Beginning of P to beginning of Q
   - QRS = 0.12 s
   - QT interval = 0.3–0.4 s (depends on HR) (*Box 4.10*)

Box 4.10 QT interval

Increased QT interval	Decreased QT Interval
• Hypokalaemia	• Hyperkalaemia
• Hypocalcaemia	• Hypercalcaemia
• Quinidine	• Digoxin

7. **Cardiac chambers (*Fig. 4.4*)**
   - Saturations
     - i.   Mixed venous saturation = 60%
     - ii. Left side saturation = 96%
   - Atrial pressure
     - i.   Right = 1–7 mmHg
     - ii. Left = 10–15 mmHg
   - Right ventricle pressure
     - i.   Systolic = 35 mmHg
     - ii. Diastolic = 4 mmHg

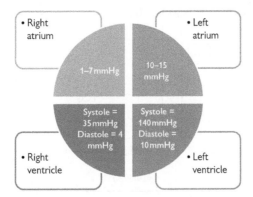

Figure 4.4 Cardiac chamber pressures

- Left ventricle pressure
  i. Systolic = 140 mmHg
  ii. Diastolic = 10 mmHg
- Pulmonary artery pressure = 35/15 mmHg

8. Stroke volume (SV)
- Is the volume ejected by the ventricles during systole
- SV = end systolic volume (ESV) − end diastolic volume (EDV)
  i. ESV = 120 mL
  ii. EDV = 40 mL
- Is 80 mL
- Ejection fraction (EF)
  i. Is 0.67
  ii. EF = SV/ESV

9. Cardiac output (CO)
- CO = SV (stroke volume) × HR
- Resting CO
  i. Male = 5.5 L/min
  ii. Female = 4.5 L/min
- Cardiac index = CO/body surface area = 3.2 L/min/m^2
- Starling's law
  i. Force of contraction is proportional to fibre length
  ii. Fibre length is proportional to stretch of ventricular muscle (ventricular dilatation)
  iii. Ventricular dilatation is proportional to venous return
- Venous return (pre-load) depends on
  i. Intrathoracic pressure
  ii. Total blood volume
  iii. Gravity
  iv. Calf muscle action
  v. Venous tone
- After-load depends on arterial resistance

10. Cardiac autonomic control is via
- Baroreceptors
  i. Are inhibitory
  ii. Are of 3 types (*Box 4.11*)

Box 4.11 Baroreceptors

Carotid sinus	Aortic body	Floor of 4th ventricle
• Located at bifurcation of common carotids • Innervated by glossopharyngeal nerve	• Located at aortic arch • Sensitive to partial pressure of O_2/CO_2 and pH	• Sensitive to CSF pressure • Cushing's reflex: ↑ CSF pressure → ↑ BP

- Chemoreceptors consist of
  i. Carotid body
    - Located at bifurcation of carotid artery
    - Sensitive to pO_2, pCO_2, and pH
  ii. Central chemoreceptor (sensitive to CO_2)

11. Coronary circulation
- Heart receives 4–5% of CO
- Coronary flow
  - i. Rate at rest = 80 mL/min
  - ii. Is greatest during diastole
- Myocardial oxygen consumption = 8 mL per 100 g of tissue

Blood vessels

1. Blood vessel wall is made up of 3 layers
- Tunica interna
- Tunica media
  - i. Thickest layer in artery
  - ii. Consist of smooth muscles
- Tunica externa – thickest layer in vein

2. Veins have valves

3. Capillaries have a single layer of tunica interna

4. Blood pressure (BP)
- BP = systemic vascular resistance (SVR) × CO
- Depends on
  - i.   Blood volume
  - ii. Viscosity
  - iii. Elasticity of vessel walls
  - iv. Length of blood vessels
  - v.   Diameter of blood vessels
  - vi. Hormones
    - Angiotensin-converting enzyme (ACE)
    - ADH
    - Adrenaline

5. Mean arterial pressure (MAP)

$$MAP = \text{Diastolic pressure} + \frac{1}{3} \times (\text{systolic pressure} - \text{diastolic pressure})$$

6. SVR depends on the following factors:
- Neurogenic (via the central sympathetic outflow paths)
- Metabolic
  - i. H^+
  - ii. O_2
  - iii. CO_2
  - iv. K^+
- Endocrine
  - i.   Adenosine
  - ii. Prostaglandin
  - iii. Serotonin
  - iv. Kinin
  - v.   Catecholamines

7. Blood flow
- Follows Poiseuille's law
- Is proportional to
  - i. Pressure

ii.   Radius

iii. 1/viscosity

iv. 1/length

- Viscosity increases when haematocrit >45%

Blood

1. **Blood is composed of**
   - Plasma (55%)
   - Blood cells (45%)

2. **Blood cells**
   - There are 3 types
     i.   Erythrocytes
     ii. Leucocytes
     iii. Thrombocytes
   - Are formed by haemopoiesis
   - Are derived from stem cells

3. **Erythrocytes**
   - Structure
     i.   Biconcave disc
     ii. Diameter = 8 mm
     iii. Do not have nucleus
   - Lifespan = 120 days
   - Contain haemoglobin

4. **Blood groups**
   - Is the classification of blood based on the presence or absence of inherited antigenic substance on the surface of RBCs
   - 2 main systems
     i.   ABO – has 4 groups (*Table 4.1*)
     ii. Rhesus – 80% of Caucasians are Rhesus positive
   - Other blood groups include
     i.   Kell system
     ii. Lewis system

Table 4.1 ABO system

Blood group	O	A	B	AB
Antigen	–	a	b	a/b
Antibody in plasma	a/b	b	a	–
Compatible donor	O	A, O	B, O	A, B, AB, O
Incompatible donor	A, B, AB	AB, B	AB, A	–

5. **Leucocytes**
   - Make up 1% of blood cells
   - Contain nuclei

6. **Thrombocytes**
   - Release serotonin, which causes vasoconstriction
   - Form a platelet plug

T. in
Obs
Gyn
Chpt 6.1

Cardiovascular changes in pregnancy

1. **Cardiac changes in pregnancy**
   - Cardiac output rises by 40%
     i. From 4.5 to 6 L/min
     ii. Plateaus at 24–30 weeks
   - Heart rate increases by 20%
   - Stroke volume increases by 30%
   - Peripheral vascular resistance decreases by 5%
   - BP decreases 10%
   - Vasodilation (due to progesterone)

2. **Distribution of CO in pregnancy**
   - Uterus – 400 mL/min
   - Kidney – 300 mL/min
   - Skin – 500 mL/min
   - GI/breast – 300 mL/min
   - In labour CO increases by 2 L/min

3. **ECG changes in pregnancy**
   - Left ventricular hypertrophy and dilatation
   - The apex is shifted anteriorly and to the left
   - Left axis deviation 15°
   - Inverted T-waves in lead 3
   - Q-wave in lead 3 and aVF
   - Non-specific ST changes

4. **Haematological changes in pregnancy**
   - Plasma volume rises by 50%
     i. From 2600 to 3800 mL
     ii. No further increase after 32 weeks
   - Total volume of RBCs rises by 18% (1400 mL to 1650 mL)
   - Leucocytes increase
   - Increase in clotting factors
   - Haemodilution – physiological anaemia
   - Haematocrit decreases

5. **Endothelial changes in pregnancy**
   - Vasodilatation due to
     i.   Increased nitric oxide (NO)
     ii. Decreased asymmetrical dimethylarginine (ADMA)
     iii. Increased PGI_2 (prostacyclin)
   - Pro-coagulant state

6. **Puerperium**
   - Increase diuresis in the first 48 hours post delivery
   - Clotting factors remain high

Respiratory system

Respiratory tree

1. **The pharynx is divided into 3 parts**
   - Nasopharynx

- Oropharynx
- Laryngopharynx

2. **The pharynx measures 130 mm in length**

3. **Nasopharynx contains**
   - Eustachian tube opening
   - Pharyngeal tonsils (adenoids)

4. **Oropharynx**
   - Contains palatine tonsils
   - Separated from the oral cavity by
     i. Uvula
     ii. Pillars of fauces

5. **Pillars of fauces consist of**
   - Anterior fold – palatoglossal arch
   - Posterior fold – palatopharyngeal arch

6. **The larynx**
   - Also known as the voice box
   - Has 4 significant cartilages
     i. Epiglottis
     ii. Thyroid cartilage (Adam's apple)
     iii. Cricoid cartilage
     iv. Arytenoid cartilage

7. **Trachea**
   - Measures 120 mm in length
   - Has 16–20 incomplete cartilage rings

8. **Bronchi**
   - Bifurcation at carina
   - Has incomplete cartilaginous rings
   - Right bronchus is more acute in angle

9. **Lung anatomy**
   - Right lung has 3 lobes
   - Left lung has 2 lobes
   - Lobules contain alveoli
   - Alveolar and capillary wall is composed of a single layer of epithelium

10. **Pulmonary vascular resistance (PVR) depends on**
    - Lung volume
      i. Small lung volume – PVR is high
      ii. Initial increase in lung volume – PVR falls
      iii. Further increase in lung volume – PVR rises exponentially
    - Pulmonary vascular tone (via nitric oxide action)
    - Hypoxia leads to pulmonary vasoconstriction
    - Pulmonary artery and venous pressure

11. **Muscles of ventilation**
    - Consist of
      i. Diaphragm
      ii. Intercostals muscles (11 pairs)
      iii. Accessory muscles (sternocleidomastoid, platysma, and scalene muscles)
    - Supplied by phrenic nerve from C3, C4, and C5

Mechanics of breathing

1. **Air is a mixture of**
   - O_2 = 21%
   - N_2 = 78%

2. **Types of respiration**
   - Physiological respiration
   - Cellular respiration
     - i.   Is metabolic process in which an organism obtains energy
     - ii. O_2 + Glucose $\rightarrow CO_2 + H_2O$ + ATP

Chpt 5

3. **Physiological respiration consist of**
   - Ventilation
   - Pulmonary gas exchange
   - Gas transport
   - Peripheral gas exchange

4. **Ventilation**
   - Is movement of air into and out of the lungs
   - Occurs as a result of pressure difference
   - Consists of
     - i.   Inspiration (an active process)
     - ii. Expiration (a passive process)
   - Factors affecting ventilation
     - i.   Airway compliance
     - ii. Airway resistance
   - Minute ventilation (MV) is
     - i.   Tidal volume (TV) × respiratory rate (RR)
     - ii. The total volume of gas entering the lung per minute
   - Alveolar ventilation (AV) is
     - i.   (TV – dead space volume) × RR
     - ii. 4.2 L/min
     - iii. The volume of gas per minute that reaches the alveoli
   - Dead space ventilation (DSV) is
     - i.   The volume of gas per minute that remain in the airways
     - ii. The volume of gas per minute not involved with gaseous exchange

5. **Inspiration**
   - Is based on Boyle's law
   - Occurs as follows (**Fig. 4.5**)

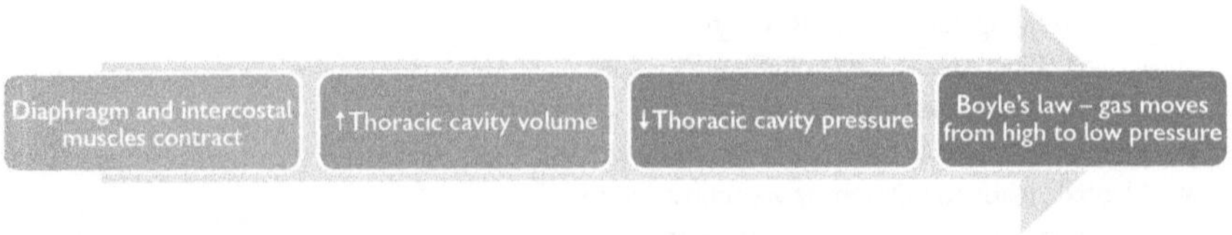

Diaphragm and intercostal muscles contract → ↑Thoracic cavity volume → ↓Thoracic cavity pressure → Boyle's law – gas moves from high to low pressure

Figure 4.5 Mechanism of inspiration

6. **Intrapleural pressure (IP)**
   - Prevents the tendency of the lung to collapse due to its elastic recoil
   - Resting IP = −5 cmH$_2$O

- Falls during inspiration
- Becomes positive during forced expiration (can reach up to $+30\,cmH_2O$)

7. **Control of ventilation is under**
   - Nervous control – respiratory centre in brainstem
   - Chemical control
     i. Central – medulla oblongata
     ii. Peripheral (aortic and carotid body)
   - Bezold–Jarisch reflex
     i. Causes hypopnoea and bradycardia
     ii. Is due to increase in parasympathetic activity
     iii. Is caused by veratrum alkaloids, nicotine, and antihistamines
   - J-receptors (proprioceptors)
     i. Are innervated by vagus nerve
     ii. Stimulation causes a reflex increase in breathing

8. **Gaseous exchange**
   - Takes place at the respiratory surface
   - Is governed by Fick's law (describes diffusion), which states that respiratory surfaces must have a
     i. Large surface area
     ii. Thin permeable surface
     iii. Moist exchange surface

9. **Factors affecting gaseous exchange**
   - Temperature (Charles' law – high temperature causes increase in velocity; increased velocity causes increased pressure)
   - Composition (Dalton's law – the total pressure of a mixture is that of all the partial pressures added together)
   - Diffusion gradient
     i. pO_2 (**Box 4.12**)
     ii. pCO_2 (**Box 4.13**)

Box 4.12 pO_2 diffusion gradient

Atmospheric	Trachea	Alveoli	Arterial
• 160 mmHg • 21 kPa	• 150 mmHg • 19.8 kPa	• 100 mmHg • 14 kPa	• 13.3 kPa

Venous			
• 40 mmHg			

Box 4.13 pCO_2 diffusion gradient

Atmospheric	Alveoli	Arterial	Venous
• 0.3 mmHg • 0.03 kPa	• 40 mmHg • 5.3 kPa	• 5.3 kPa	• 45 mmHg • 6.1 kPa

Exhaled air			
• 4 kPa			

Box 4.14 Lung compliance changes

Lung complicance is increased in	Lung compliance is decreased in
• Obstructive lung disease	• Restrictive lung disease
• Expiration	• Pulmonary oedema
• Old age	• Acute respiratory syndrome (ARDS)

10. Lung compliance (*Box 4.14*)
- Is defined as the change in lung volume per unit change in pressure
- Is $200\,mL/cmH_2O$
- Governed by Laplace's law ($P = 2T/r$)
    i.   Transpulmonary pressure (P) is proportional to wall tension (T)
    ii. Transpulmonary pressure (P) is inversely proportional to radius (r)
    iii. Transpulmonary pressure is required to prevent alveolar collapse
- Pulmonary surfactant
    i.   Reduces wall tension and thus compliance
    ii. Secreted by lung type 2 pneumocytes
    iii. Composed of dipalmitylphosphatidylcholine and cholesterol
- Elastance
    i.   Is defined as 1/compliance
    ii. Measures elastic recoil of lung

11. Airway resistance
- Is governed by Poiseuille's law ($R = 8l/\pi r4$)
    i.   Resistance (R) is proportional to length (l) of tube
    ii. Resistance (R) is inversely proportional to radius (r) of tube
- Factors that influence diameter of airways
    i.   Respiratory secretions
    ii. Lung volumes (high volumes cause decreased resistance due to radial traction)
    iii. Smooth muscles of respiratory tree
- Closing volume is
    i.   The volume at which airways collapse
    ii. Between FRC and RV
    iii. Increases with age

Respiratory function

1. Lung volumes
- Residual volume (RV) is
    i.   The volume that remains in the lungs following maximal expiration
    ii. 1.5 L
- TV is
    i.   7 mL/kg
    ii. or approximately 500 mL
- Inspiratory reserve volume (IRV) is
    i.   The volume that can be inspired above the TV
    ii. 1.5 L
- Expiratory reserve volume (ERV) = 1.5 L
- Vital capacity (VC)
    i.   Is the volume of gas that can be inhaled from forced expiration to inhalation
    ii. VC = IRV + ERV + TV
    iii. VC = 3.5 L

- Inspiratory capacity (IC) = TV + IRV
- Functional residual capacity (FRC) (*Box 4.15*)
  - i.   Is the volume of gas left in the lung at the end of quiet respiration
  - ii. FRC = RV + ERV
  - iii. FRC = 2.5–3 L
- Total lung volume (TLV)
  - i. TLV = VC + RV
  - ii. TLV = 5 L

Box 4.15 FRC changes

FRC is increased by	FRC is decreased by
• Obstructive lung disease • Continuous positive airway pressure (CPAP)	• Restrictive lung disease • Pregnancy • Anaesthesia • Following surgery

2. **Alveoli**
   - Total alveolar volume = 2 L
   - Alveolar ventilation = 350 mL
   - Basal O_2 consumption = 250 mL/min
   - O_2 capacity = 20 mL/100 mL blood

3. **Spirometry** (*Box 4.16*)
   - Forced vital capacity (FVC) is the total amount of air that can be forcibly exhaled after inspiration
   - Forced expiratory volume in 1 second (FEV_1) = 3 L
   - FEV_1/FVC = 75%–80%
   - Peak expiratory flow rate (PEFR) = 600 mL/breath
   - Respiratory rate = 10–18 breaths/min

Box 4.16 Spirometry changes in lung disease

Obstructive lung disease	Restrictive lung disease
• Total lung volume ↑ • FRC ↑ • RV ↑ • PEFR ↓ • FEV1/FVC ↓	• All lung volumes are reduced • FEV1/FVC ↑ or normal

4. **Dead space**
   - Is the volume of inspired air that is not involved in gaseous exchange
   - 3 types
     - i.   Anatomical (is approximately equal to body weight in pounds) = 150 mL
     - ii. Alveolar (those ventilated but not perfused)
     - iii. Physiological
   - Physiological dead space (PDS) is
     - i. Anatomical dead space + alveolar dead space
     - ii. 2–3 mL/kg

Respiratory changes in pregnancy

Chpt 6.1 1. **Respiratory changes in pregnancy are due to progesterone (*Fig. 4.6*)**

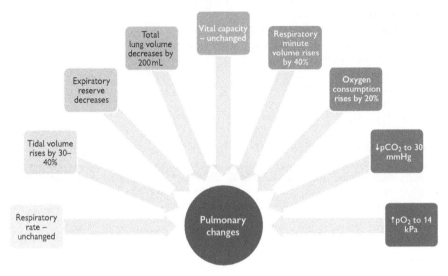

Figure 4.6 Pulmonary changes in pregnancy

- Anatomical
  i. Engorged turbinates
  ii. Bronchiole relaxation
  iii. Decreased airway resistance
- Mechanical
  i. Oxygen demand increases by 20%
  ii. Increased TV
  iii. VC = same
  iv. RR = same
  v. Lung compliance = same
  vi. Decreased chest compliance
  vii. Decreased RV by 200 mL
  viii. Decreased ERV
  ix. Decreased total lung volume by 200 mL
  x. Increased IRV
  xi. Breathing more diaphragmatic than thoracic
  xii. FEV_1 = same
  xiii. PEFR = same
- Gases
  i. Decreased pCO_2 to 30 mmHg
  ii. Increased pO_2 to 14 kPa

Maternal and fetal oxygen transport

1. **General facts**
   - Cyanosis occurs when deoxyhaemoglobin >5 g/dL
   - Decrease in O_2 saturation by 1% causes an increase in ventilation by 600 mL/min
   - Only 1% of O_2 in blood is dissolved in plasma
   - Haematocrit of venous blood is 3% higher than that of arterial blood
   - Carbon monoxide has 240 times more affinity for haemoglobin than oxygen

2. **Fetal and maternal values** (*Table 4.2*)

Table 4.2 Fetal and maternal gas values

		Maternal	Fetal
pO_2 (mmHg)	Artery	80–100 (9–13 kPa)	25
	Placental pool	45	
	Venous		35
pCO_2(kPa)	Artery	4.7–6.0 (35–45 mmHg)	4.9–10.7
	Venous		3.5–7.9
pH	Artery	7.34–7.44	7.05–7.38
	Venous		7.17–7.48
Base excess (mmol/L)	Artery	−3 to 3	−2.5 to 10
	Venous		−1 to 9
Hb (g/dL)		12	17
Blood O_2 content (mL/100 mL)		15	25
O_2 saturation (%)	Artery	>97%	25
	Venous		75

3. **O_2 dissociation curve**
   - Is sigmoid shaped
     i. At pO_2 >60 mmHg the curve is flat (which means O_2 content of blood does not change significantly with increase in pO_2)
   - P_{50} is
     i. The pO_2 in blood at which the Hb is 50% saturated
     ii. 26.6 mmHg
   - Left shift, indicating higher affinity for O_2 (decrease in P_{50}), is caused by
     i. Carbon monoxide
     ii. Fetal Hb
     iii. Decreased 2,3-DPG
   - Right shift, indicating decreased affinity for O_2 (increase in P_{50} – which means that larger pressures are required to maintain an O_2 saturation of 50%), is caused by
     i. Hyperthermia
     ii. Acidosis
     iii. Hypercapnia

4. **Properties of haemoglobin**
   - Bohr effect
     i. States that in the presence of CO_2, the O_2 affinity for dissociation of respiratory pigment decreases
     ii. Shift of the oxyhaemoglobin dissociation curve to the right when the pH is low even with a relatively high PO_2
   - Haldane effect – states that deoxygenation of blood increases its ability to carry CO_2

5. **CO_2 transport**
   - In 3 forms
     i. Solution (10%) – CO_2 is 24 times more water-soluble than O_2
     ii. Hydration (60%): $CO_2 + H_2O \rightarrow H_2CO_3 \rightarrow H^+ + HCO_3^-$ – occurs in RBCs
     iii. Carbamino compounds (30%)
   - RBCs have carbonic anhydrase
   - Plasma has no carbonic anhydrase

- Chloride shift
  i. HCO_3^- leaves the RBCs and moves into plasma
  ii. Cl^- moves into RBCs from plasma to maintain electrical neutrality
- Majority of CO_2 is transported in plasma as HCO_3^-
- H^+ is buffered in RBCs

6. **2,3-diphosphoglycerate (2,3-DPG)** *(Box 4.17)*
   - Is a product of glycolysis

Box 4.17 2,3-DPG changes

2,3-DPG increases in	2,3-DPG decreases in
• Exercise • High altitude • Elevated androgens • Elevated thyroxine • Elevated growth hormones	• Acidosis

Digestive tract and nutrition

Digestive tract

1. **Two sets of teeth develop in the course of a lifetime**
   - Deciduous ('milk' teeth) – total of 20 (start to erupt at 6 months of age)
   - Permanent teeth – total of 32 (start to erupt at 6 years of age)

2. **Salivary glands**
   - 3 pairs of exocrine glands empty into the mouth
     i.   Parotid (duct opens at 2nd upper molar)
     ii. Submandibular (ducts open on either side of frenulum of tongue)
     iii. Sublingual (ducts open on floor of mouth)
   - Produce 1.5 L of saliva per day
   - Saliva contains amylase

3. **Digestive tract is made up of 4 layers**
   - Mucosa
   - Submucosa
     i.   Contains blood vessels, nerves, and lymph
     ii. Has Meissner's (submucosal) plexus
     iii. Responsible for secretions
   - Muscular layer
     i.   Has Auerbach's (mesenteric) plexus
     ii. Responsible for contractions
   - Serosa – is a continuation of the peritoneum

4. **Gastric secretions**
   - 3 L are produced per day
   - Consist of
     i.   HCl (pH 1.5–3.5)
     ii. Pepsinogen
     iii. Intrinsic factor (for the absorption of vitamin B_{12})

5. **Digestion has 3 phases**
   - Cephalic phase
   - Gastric phase
     i.   Gastrin is secreted
     ii. Continues until stomach is emptied and pH falls to 1.5
   - Intestinal phase causes the production of 3 hormones
     i.   Gastric inhibitory peptide (GIP) – inhibits gastric motility and secretion
     ii. Secretin – inhibits gastric secretion
     iii. Cholecystokinin (CCK) – inhibits gastric emptying
   - Gastric emptying
     i.   Takes 2–6 hours
     ii. Protein stays the longest period of time in the stomach
   - Intestinal emptying takes 3–5 hours
   - Chyme is digested food

6. **Small Intestine**
   - Epithelium contains microvilli (brush border)
   - pH = 7.5
   - Produces 3 L of intestinal secretions per day
   - Food movement is via
     i.   Peristalsis
     ii. Segmentation
   - Ileum is
     i.   The only site of absorption of vitamin B_{12} and bile salts
     ii. Critical in fluid and Na^+ conservation
   - Jejunal contents are isotonic
   - Small bowel motility is 3 times slower in ileum compared to the jejunum

7. **Resection of ileum causes**
   - Loss of bile salts that is not met by increased synthesis
   - Reduction in bile salt pool
   - Bile salts loss into the colon causes
     i.   Reduction in salt and water reabsorption
     ii. Diarrhoea (which may be treated with cholestyramine)
   - Increased intestinal transit
   - Short gut syndrome
   - Renal calculi
   - Cholelithiasis

8. **Large intestines**
   - Secretes mucus
   - Does not produce enzymes
   - Has commensal bacteria that produce
     i.   Some vitamins of the vitamin B family
     ii. Vitamin K
   - Efficiency of salt and water resorption = 90%
   - Transit time = 24–150 h
   - Flatus is made up of
     i.   Hydrogen
     ii. Methane
     iii. CO_2

9. **Bile**
   - 1 L produced per day
   - Is alkaline
   - Contains
     i.   Bile salts
     ii. Bile pigments
     iii. Cholesterol
   - Bile salts
     i.   Are essential for absorption of fat and fat-soluble vitamins
     ii. Are bile acids conjugated to glycine or taurine
     iii. The 2 major bile acids are
        - Cholic acid
        - Chenodeoxycholic acid
   - Enterohepatic circulation of bile salts is essential to maintain bile salt pool

10. **Bilirubin**
    - Is a bile salt
    - Product of haemoglobin breakdown
    - Lipophilic
    - Converted to
      i. Stercobilin (excreted in faeces)
      ii. Urobilinogen (excreted in urine)

11. **Physiological jaundice**
    - Common between day 3 and 7 of life
    - Due to
      i. Immature liver enzymes
      ii. Haemolysis of fetal RBCs
    - Can cause kernicterus (deposition of bilirubin in basal ganglia)

12. **Pancreatic juices**
    - 1.5 L produced per day
    - Contain
      i.   Water
      ii. Sodium chloride
      iii. Sodium bicarbonate
      iv. Enzymes
         - Trypsinogen
         - Chymotrypsinogen
         - Proelastase
         - Amylase
         - Lipase
    - Are alkaline

Nutrition

1. **Calories**
   - Energy provided
     i.   Carbohydrate = 4.2 kcal/g
     ii. Protein = 4.2 kcal/g
     iii. Fat = 9 kcal/g

- Requirement (is about 30 kcal/kg/day)
  - i.   Non-pregnant = 2200 kcal/day
  - ii. Pregnant = 2400 kcal/day
  - iii. Lactating = 2800 kcal/day

2. **Daily recommended intake**
   - Carbohydrate = 400 g/day
   - Fat = 100 g/day
   - Salt = 6 g/day
   - Folic acid = 400 µg/day
   - Protein
     - i. Non-pregnant = 1.5 g/kg body weight/day
     - ii. Pregnant = 2 g/kg body weight/day

3. **Nitrogen requirements**
   - 1 g of nitrogen is contained within 6.25 g of protein
   - 6.25 g of protein is contained within 36 g of wet weight tissue
   - Normal urinary nitrogen excretion is 14 g/day
   - Nitrogen intake
     - i.   Basic nitrogen requirements – 0.1 g/kg/day
     - ii. Nitrogen requirements in hypermetabolic state – 0.2 g/kg/day
     - iii. Nitrogen intake of >14 g/day has no benefit
   - Nitrogen loss
     - i. Daily = 2 g/day
     - ii. Menstruation = 2 g/month

4. **Iron**
   - Iron requirement
     - i. Non-pregnant = 2.8 mg/day
     - ii. Pregnant = 6 mg/day
   - Iron deficiency anaemia is characterized by
     - i.   Iron <12 µmol/L
     - ii. TIBC saturation <15%
     - iii. Microcytic
     - iv. Microchromic
   - Total body iron = 40 mg/kg body weight

5. **Vitamins and minerals**
   - Vitamins A, D, E, and K (the ADEK group of vitamins) are fat soluble
   - Vitamin and mineral daily recommended requirements (*Table 4.3*)
   - Vitamin deficiencies and overdoses (*Table 4.4*)

GIT changes in pregnancy

1. **Changes in pregnancy**
   - Vomiting
   - Heartburn/reflux (due to the relaxation of gastro-oesophageal sphincter)
   - Delayed gastric emptying
   - Constipation (due to relaxation of intestinal smooth muscles by progesterone)
   - Gingivitis (due to increased vascularity in gums)

Table 4.3

Vitamin	Requirement/day (µg/day)	Minerals	Requirement/day (µg/day)
A (retinol)	800	Ca^{2+}	800
B_1 (thiamine)	1000	Iron	12
B_2 (riboflavin)	1500	Na^+	3000
B_3 (niacin)	15 000	Cl^-	3500
B_6 (pyridoxine)	2000	K^+	1000
B_{12} (cobalamin)	2	Iodide	0.1
C (ascorbic acid)	30 000	Zinc	150
D (calciferol)	10	Mg^{2+}	300
E (tocopherol)	10 000		

Table 4.4

Vitamin		Deficiency	Toxicity
A		Keratomalacia Night blindness	(at dose >3000 µg/day) Hypervitaminosis A
B	B_1	Beriberi Wernicke–Korsakoff syndrome	No known toxicity
	B_2	Ariboflavinosis	No known toxicity
	B_3	Pellagra	Liver damage
	B_5 (pantothenic acid)	Paraesthesia	No known toxicity
	B_6	Microcytic anaemia Peripheral neuropathy	(at dose >100 mg/day) Impairment of proprioception
	B_7 (biotin)	Dermatitis Enteritis	No known toxicity
	B_9 (folic acid)	Macrocytic anaemia	No known toxicity
	B_{12}	Megaloblastic anaemia	No known toxicity
C		Scurvy	(at dose >2 g/day) Vitamin C megadosage
D		Rickets Osteomalacia	(at dose >50 µg/day) Hypervitaminosis D
E		Haemolytic anaemia in newborn infants	
K (phylloquinone)		Bleeding diathesis	No known toxicity

Urinary system

Urinary tract

1. **Kidney consist of**
   - Functional units – nephrons
   - Collecting ducts (collect urine from nephrons)

2. **Nephrons**
   - Each kidney contains about 1 million nephrons
   - Is made up of 4 regions
     i. Bowman's capsule (surrounds glomerulus)
     ii. PCT
     iii. Loop of Henle
     iv. DCT

3. **Urine is formed by 3 processes**
   - Glomerular filtration
   - Selective tubular reabsorption
   - Tubular secretion (secretion of H^+ and K^+ ions)

4. **Glomerulus**
   - Is a mass of capillaries in Bowman's capsule
   - Contains 2 arterioles
     i. Afferent
     ii. Efferent (smaller in size)

5. **PCT**
   - Reabsorbs
     i. Water (passively)
     ii. Solutes (actively)
   - 80% filtrate is reabsorbed
   - Glucose (when plasma levels are in the physiological range) is completely reabsorbed
   - Renal threshold (the maximum limit of solute that can be reabsorbed) reduces in pregnancy

6. **Loop of Henle**
   - Solute reabsorption occurs at ascending loop
   - Water reabsorption occurs at descending loop
   - Ascending limb is impermeable to water
   - Concentrates urine

7. **DCT**
   - Only 5% of filtrates reach the DCT
   - Plays a role in water absorption
   - Is under the influence of
     i. ADH
     ii. Aldosterone

8. **The juxtaglomerular apparatus is composed of specialized cells situated in**
   - Ascending loop of Henle (macula densa) – measures Na^+ concentration
   - Afferent arteriole (juxtaglomerular cells) – modified endothelial cells, which are pressure sensitive

9. **Renal functions**
   - Urine production

- Synthesis of
  i.   Glucose
  ii. Erythropoietin (EPO)
  iii. Vitamin D

10. General functional measurements

- Renal blood supply
  i.   Receives 25% of CO
  ii. 1.2 L/min
- Renal plasma flow (RPF) = 660 mL/min
- Creatinine clearance = 120 mL/min
- GFR = 120 mL/min
  i.   Proportional to body surface area
  ii. Is 10% less in females
- Filtration fraction = GFR/RPF = 0.18

11. Ureter has 3 layers

- Outer fibrous
- Middle muscular
- Inner transitional epithelium

12. Bladder

- Stimulated at 300 mL of volume
- Nerve supply via Lee–Frankenhauser plexus

13. Micturition

- Voiding is under voluntary control mediated by the pontine reticular formation in the cerebellum
- Bladder contractility is dependent on sacral spinal reflex
- Urethral function is controlled by pudendal nerve
- Micturition cycle involves 3 phases
  i.   Storage
  ii. Initiation
  iii. Voiding
- In bladder filling
  i.   Ascending impulses pass from (*Fig. 4.7*)

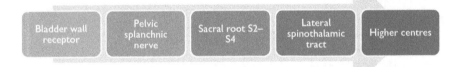

Bladder wall receptor → Pelvic splanchnic nerve → Sacral root S2–S4 → Lateral spinothalamic tract → Higher centres

Figure 4.7 Ascending impulses from bladder during bladder filling

  ii. Descending impulses inhibit detrusor contraction via the sympathetic nervous system (*Box 4.18*)
- Bladder initiation phase begins with
  i.   Relaxation of pelvic floor

ii. Suppression of descending inhibitory impulses via parasympathetic system (acting on M2 and M3 muscarinic receptors in the bladder)
  ● Voiding phase begins when rising intravesical and falling urethral pressures equalize

Chpt 14.8

4. Normal urodynamic values
  ● Residual volume = <50 mL
  ● 1st sensation = 200 mL
  ● Voiding volume = 400 mL
  ● Bladder capacity = 600 mL
  ● Flow rate > 15mL/s
  ● Pressures
   i. Negligible rise in detrusor pressure on filling (< 15cmH$_2$O)
   ii. Maximum voiding detrusor pressure < 50cmH$_2$O
   iii. Intraurethral at rest (with sphincter contracted) = 50–100 cmH$_2$O
   iv. Absence of systolic detrusor pressure during filling

Urinary system changes in pregnancy

1. Changes of urinary system in pregnancy
  ● Increase uterine size causes
   i. Increased frequency
   ii. Nocturia
  ● Lowered renal threshold leads to glycosuria
  ● Increased kidney size by 1 cm
   i. Due to renal hypertrophy
   ii. No hyperplasia
  ● Mild renal pelvis and ureteric dilatation (due to progesterone and obstruction by gravid uterus)
  ● Increased renal blood flow (from 1.2 to 1.5 L/min)
  ● Increased GFR (from 140 to 170 mL/min)
  ● Decreased filtration fraction (GFR/RPF)

2. Renal metabolic changes in pregnancy
  ● Decreased HCO$_3^-$ (in response to decreased CO$_2$)
  ● Decreased Na$^+$ (in response to fall in HCO$_3^-$)
  ● Decreased osmolarity by 10 mmol/L (in response to progesterone)
  ● Decreased urea (from 4.3 to 3.1 mmol/L)
  ● Decreased creatinine (from 73 to 47 µmol/L)

3. Retention of urine is common in labour

4. Postnatal changes
  ● Urine output increases for 7 days postpartum
  ● Urinary tract infection (UTI) occurs in 2–4% of women in the puerperium

5. Neonate – passage of urine is expected within 24 hours post delivery

Box 4.18 Detrusor inhibitory sympathetic impulses

α-receptors	β-receptors
● Located in bladder neck and urethra ● Increase outlet urethral resistance	● Located on detrusor muscle ● Cause detrusor smooth muscle relaxation

Female reproductive system

Folliculogenesis

1. **Folliculogenesis**
   - Defined as growth and development of follicle from the earliest 'resting' stages through to ovulation
   - 2 main phases
     i.   Pre-antral – independent of FSH
     ii. Antral (Graafian) – dependent on FSH
   - Is based on 2-cell 2-gonadotrophin hypothesis for oestrogen production
     i.   In response to LH, thecal tissues produce androgens, which can then be converted to oestrogen in granulosa cells via FSH-induced aromatization
     ii. Granulosa cells are dependent on androgens from theca cells to make oestrogens
     iii. FSH is important in early folliculogenesis
     iv. LH optimizes final stages of follicle maturation and promotes growth of dominant follicle

2. **Theca cells**
   - Secrete
     i.   Androgens
     ii. Progesterone
   - Do not secrete testosterone as they lacks 17β-HSD
   - Have **only** LH receptors

3. **Granulosa cells**
   - Secrete
     i.   Oestrogen
     ii. Progesterone
   - Contain P450 aromatase
   - Have LH and FSH receptors

4. **Stages of ovarian follicle development (*Fig. 4.8*)**

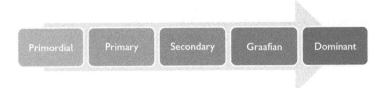

Figure 4.8 Ovarian follicle developmental stages

5. **Primordial follicles**
   - Consist of a primary oocyte surrounded by
     i.   A single layer of granulosa cells
     ii. Basal lamina
   - Formed at 6 months gestation
   - Number of primordial follicles at
     i.   6 months gestation = 5–7 million
     ii. Birth = 2 million
     iii. Puberty = 300 000 to 500 000 (only about 500 will be selected to ovulate)

6. **Primary follicle**
   - Is the stage when the granulosa cells in the primordial follicle change from flat to cuboidal
   - Zona pellucida forms around the ovum
   - FSH receptors develop
   - Is independent of gonadotrophin stimulation

7. **Secondary follicle**
   - Is the stage when primary follicle attains a second layer of granulosa cells
   - Occurs at day 5 of cycle
   - Follicle mitotic activity is high
   - Theca cells are recruited to surround the granulosa cells and form 2 layers
     i.   Theca interna
     ii. Theca externa
   - A capillary network exists between the 2 theca layers

8. **Pre-antral follicle**
   - Is a secondary follicle in its late stages of development
   - Histologically contains
     i.   Oocyte
     ii.   Zona pellucida
     iii. 9 layers of granulosa cells
     iv.   Basal lamina
     v.   Theca interna
     vi.   Capillary network
     vii. Theca externa

9. **Graafian follicle**
   - Also known as
     i.   Tertiary follicle
     ii. Antral follicle
   - Is marked by the formation of a fluid-filled cavity between the granulosa cells
   - Corona radiata = granulosa cells immediately surrounding the ovum
   - Dependent on FSH
   - Grows to a size of >1 cm
   - Secretes oestrogen

10. **Preovulatory follicle**
    - Is a Graafian follicle in its late stages of development
    - 5 to 7 preovulatory follicles will enter the menstrual cycle and compete to become the dominant follicle
    - Follicles with low FSH receptors will stop developing and undergo atresia
    - Dominant follicle will undergo ovulation
    - Usually only 1 follicle per cycle undergoes ovulation while the rest will undergo atresia

11. **Size of follicle at ovulation ≈ 20 mm**

12. **Time length of folliculogenesis**
    - Lasts for about 375 days (i.e. from resting follicle stage to ovulation)
    - Coincides with 13 menstrual cycles
    - Follicular growth (from pre-antral follicle stage to ovulation) takes 90 days

Oogenesis

1. **Oogenesis**
   - Process by which mature ova are formed

- Consist of
  - i.   Oocytogenesis
  - ii. Ootidogenesis
  - iii. Maturation
- Stages of development (**Fig. 4.9**)

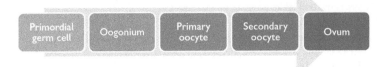

Figure 4.9 Stages of ovum development

2. **Primordial germ cells**
   - Migrate from yolk sac to the ovaries
   - Mature to oogonia

3. **Oogonia**
   - Consist of 46 chromosomes (diploid)
   - Reach a maximum of 6–7 million by 16–20 weeks of intrauterine life
   - Divide by mitosis
     - i. To form primary oocyte
     - ii. At 3rd month of gestation (2nd trimester of pregnancy)

4. **Primary oocyte**
   - Contains 46 chromosomes (diploid)
   - Surrounded by primordial follicle
   - Undergoes meiosis 1 at 5th month gestation
   - Meiosis 1 is not completed until ovulation (arrested at prophase 1)
   - At ovulation primary oocyte completes meiosis 1 forming
     - i. Secondary oocyte
     - ii. 1st polar body

5. **Dictyate**
   - Is a prolonged resting phase in oogenesis
   - Starts late in fetal life and ends (due to LH surge) before ovulation

6. **Secondary oocyte**
   - Contains 23 chromosomes (haploid)
   - Is the primitive ovum
   - Surrounded by secondary follicle
   - Enters meiosis 2
   - Meiosis 2 is not completed until fertilization occurs (arrested at metaphase 2)
   - At fertilization secondary oocyte completes meiosis 2 forming
     - i. Ovum
     - ii. 2nd polar body

Reproductive cycle

1. **Reproductive cycle**
   - Lasts 28–30 days

- 1st day
    i.   Is the onset of menstruation
    ii. Oestrogen and progesterone levels are at their lowest

2. Menstrual cycle
- Is the proliferation and shedding of the functional layer of endometrium
- Has 3 phases
    i.   Menstruation (day 1–5)
    ii. Proliferation (day 6–15)
    iii. Secretion (day 16–28)
- Menstruation
    i.   Blood loss is 50–150 mL
    ii. Is due to withdrawal of progesterone
- Proliferative phase
    i.   Also known as the follicular phase
    ii. Is under the influence of oestrogen produced from the Graafian follicle
- Secretory phase
    i.   Also known as luteal phase
    ii. Is under the influence of the corpus luteum
    iii. Is the interval between ovulation and menstruation
    iv. Is relatively constant and lasts approximately 14 days

3. Hormonal changes during the ovarian cycle
- Day 1
    i.   Low levels of oestrogen/progesterone stimulate gonadotrophin-releasing hormone (GnRH) increase
    ii. GnRH stimulates FSH increase
    iii. FSH stimulates secondary follicle to secrete oestrogen
- Day 14
    i.   High oestrogen
        - Inhibits release of FSH
        - Initiates release of LH
    ii. LH initiates ovulation
- Post-ovulation
    i.   Corpus luteum secretes progesterone
    ii. Increased progesterone levels cause decreased LH levels
- Dominant follicle survives fall in FSH by responding to LH

4. Rules for hormones through ovarian/menstrual cycle
- FSH – intercycle rise
- LH
    i.   Rises slowly through follicular phase
    ii. Has a mid-cycle surge
    iii. Then rapidly declines to low levels
- Oestradiol rises up to mid-cycle, falls, then peaks in the luteal phase
- Progesterone levels start low then has one peak in the luteal phase

5. Ovulation
- Is the process in which an ovarian follicle ruptures and releases an ovum
- Defines the transition from follicular to luteal phase
- Occurs 18 hours after peak of LH
- Signs
    i.   Mid-cycle pelvic pain (Mittelschmerz)

ii.   Fluid in the pouch of Douglas
● Ruptured follicle becomes the corpus luteum

6. **Corpus luteum**
   ● Develops
     i.   From ruptured Graafian follicle
     ii. During luteal phase of menstrual cycle
   ● Produces oestrogen and progesterone
   ● Has LH receptors
   ● Fate if fertilization occurs (**Fig. 4.10**)

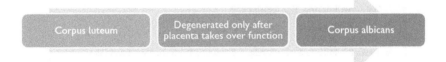

Figure 4.10 Fate of corpus luteum if fertilization occurs

     i.   Persists for 6 months
     ii. Function is replaced by placenta at 3rd month
   ● If fertilization does not occur, corpus luteum becomes corpus albicans and menstruation
     begins (**Fig. 4.11**)

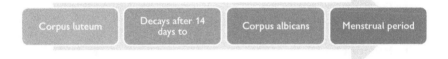

Figure 4.11 Fate of corpus luteum if fertilization does not occur

7. **Corpus albicans**
   ● Is a mass of fibrous scar tissue
   ● Is the degenerated corpus luteum if fertilization does not occur

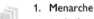
T. in
Obs
Gyn

Chpts 2.6
& 2.10   *Menarche and menopause*

1. **Menarche**
   ● Is the time of first menstruation
   ● Occurs around the age of 10–16
Chpt 6
   ● Average age is 12.3 years in African girls and 12.8 in Western (Caucasian) girls
   ● Occurs due to changes in puberty
     i.   Sufficient body mass has to be achieved (minimum of 48 kg with 17% of it being fat)
     ii. Activation of the GnRH pulse generator
     iii. Ovarian oestrogen-induced growth of uterus
     iv. Fluctuating oestrogen levels
   ● Does not signal that ovulation has occurred
     i.   1st year post-menarche – 80% of cycles are anovulatory
     ii. 3rd year post-menarche – 50% of cycles are anovulatory
     iii. 5th year post-menarche – 10% of cycles are anovulatory

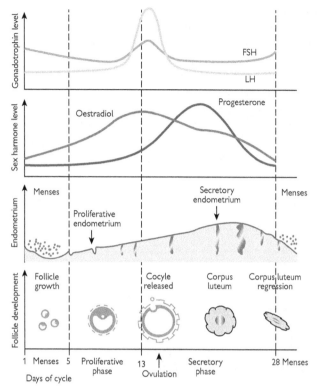

Figure 4.12 The hormonal and endometrial axis of the human menstrual cycle

Reproduced from *Training in Obstetrics and Gynaecology*, by Sarris, Bewley, and Agnihotri, © Oxford University Press, (2009).

- Nubility = anthropological term for a state of regular ovulation
- Primary amenorrhoea is diagnosed when menarche fails to occur
    i.   3 years after thelarche (beginning of breast development)
    ii. by the age of 16 in the presence of normal secondary sexual characteristics
    iii. by the age of 14 in the absence of other secondary sexual characteristics

2. Menopause
- Occurs between 45 and 55 years of age
- Average age in the UK is 51 years
- Age of menopause is reduced by
    i.   Cigarette smoking (by 12 months)
    ii. Hysterectomy with ovarian conservation (believed to be by about 4 years)
    iii. Uterine artery embolization (5% risk of premature menopause)
- Premature menopause
    i.   Occurs in approximately 1% of women
    ii. Occurs before the age of 40
    iii. Incidence is higher in identical twins
    iv. 5% of identical twins reach menopause by the age of 40
- The process can take between 6 months to 3 years to complete
- Biochemical changes
    i.   Fall in oestradiol

ii. Decreased levels of inhibin

iii. Rise in LH and FSH (FSH >30 IU/dL)

- The predominant oestrogen during the menopausal years is oestrone
- Symptoms (*Box 4.19*)

Box 4.19 Symptoms of the menopause

Vasomotor	Urogenital tract	Skeletal	Psychological
• Hot flushes	• Urinary urgency	• Osteopenia	• Mood disturbance
• Migraine	• Urinary frequency	• Osteoporosis	• Memory loss
	• Urethral syndrome		• Insomnia
	• Vaginal atrophy		

Sexual
• Decreased libido
• Dyspareunia

Male reproductive system

1. **Spermatogenesis** (*Fig. 4.13*)
    - Spermatozoa are produced in the seminiferous tubules
    - Mature spermatozoa move into the lumen
    - Takes 70–80 days to produce
    - New cycle every 16 days
    - Under the influence of FSH
    - Consists of
        i. Spermatocytogenesis (creation of secondary spermatocyte from spermatogonium)
        ii. Spermatidogenesis (creation of spermatid from secondary spermatocyte)
        iii. Spermiogenesis

2. **Spermatocytogenesis**
    - Spermatogonium undergoes mitosis to produce primary spermatocyte
    - Primary spermatocyte
        i. Contains 46 chromosomes (diploid)
        ii. Undergoes meiosis 1 to produce secondary spermatocyte

3. **Secondary spermatocyte**
    - Contains 23 chromosomes (haploid)
    - Undergoes meiosis 2 to produce 4 spermatids

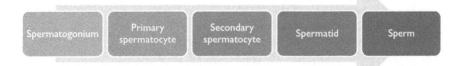

Figure 4.13 Developmental stages of sperm

4. **Spermiogenesis**
   - Is the maturation of spermatids
   - Under the influence of testosterone
   - Spermatid structural changes
     i.   Axoneme forms
     ii. Golgi apparatus becomes the acrosome
     iii. Centriole of cell becomes the tail of sperm
     iv. DNA becomes highly condensed
     v.   Excessive cytoplasm is removed as residual bodies
   - Spermiation = release of mature spermatozoa from Sertoli cells into the lumen of the seminiferous tubule

5. **Spermatozoa structure**
   - Head (contains acrosome)
   - Body (contains mitochondria)
   - Tail

6. **Hormonal control**
   - GnRH
     i.   Released at the age of 10
     ii. Produces FSH and LH
   - FSH
     i.   Acts on seminiferous tubules
     ii. Stimulates spermatogenesis
   - LH
     i.   Acts on Leydig cells
     ii. Stimulates testosterone production
   - Testosterone – inhibits GnRH and LH
   - Inhibin
     i.   Produced by Sertoli cells in response to increased spermatozoa
     ii. Inhibits FSH

7. **Semen**
   - Combination of secretions from
     i.   Seminal vesicles
     ii. Prostate
     iii. Bulbourethral (Cowper's) glands
     iv. Hyaluronidase – aids passage of sperm through cervical mucus
   - Normal semen analysis values (based on WHO 2010 criteria)
     i.   Volume = 1.5mL (range = 1.4–1.7mL)
     ii.   Each mL contains 50–150 million spermatozoa (normal ≥15 million/mL) (range = 12–16 million/mL)
     iii. Total sperm per ejaculate = 39 million (range = 33–46 million)
     iv.   Vitality is > 55%
     v.   Leukocyte: < 1 million/mL
     vi.   300 million sperm produced/day
     vii. pH = 7.2–7.6
     viii. Spermatozoa survive for 3–4 days
     ix.   Total motility: > 38% (with progressive motility > 31%)
     x.   Normal morphology: > 3%
   - Seminal fluid composition
     i.   Carnithine
     ii. Inositol
     iii. Glycerophosphocholine

    iv. Phosphatase

    v. Fructose

    vi. Citric acid

8. **Spermatozoa journey**
   - Semen coagulates in vagina
   - Cervical passage
     i. Glycoprotein molecules arrange in parallel lines
     ii. Sperm form reservoir in cervical crypt
   - Capacitation
     i. Is the biochemical removal of sperm surface glycoprotein
     ii. Initiates whiplash movement of sperm tail
     iii. Occurs in uterus via uterine fluid
   - Acrosome reaction – allows sperm to penetrate the zona pellucida

Musculoskeletal system

1. **The musculoskeletal system consists of**
   - Bones (206)
   - Joints (230)
   - Ligaments (900)
   - Muscles (639)
   - Tendons (about 4000)

Bone

1. **Bones are formed from**
   - Collagen
   - Inorganic materials
     i. Collagen
     ii. Phosphate
   - Water

2. **Hormones responsible for bone development**
   - Growth hormone
   - Thyroid
   - Parathyroid
   - Oestrogen
   - Testosterone

3. **Bone ossification**
   - 2 types
     i. Membranous
     ii. Direct
   - Primary centre is in the diaphysis
   - Secondary centres in epiphysis

4. **Bone has 2 types of tissue**
   - Compact (also known as cortical)
     i. Hard and dense
     ii. Composed of sheets (lamellae)
     iii. Arranges in concentric cylinders called Haversian systems
     iv. At the centre of the cylinder is the Haversian canal
     v. Osteocytes lie in the lacunae within the lamellae

    vi. Canaliculi (small canals) radiates from the lacunae
- Cancellous
  - i. Composed of an irregular honeycomb of thin plates (trabeculae)
  - ii. Contains red bone marrow

5. **There are 5 main types of bone**
   - Long
     - i. Shaft has compact bone
     - ii. Epiphysis has cancellous bone
   - Short
     - i. Mainly cancellous bone
     - ii. Cortex (outer shell) is compact bone
   - Flat – made up of 2 parallel plates of compact bone surrounding a layer of cancellous bone
   - Irregular
   - Sesamoid
     - i. Forms in areas of pressure
     - ii. Found in tendons

6. **Bone healing**
   - Haematoma forms initially
   - Macrophages phagocytose the haematoma
   - Osteoblast lay down new bone (callus)
   - Osteoclast reshape bone and form a central medullary canal

Muscles

1. **Muscles – there are 3 groups**
   - Skeletal – voluntary/striated muscle
   - Smooth
     - i. Involuntary/visceral muscles
     - ii. Spindle shaped cells
     - iii. Cells are connected by gap junctions
   - Cardiac
     - i. Branched fibres
     - ii. Cells are connected via intercalated disc

2. **Skeletal muscle**
   - There are 2 types of skeletal muscle fibre (*Box 4.20*)

Box 4.20 Types of skeletal muscle fibre

Type 1	Type 2
• Slow twitch fibre	• Fast twitch fibre
• Red	• White
• Contains high levels of myoglobin	• Contains large reserve of glycogen
• Aerobic	• Anaerobic

   - Architecture (*Fig. 4.14*)

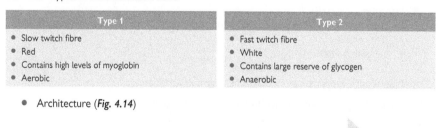

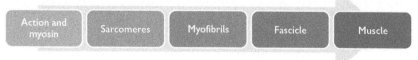

Figure 4.14 Architecture of a muscle fibre

3. **Myofibrils**
   - Contains
     - i. Actin (thin filament)
     - ii. Myosin (thick filament)
   - Are enclosed in
     - i. Epimysium (covers the whole muscle)
     - ii. Perimysium (covers the bundle)
   - iii. Endomysium (covers a single muscle cell)

4. **Muscle contraction**
   - Skeletal muscle contraction is associated with troponin (*Fig. 4.15*)
   - Smooth muscle contraction is associated with calmodulin – contraction occurs following phosphorylation of myosin

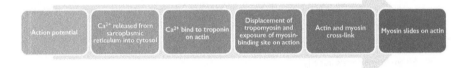

Figure 4.15 Skeletal muscle contraction mechanism

5. **Muscle fuels**
   - Phosphocreatine
   - Glycogen
   - Blood glucose
   - Fatty acids

Musculoskeletal changes in pregnancy

1. **Muscle relaxation**

2. **Relaxation of sacroiliac joints**

3. **Separation of pubic symphysis**
   - Normally, space between joint in pregnancy is up to 9 mm
   - If >10 mm there is significant separation

4. **Muscle relaxation in pregnancy occurs via**
   - Progesterone through
     - i. Suppression of mRNA production for oxytocin, oxytocin receptor, and prostaglandin F (FP) receptor
     - ii. Increase in cAMP
     - iii. Decrease in number of gap junctions
   - NO through expression of eNOS by the syncytiotrophoblast

Chpt 5

5. **Postnatal changes – it takes 3 months for muscle tone to normalize**

Nervous system

Chpt 3

Nervous tissue

1. **Nervous system is divided into**
   - Anatomical divisions

    i.   Central nervous system (CNS) – includes brain and spinal cord

    ii. Peripheral nervous system (PNS) – consist of cranial and spinal nerves

- Physiological divisions
  - i.   Autonomic nervous system (ANS)
  - ii. Somatic nervous system (SNS)

2. Cells of the nervous system consist of

- Neurones
- Glial cells

3. Neuronal structure consists of

- Cell body (contains Nissl bodies – characteristic of neurones)
- Dendrites
- Axon
- Presynaptic terminal

4. Glial cells

- Are
  - i.   Non-neuronal cells
  - ii. Non-excitable cells
- Functions
  - i.   Provide support and nutrients to neurones
  - ii. Forms myelin
- There are 4 types of glial cell in the CNS
  - i.   Astrocytes
  - ii. Oligodendrocytes
  - iii. Microglia
  - iv. Ependyma
- There are 3 types of glial cell in the PNS
  - i.   Schwann
  - ii. Satellite
  - iii. Enteric glial

5. Ependyma

- Is an epithelial membrane lining the cavities in the brain and spinal cord
- Formed of ependymal cells
- Includes choroidal epithelial cells

6. Nerve fibre

- Is the name given to an axon of a nerve cell
- 2 types of fibre are present
  - i.   Myelinated
  - ii. Non-myelinated
- Divided into A, B, and C fibres (*Box 4.21*)
- Myelin sheath is formed by
  - i.   Oligodendrocytes in the CNS
  - ii. Schwann cells in the PNS
- Architecture
  - i.   Axons are organized into bundles called fascicles
  - ii. Nerves consist of grouped fascicles
- Covering
  - i.   Endoneurium – covers individual groups of axons
  - ii. Perineurium – covers groups of fascicles
  - iii. Epineurium – covers the nerve

Box 4.21 Nerve fibres

A fibre	B fibre	C fibre
• Largest diameter fibre • Has shortest absolute refractory period • Myelinated • Conductance speed = 12–130 m/s • Associated with touch, pressure, joint position, and temperature • Motor innervation to skeletal muscles	• Myelinated • Conductance speed = 15 m/s • Found in ANS	• Has smallest diameter • Unmyelinated • Has longest absolute refractory period • Conductance speed = 2 m/s • Associated with pain • Visceral motor fibres to heart and smooth muscles

7. **Axonal degradation pathway** (*Fig. 4.16*)

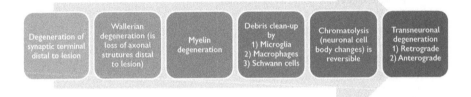

Figure 4.16 Axonal degradation pathway

Action potential

1. **Plasma membranes**
   - Exhibit membrane potential
     i. Membrane potential is an electrical voltage difference across the membrane
     ii. Resting membrane potential is – 70 mV (the minus sign indicates that the inside of the cell is negative in relation to the outside)
   - Is a good electric insulator (impermeable to ions)
   - Has 2 structures to transfer ions
     i. Ion pump
     ii. Ion channel

2. **Ion channels**
   - There are 2 types
     i. Leak (age) channels (always open)
     ii. Gated channels
   - Gated channels depend on 4 stimuli
     i. Voltage
     ii. Chemicals

iii. Mechanical pressure

iv. Light

3. **Resting membrane potential**
   - Arises due to
     - i. Unequal distribution of ions across plasma membrane
     - ii. Permeability of plasma membrane to K^+ is higher than to Na^+
   - Is calculated by the Goldman equation

4. **Potential**
   - There are 2 types
     - i. Graded potential (due to the presence of chemical, mechanical, or light-gated ion channels)
     - ii. Action potential
   - It can cause the plasma membrane to be
     - i. Hyperpolarized = membrane potential more negative
     - ii. Depolarized = membrane potential less negative

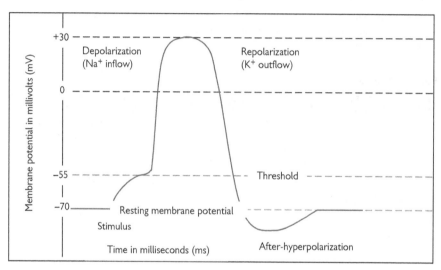

Figure 4.17 Action potential

5. **Action potential (*Fig. 4.17*)**
   - Is generated on an all-or-none principle
   - Consists of
     - i. Depolarization
     - ii. Repolarization
   - Lasts 1 ms
   - Involves 2 types of voltage-gated ion channel (Na^+ and K^+ channels)
   - Depolarization is due to rapid opening of voltage-gated Na^+ channels
   - Repolarization is due to
     - i. Slow opening of voltage-gated K^+ channels
     - ii. Closure of voltage-gated Na^+ channels
   - After-hyperpolarization
     - i. Is hyperpolarization that occurs after the repolarization phase of an action potential
     - ii. Due to open voltage-gated K^+ channels

6. **Refractory periods**
   - Is the time in which an excitable cell cannot generate another action potential
   - There are 2 types
     i.   Absolute – refers to the time period during which a second action potential cannot be created irrespective of stimulus
     ii. Relative – refers to time during which a second action potential can be created only by a large stimulus

7. **Propagation of action potentials**
   - Types of impulse conduction
     i.   Non-myelinated = continuous propagation
     ii. Myelinated = saltatory conduction (jumps from one node of Ranvier to another)
   - Speed of propagation depends on
     i.   Fibre size (large fibres conduct at faster speeds)
     ii. Presence of myelin

Neurotransmitters

Chpt 5

1. **Neurotransmitters**
   - Are stored in vesicles in the presynaptic terminals
   - Include (**Box 4.22**)

Box 4.22 Neurotransmitters

Acetylcholine	Amino acids	Catecholamines	Neuropeptides
	• Excitatory (glutamate and aspartate) • Inhibitory (GABA and glycine)	• Noradrenaline • Adrenaline • Dopamine • Serotonin	• Endorphins • Enkephalins • Substance P • CCK • Gastrin

Gases
• Nitric oxide • Carbon monoxide

2. **Transmission at synapses**
   - Release of neurotransmitters is as follows (**Fig. 4.18**)

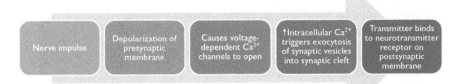

Figure 4.18 Neurotransmitter release pathway

- Removal of neurotransmitter from synaptic cleft is via
  - i.   Diffusion
  - ii. Enzymatic degradation
  - iii. Reuptake into cells

3. **Impulse conduction and synaptic transmission is altered by**
   - pH
     - i.   Alkalosis – increases excitability of neurones
     - ii. Acidosis – results in depression of neuronal activity
   - Neurotransmitter agonists/antagonists
   - Receptor site antagonists (e.g. curare)
   - Anticholinesterase agents
     - i.   Neostigmine
     - ii. Physostigmine

Brain

1. **Brain**
   - Cerebral blood flow is
     - i.   50 mL per 100 g of brain tissue
     - ii. 15% of cardiac output
     - iii. 750 mL/min
   - Comprises 2% of body weight
   - Consumes 20% of oxygen at rest
   - Fuels
     - i.   Glucose
     - ii. Liver glycogen – only after conversion to glucose via glycogenolysis
     - iii. Muscle protein – only after gluconeogenesis
     - iv. Ketone bodies
   - **Cannot** use fatty acids
   - Has an absolute requirement for glucose
     - i.   During normal food intake uses 100 g/day
     - ii. During starvation needs 25 g/day
   - Does not have receptors for insulin
   - For adequate cerebral perfusion MAP must be >70 mmHg

Reflexes

1. **Reflexes**
   - Are involuntary (autonomic) response(s) to (a) stimuli(us)
   - 2 types
     - i.   Somatic
     - ii. Autonomic

2. **Reflex arc**
   - Is a neural pathway that mediates a reflex action
   - Includes 5 functional components (**Fig. 4.19**)

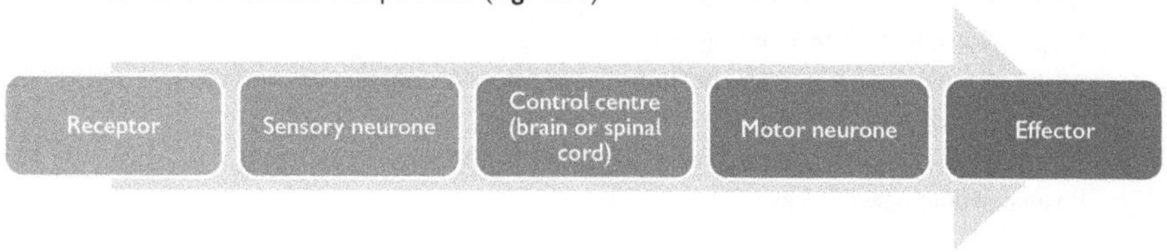

Receptor → Sensory neurone → Control centre (brain or spinal cord) → Motor neurone → Effector

Figure 4.19 Reflex arc

3. **2 types of reflex arc**
   - Monosynaptic (always ipsilateral) include
     - i.   Stretch reflex
     - ii. Tendon reflex
   - Polysynaptic
     - i.   Flexor reflex
     - ii. Crossed extensor reflex

4. **Reflex receptors**
   - Stretch reflex receptor = muscle spindles
     - i.   Causes muscle contraction
     - ii. Muscle spindle monitors change in muscle length
   - Tendon reflex receptor = Golgi tendon organ
     - i.   Causes muscle relaxation
     - ii. Golgi organ monitors change in muscle tension

Autonomic nervous system

Chpt 5

1. **General characteristics**
   - All preganglionic fibres are cholinergic
   - Postganglionic fibres
     - i.   Parasympathetic = cholinergic
     - ii. Sympathetic = adrenergic except for the sweat glands, which are cholinergic
     - iii. Absent in adrenal gland because the chromaffin cells of the adrenal medulla are in a developmental sense postganglionic cells

2. **Sympathetic system is composed of**
   - Preganglionic nerve fibres arising from vertebral levels T1 to L2
   - Sympathetic ganglia
     - i.   Paravertebral (also known as sympathetic trunk)
     - ii. Prevertebral
   - Postganglionic nerve fibres

3. **Sympathetic trunk**
   - Is a paired structure lying on either side of the spinal cord
   - Each chain has 22 ganglia
     - i.   Cervical – 3
     - ii.   Thoracic – 11
     - iii. Lumbar – 4
     - iv.   Sacral – 4

4. **Sympathetic prevertebral ganglion consists of**
   - Coeliac ganglion
   - Superior mesenteric ganglion
   - Inferior mesenteric ganglion

5. **Parasympathetic system consists of**
   - Preganglionic nerve fibres arising from
     - i.   Cranial nerves – 4 in total (oculomotor, facial, glossopharyngeal, and vagus)
     - ii. Vertebral levels S2–S4
   - Parasympathetic ganglia (contained within the wall of the visceral organs)
   - Postganglionic nerve fibres

Lymphatic system

1. The lymphatic system is composed of
- Lymphatic capillaries
- Lymphatic vessels
- Lymphatic tissues
- Lymphatic ducts (thoracic duct and right lymphatic duct)

2. Flow of lymph is
- Always towards the heart
- Directed to at least one lymph node before reaching a lymphatic duct
- Maintained by
  i. Valves
  ii. Pressure
     - Muscular contraction
     - Pulsating artery
  iii. Suction – negative pressure created by the contracting heart

3. The composition of lymph is comparable with that of plasma

4. Lymphatic tissue is found in
- Lymphatic nodes
- Spleen
- Thymus

5. Lymph nodes
- Have several afferent vessels
- Have only one efferent vessel
- Contains
  i. Lymphocytes
  ii. Macrophages

6. Lymphatic functions
- Immune system
- Collect excessive fluid
- Transport of fat-soluble (digested) food (fatty acids)

Skin

1. The skin is composed of 2 layers
- Epidermis
- Dermis

2. Epidermis
- Composed of stratified squamous epithelium
- Consists of 4 cell types
  i. Keratinocytes – formation cycle last 3–4 weeks
  ii. Melanocytes
  iii. Langerhans cells
     - Produced by bone marrow
     - Are a type of immune cell
  iv. Merkel cells – involved in sensation of touch
- Consists of 4 layers (*Fig. 4.20*)

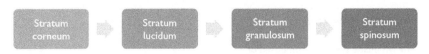

Figure 4.20 Layers of the epidermis from superficial to deep

3. **Dermis**
   - Contains
      i.   Hair follicles
      ii. Blood vessels
      iii. Glands
      iv. Nerves
   - Papillae in the dermis give rise to surface ridges such as fingerprints

4. **Skin gets its colour from 3 pigments**
   - Melanin
   - Carotene
   - Haemoglobin

5. **The skin contains 2 types of glands**
   - Sebaceous (associated with hair follicles)
   - Sweat

6. **Sweat glands are of 2 types (*Box 4.23*)**

Box 4.23 Types of sweat glands

Eccrine (also known as merocrine)	Apocrine
• Produce watery secretions • Present all over body	• Produce viscous secretions • Associated with sexual excitement • Present in axilla; pubic area; areola

T. in
Obs
Gyn

Chpt 8.23

7. **Changes in pregnancy (*Fig. 4.21*).**

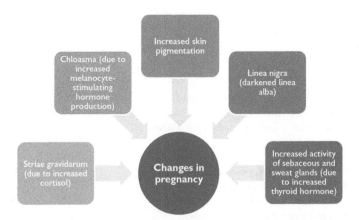

Figure 4.21 Skin changes in pregnancy

Special senses

1. **Sight**
   - The eye is composed of 3 layers
     i. Sclera
     ii. Choroids
     iii. Retina
   - Retina has 2 types of cells
     i. Rods – mainly located at the peripheries
     ii. Cones
        - Sensitive to bright light and colour
        - Make up the macula densa

2. **Hearing**
   - The ear is enclosed in the temporal bone
   - Divided in to 3 parts
     i. Outer ear
     ii. Middle ear
     iii. Inner ear
   - Middle ear consists of
     i. Tympanic cavity
     ii. Eustachian tube
   - Tympanic cavity contain 3 bones
     i. Malleus
     ii. Incus
     iii. Stapes
   - Inner ear has 2 openings to the middle ear
     i. Oval window
     ii. Round window
   - Stapes attaches to the oval window
   - Inner ear consist of
     i. Labyrinth
        - Bony
        - Membranous
     ii. Semicircular canals
   - Labyrinth is filled with
     i. Perilymph – contained between bony and membranous labyrinth
     ii. Endolymph – contained within the membranous labyrinth

3. **Taste**
   - The tongue is divided into 3 zones
     i. Front
        - Sweet
        - Salt
     ii. Lateral – Sour
     iii. Rear – Bitter
   - Innervation supplied by 3 nerves
     i. Facial
     ii. Vagus
     iii. Glossopharyngeal

4. **Olfaction**
   - Smell is detected by olfactory sensory neurones in the roof of the nasal cavity, known as the olfactory epithelium

- Olfactory sensitivity is dependent on the proportion of olfactory epithelium to respiratory epithelium in the nasal cavity
  i.   Humans have about $10\,cm^2$ of olfactory epithelium
  ii. Dogs have $170\,cm^2$ of olfactory epithelium
- Journey of an odour molecule (*Fig. 4.22*)

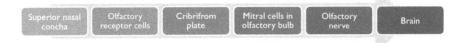

Figure 4.22 Journey of an odour molecule via the nasal passage

5. Touch
- Has 2 main components
  i.   Touch
  ii. Pressure
- There are 4 main mechanoreceptors in humans
  i.   Meissner's corpuscles
  ii. Pacinian corpuscles
  iii. Merkel's disc (detects pressure and sustained touch)
  iv. Ruffini corpuscles (sensitive to skin stretch)
- Meissner's corpuscles
  i.   Are encapsulated unmyelinated nerve endings
  ii. Sensitive to light touch
  iii. Do not detect pain (pain is exclusively detected by free nerve endings)
  iv. Situated in the papillae of skin
  v.   Also found in genital area
- Pacinian corpuscles
  i.   Are sensitive to pressure and vibrations
  ii. Situated deep in the skin

6. Pain
- Is defined as an unpleasant sensory or emotional experience associated with actual or potential tissue damage
- Can be classified into 2 groups
  i.   Somatogenic
  ii. Psychogenic
- Somatogenic pain can be further divided into
  i.   Nociceptive
  ii. Neuropathic
- Nociceptive pain
  i.   Can be divided into superficial and deep pains
  ii. Superficial nociceptive pain is localized pain arising from skin or superficial tissues
  iii. Deep pain can be divided into deep somatic and visceral pain
- Deep somatic pain is
  i.   Poorly localized
  ii. Dull and aching in nature
  iii. Initiated by stimulation of nociceptors in ligaments, tendons, muscles, bones, fasciae, and blood vessels

7. Changes in pregnancy (*Fig. 4.23*)

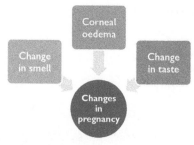

Figure 4.23 Special senses changes in pregnancy

Fetal and placental tissues

Amniotic fluid

1. **Amniotic fluid volumes**
   - 10 weeks = 30 mL
   - 12 weeks = 50 mL
   - 16 weeks = 190 mL
   - 35 weeks = 900 mL
   - >35 weeks volume decreases

2. **Amniotic fluid measurements**
   - Osmolality = 275 mOsm/L
   - Fluid exchange = 500 mL/day
   - Gases
     - i.   pH = 7 (acidic)
     - ii. pO_2 = 2–15 mmHg
     - iii. pCO_2 = 50–60 mmHg

3. **Formation and clearance of amniotic fluid depends on (Box 4.24)**

Box 4.24 Amniotic fluid formation and clearance

In the 1st trimester	In the 2nd trimester
• Placenta	• Fetal swallowing
• Transport across fetal skin (fetal skin keratinises at 22–25 weeks gestation)	• Fetal urine
	• Fetal lung secretions (200–400 mL/day)
	• Placenta (intramembranous pathway)

4. **Fetal urine**
   - Urine first enters amniotic space at 8–11 weeks gestation
   - Urine production at
     - i. 25 weeks = 110 mL/kg/day
     - ii. Term = 700–900 mL/day
   - Full development of renal system does not occur until several months post delivery

5. **Fetal swallowing**
   - Starts at 12 weeks
   - 250 mL/day

6. **Amniotic fluid composition** (*Fig. 4.24*)
   - α-fetoprotein
     i. Less than in fetal blood
     ii. Peaks at 10–12 weeks
   - There is no fibrinogen
   - Bilirubin, which decreases in 3rd trimester

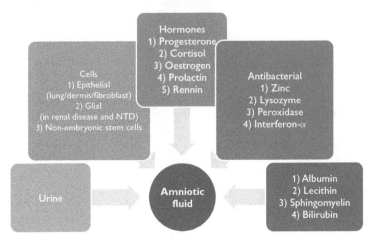

Figure 4.24 Composition of amniotic fluid

Fetal membranes

1. **The membranes consist of 2 layers**
   - Amnion
   - Chorion

2. **Amnion**
   - Amniotic cavity is formed by day 7
   - Has 5 layers
     i. Cuboidal epithelium
     ii. Basement membrane
     iii. Compact layer
     iv. Fibroblast layer
     v. Spongy layer (remnant of extra-embryonic coelom)
   - Does not contain blood vessels, lymphatics, or nerves

3. **Chorion has 4 layers**
   - Cellular layer
   - Basement membrane
   - Reticular layer
   - Trophoblast

Fetal lungs

1. **Fetal respiration**
   - Measurements
     i. First breath = 10–60 mL
     ii. Tidal volume = 6 mL/kg
     iii. Functional residual capacity = 30 mL/kg
   - Fetal lung development has 4 phases (*Box 4.25*)

Box 4.25 Phases of fetal lung development

Pseudoglandular period	Canalicular period	Terminal sac period	Alveolar period
• 5–17 weeks gestation	• 16–25 weeks gestation • Primitive alveoli • Low diffusing capacity at 24 weeks (due to huge separation from respiratory tissue and capillaries)	• 24 weeks to birth • Potential for gaseous exchange improves • Surfactant synthesis by type 2 pneumocytes	• Late fetal life to 8 years of age • Final alveolar growth • Alveolar-like structures present at 32 weeks gestation • At 34 weeks 15% of adult number of alveoli are present

2. **Surfactant**
   - Increases lung compliance
   - Predominant phospholipid is dipalmitoyl phosphatidylcholine (DPPC)
   - Produced by type 2 pneumocytes
   - Triggers to surfactant biosynthesis
     i.   Increase in cortisol at 32 weeks gestation
     ii. Thyroid hormone
     iii. Thyrotropin-releasing hormone
     iv. Prolactin

3. **First breath following delivery**
   - For lung inflation to occur
     i. First inspiratory effort requires a transpulmonary pressure of $60\,cmH_2O$
     ii. Second inspiratory effort requires transpulmonary pressure of $40\,cmH_2O$
   - Triggered by hypercapnia and hypoxia resulting from partial occlusion of umbilical cord
   - Is promoted by
     i. Tactile stimulation
     ii. Decreased skin temperature

4. **Respiratory distress syndrome (RDS)**
   - Affects 10–15% premature babies
   - Aetiology = surfactant deficiency
   - Risk factors
     i.   Male sex
     ii. Caesarean section
     iii. Perinatal asphyxia
     iv. Maternal diabetes
     v.   2nd twin in a twin pregnancy

5. **Lung maturity is confirmed by amniotic fluid levels of**
   - Lecithin : sphingomyelin ratio of 2 : 1
   - Lecithin = $10\,mg/100mL$

Fetal circulation

1. **Fetal circulation**
   - Only 10% of the CO enters the lungs
   - Pathway
     i.   Umbilical vein to right atrium (**Fig. 4.25**)
     ii. Right atrium to aorta can follow 2 pathways (**Figs 4.26 and 4.27**)
     iii. Aorta to umbilical artery

- Therefore, 4 shunts are present in the fetal maternal circulation
  i.   Placenta – the entire placenta acts as a shunt to the maternal circulation as it is an 'external' unit not present in the non-pregnant woman
  ii. Ductus venosus
  iii. Foramen ovale
  iv. Ductus arteriosus
- Ductus arteriosus patency is mediated by prostaglandins

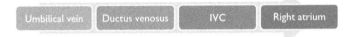

Figure 4.25 Fetal circulation – umbilical vein to right atrium

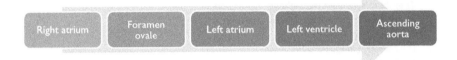

Figure 4.26 Fetal circulation – right atrium to ascending aorta

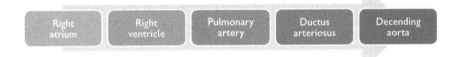

Figure 4.27 Fetal circulation – right atrium to descending aorta

2. **Cardiopulmonary adjustments at birth**
   - Vasoconstriction of umbilical arteries
   - Autotransfusion: blood from the fetal side of the placental system enters baby because umbilical veins (which return blood from the placenta to the baby) do no constrict – contributes 75–100 mL
   - Opening of pulmonary circulation due to decreased pulmonary vascular resistance by
     i. Expansion of lungs at birth
     ii. Pulmonary vasodilation
   - Closure of ductus venosus within 3 hours of birth
   - Closure of foramen ovale due to
     i.   Increased left atrial pressure
     ii. Decreased right atrial pressure
     iii. Both of these changes in atrial pressure is due to decreased pulmonary vascular resistance
   - Closure of ductus arteriosus

3. **Ductus arteriosus**
   - Functional closure
     i. Occurs within a few hours of birth
     ii. Functional closure is due to rapid rise in pO_2 at birth causing smooth muscle contraction and fall in prostaglandin levels
   - Permanent closure occurs at 1 week of infant life

4. **Hypoxia has 3 effects on the newborn**
   - Pulmonary vascular resistance remains high
   - Ductus arteriosus remains patent
   - The patent ductus arteriosus maintains a right-to-left shunt

5. **Fetal erythropoiesis**
   - Begins at 3 weeks gestation
   - At 3 weeks gestation it occurs in
     i. Placenta
     ii. Yolk sac
   - At 4 weeks gestation it occurs in
     i. Endothelium of blood vessels
     ii. Liver
   - At end of 1st trimester it occurs in
     i. Bone marrow
     ii. Spleen

6. **Fetal erythrocytes**
   - Early fetal erythrocytes are nucleated
   - Reticulocyte count at term is 5% (in adults this is 1%)
   - Life span
     i. Depends on fetal gestation
     ii. At term = 80 days

Placenta

1. **Structure**
   - It is a discoid organ
   - Weighs approximately 600 g at term
   - Diameter = 25 cm
   - Thickness = 3 cm
   - Surface area is
     i. $5 \, m^2$ at 28 weeks of fetal life
     ii. $14 \, m^2$ at term
   - Blood flow = 1.5 L/min
   - Consumes 1/3 of O_2 supplied

2. **Extravillous trophoblast invasion and conversion of spiral arterioles**
   - Trophoblasts differentiate from day 12
   - Wave 1 occurs between 8 and 10 weeks gestation
     i. Interstitial cells migrate to inner 1/3 of myometrium and form giant cells
     ii. Endovascular migration down spiral arteries
   - Wave 2 occurs between 16 and 18 weeks gestation
   - Leads to
     i.   Loss of smooth muscle of spiral arterioles
     ii. Dilatation
     iii. Loss of vasoreactivity

iv. Low-pressure vessels

v. High-capacity vessels

3. **Villi**
    - Consists of
      i. Syncytiotrophoblast
      ii. Cytotrophoblast (is uninucleated)
      iii. Mesenchyme
    - Types
      i. Stem
      ii. Intermediate
      iii. Terminal (which is the functional unit)

4. **Syncytiotrophoblast**
    - Has no mitotic activity
    - Multinucleated
    - Involved in hormonal synthesis

5. **Mature placenta**
    - Villi are arranged as lobules
    - There are 40–60 lobules (cotyledons)
    - Each lobule receives a spiral artery

6. **Placental blood circulation**
    - Pressures at the fetal maternal interface
      i. Umbilical artery – 50 mmHg
      ii. Umbilical vein – 20 mmHg
      iii. Maternal spiral artery – 70 mmHg
      iv. Intervillous space – 10 mmHg
    - Placental barrier is composed of (outermost to innermost part)
      i. Syncytiotrophoblast (the only layer that comes into contact with maternal blood)
      ii. Cytotrophoblast
      iii. Extra-embryonic mesoblast – contains Hofbauer cells (these are macrophages that are involved in restructuring of the stroma, in order to ensure plasticity during the development of the villi)
      iv. Fetal capillaries

7. **Functions**
    - Maternal–fetal transport (*Box 4.26*)
    - Hormone synthesis
      i. human chorionic gonadotrophin (hCG)
      ii. human placental lactogen (hPL)
      iii. Placental growth hormone (secreted between 10 and 20 weeks)
      iv. Progesterone
    - Barrier to pathogens
    - Immunological interface

Box 4.26 Materno-fetal transport

Passive diffusion	Facilitated	Active	Receptor mediated endocytosis
• Urea • Free fatty acids • Respiratory gases	• Glucose	• Amino acid	• IgG (occurs from 35 weeks)

8. **Placenta cannot synthesize oestrogen de novo**
   - Works with fetal adrenals to synthesize dehydroepiandrosterone (DHEA)
   - Fetal liver : DHEA → oestriol (utilized as a measure of fetal well being)
   - Placenta : DHEA → oestradiol and oestrone

Miscellaneous fetal facts

1. **The length of a twin pregnancy is 3 weeks shorter than in a singleton pregnancy**

2. **Fetal adrenal glands**
   - Have a fetal zone (occupying 80–90% of the volume of the cortex), which disappears soon after birth
   - Are involved in the maturation (via cortisol production) of the lungs, liver, thyroid, and GIT
   - Are involved in the development of
     - i.   Hypothalamic function
     - ii. Pituitary–thyroid axis
     - iii. Hepatic enzymes
   - Are involved in the sequential change of placental structure
   - Promote thymic involution
   - In some mammals are involved in the initiation of parturition, however, the contribution in humans is unclear

3. **Fetal movements are first felt (quickening) in**
   - Primips at 18 weeks
   - Multips at 16 weeks

4. **Meconium**
   - Is a thick greenish-black substance
   - Formed during intrauterine life
   - Consists of
     - i.   Amniotic fluid
     - ii. Mucus
     - iii. Desquamated gastrointestinal mucosa cells (approximately 60% of meconium mass)
     - iv. Fatty acids
     - v.   Bile salts
   - Usually passed from GIT within 48 hours of delivery
   - In ≈ 12% of births, meconium is present intrapartum due to
     - i.   Post-dates
     - ii. Fetal distress which possibly causes fetal intestinal contraction and anal sphincter relaxation (although this is widely believed, it has never been proven)
   - Meconium in the lungs (meconium aspiration syndrome) occurs in 0.5–2 per 1000 live births and causes
     - i.   Mechanical lung obstruction
     - ii. Displacement of surfactant
     - iii. Pneumonitis (chemical inflammation)
     - iv. Decreased efficiency of gaseous exchange
   - Complications of meconium aspiration syndrome include
     - i.   Pneumothorax
     - ii. Persistent pulmonary hypertension of the newborn

5. **Neonatal skin**
   - 2 structures protect the neonatal skin during intrauterine life (**Box 4.27**)
   - Is sterile *in utero*

- Milia
  - i. Are enlarged sebaceous glands
  - ii. Seen on nose and cheek

Box 4.27 Protective neonatal skin structures

Vernix caseosa	Lanugo
• Is a fatty film that develops over the skin	• Fine covering of hairs
• Develops from week 20 of intrauterine life	• Develops from week 20 of intrauterine life
	• It is shed at week 36 of intrauterine life

6. **Fetal weight** (*Table 4.5*)
   - Average fetal weight gain
     - i. Before 28 weeks = 100 g/week
     - ii. After 28 weeks = 200 g/week

Table 4.5

Gestational age (weeks)	Approximate fetal weight if on the 50th centile (g)
16	150
18	225
20	330
22	480
24	670
26	915
28	1200
30	1550
32	1950
34	2380
36	2810
38	3240
40	3620

Physiological changes in pregnancy – quick glance

Chpts 6.1 & 6.2

1. **Cardiovascular** (*Fig. 4.28*)
   - Increased plasma volume by 40–50%
     - i. 2600 mL to 3800 mL
     - ii. No further increase after 32 weeks
   - Increased red cell mass by 18%
     - i. 1400 mL to 1650 mL
   - Increased CO by 40%
     - i. 4.5 L/min to 6 L/min
     - ii. Plateau at 24–30 weeks

- Increased HR by 20%
- Increased stroke volume by 30%
- Increased O_2 consumption by 20%
    i. Extra 30–50 mL/min
- Decreased arteriovenous O_2 gradient
- Decreased peripheral vascular resistance by 5%
    i.   Systolic BP decreases by 5 mmHg
    ii. Diastolic BP decreases by 10 mmHg
    iii. Large pulse pressure

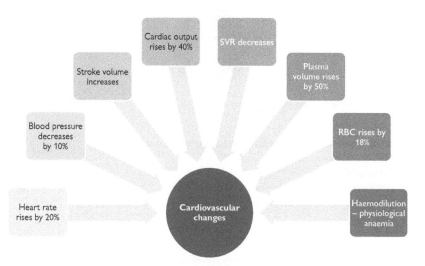

Figure 4.28 Cardiovascular changes in pregnancy

2. **Pulmonary (*Fig. 4.29*)**
    - Oxygen demand increases by 20%
    - Decreased airway resistance
    - Increased TV
    - VC = same
    - RR = same
    - FEV_1 = same
    - PEFR = same
    - Lung compliance = same
    - Decreased chest compliance
    - Decreased RV by 200 mL
    - Decreased ERV
    - Decreased total lung volume by 200 mL
    - Increased IRV
    - Decreased pCO_2 to 30 mmHg
    - Increased pO_2 to 14 kPa
    - Breathing becomes more diaphragmatic than thoracic

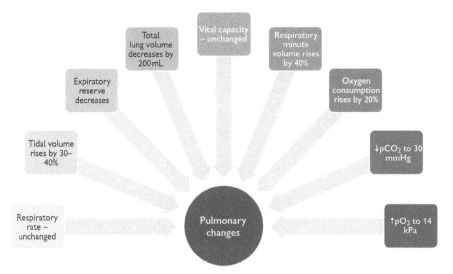

Figure 4.29 Pulmonary changes in pregnancy

3. **Distribution of increased maternal O_2 consumption in pregnancy**
   - Fetus = 20 mL/min
   - Increased CO = 6 mL/min
   - Increased renal work = 6 mL/min
   - Increased maternal metabolic rate = 18 mL/min

4. **Gastrointestinal (*Fig. 4.30*)**

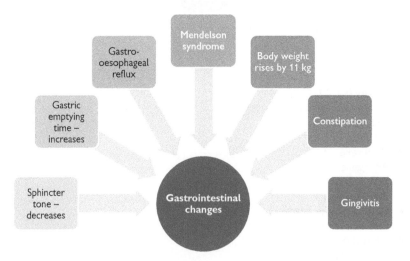

Figure 4.30 Gastrointestinal changes in pregnancy

5. **Liver (*Fig. 4.31*)**

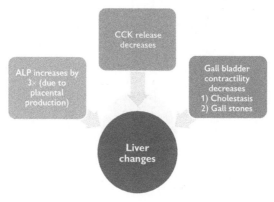

Figure 4.31 Liver changes in pregnancy

6. **Renal (*Fig. 4.32*)**
   - Increased kidney size by 1 cm
     i. Renal hypertrophy
     ii. No hyperplasia
   - Ureteric dilatation (due to progesterone and obstruction)
   - Increased renal blood flow (from 1.2 to 1.5 L/min)
   - Increased GFR (from 140 to 170 mL/min)
   - Decreased filtration fraction (GFR/RPF)
   - Decreased plasma urea (from 4.3 to 3.1 mmol/L)
   - Decreased plasma creatinine (from 73 to 47 μmol/L)

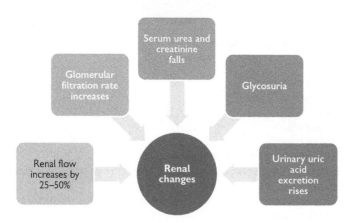

Figure 4.32 Renal changes in pregnancy

7. **Uterus (*Fig. 4.33*)**

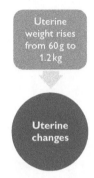

Figure 4.33 Uterine changes in pregnancy

8. **Metabolic and drug metabolism (*Fig. 4.34*)**

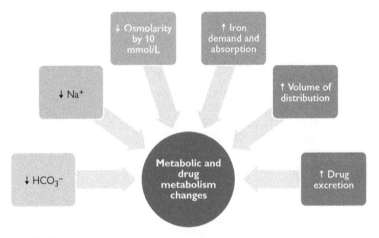

Figure 4.34 Metabolic changes in pregnancy

9. **Haematological changes**
   - Increased erythropoiesis
     i.   Increased EPO
     ii. Increased hPL
   - Physiological anaemia
   - Increased white blood cell (WBC) count
   - Gestational thrombocytopenia (due to haemodilution although increased platelet production)
   - Hypercoagulant state due to increased coagulant factors (all except for factor XI and XIII)
   - Increased fibrinogen
   - Increased erythrocyte sedimentation rate (ESR)
   - Fibrinolytic system
     i.   Increased anti-thrombin 3
     ii. Increased fibrin-degradation products (FDPs)
     iii. Activity remains low in labour
     iv. Returns to normal 1 hour after delivery of placenta
     v.   Placenta secretes plasminogen activator inhibitor (PAI-2), which inhibits fibrinolytic system

Biochemistry

CONTENTS

Cell

Cell structure

1. **The cell is the functional basic unit of all living organisms**

2. **Humans have ≈ 10^{14} cells**

3. **There are 2 types of cell (*Box 5.1*)**
   - Prokaryotic
   - Eukaryotic

Box 5.1 Types of cells

Prokaryotic cells	Eukaryotic cells
• Are mainly bacteria	• Are mainly protista, fungi, plants, and animals
• Size = 1–10 μm	• Size = 10–100 μm
• Do not contain membrane-bound organelles	• Contain membrane-bound organelles
• Lack nucleus	• Have a nucleus
• Nuclear material lies in the cytoplasm	• Chromosome is usually a linear molecule with histone proteins
• Chromosome is usually a circular molecule	• Cell wall may or may not be present
• Can carry plasmids	• Usually contain mitochondria
• Most have cell wall (except for mycoplasma and thermoplasma)	• Cell division occurs via mitosis or meiosis
• Lack mitochondria	
• Cell division occurs via binary fission	

4. **All eukaryotic cells have**
   - Plasma membrane
     i. Made of a phospholipid bilayer
     ii. It is semi-permeable
     iii. Contains receptor proteins

- Cytoplasm
  - i.   Provides cellular shape and integrity
  - ii. Contains cytoskeletons (i.e. responsible for cytokinesis and endocytosis)
  - iii. Contains organelles
- Nucleus
  - i.   Is spherical
  - ii. Is the largest cellular organelle
  - iii. Surrounded by a nuclear envelope (i.e. a double membrane)
  - iv. Contains the nucleolus (that synthesizes ribosomal RNA)
  - v.   Contains genetic material

5. **Organelles within an eukaryotic cell**
   - Endoplasmic reticulum (ER) – there are two types
     - i.   Smooth ER
     - ii. Rough ER (contains ribosomes on its surface)
   - Golgi apparatus
   - Mitochondria
     - i.   Are the power house of the cell
     - ii. Contain genetic material inherited maternally
     - iii. Are self-replicating organelles
   - Lysosomes and peroxisomes
     - i.   Are rich in digestive enzymes
     - ii. Lysosomes internal pH value is 4.8

Cell signalling

1. **Signal transduction**
   - Is the process by which an external stimulus to a cell is converted to a specific cellular response, which includes
     - i.   Activation of genes
     - ii. Metabolic alterations
     - iii. Proliferation of the cell
   - Can take milliseconds (for ion influx) to days (for gene expression)
   - Intracellular signal transduction is via second messengers

2. **Signalling molecules**
   - Can be classified in to 6 groups
     - i.   Hormones
     - ii. Growth factors
     - iii. Cytokines
     - iv. Chemokines
     - v.   Neurotransmitters
     - vi. Extracellular matrix components (e.g. fibronectin)
   - Act on cellular receptors, which can be divided into two classes
     - i.   Cell surface receptors
     - ii. Intracellular receptors

3. **There are 3 types of extracellular cell signalling**
   - Endocrine action (via bloodstream)
   - Paracrine action (acts locally on neighbouring cells)
   - Autocrine action (acts on cell producing the hormone)

Cell surface receptors

1. **There are 3 main classes of cell surface receptors**
    - Ion-channel-linked receptors – consist of 2 types
      i. Voltage gated
      ii. Ligand gated
    - Enzyme-linked receptors
      i. Consist of 6 types
      ii. Activate tyrosine protein kinase
      iii. Are receptors for growth factors
    - G protein-coupled receptors
      i. Also known as the 'seven transmembrane domain receptors' or serpentine receptors
      ii. Activate G proteins (guanine nucleotide-binding proteins)
      iii. Have 3 subunits (α, β, γ)
      iv. Found only in eukaryotes

2. **Examples of cell surface receptors (*Box 5.2*)**

Box 5.2

Ion-channel receptors	Enzyme linked receptors	G protein-coupled receptors
• Nicotinic acetylcholine receptors	• Tyrosine kinase receptors	• Rhodopsin-like receptors
• GABA receptors	• Tyrosine phosphatase receptors	• Secretin receptors
• 5-HT receptors	• Guanylyl cylase receptors	• Metabotropic glutamate receptors
• Glycine receptors	• Histidine kinase receptors	• cAMP receptors
• Voltage-gated Na^+ channel	• Serine receptors	
• Voltage-gated Ca^{2+} channel		
• Voltage-gated K^+ channel		

3. **Examples of G protein-coupled receptor subclasses (*Box 5.3*)**

Adrenergic receptors

1. **Adrenergic receptors (*Table 5.1*)**
    - Are members of the G protein-coupled receptor superfamily
    - Promote glycogenolysis and gluconeogenesis from adipose tissue and liver
    - There are 2 adrenergic receptor subgroups: α and β

2. **β-antagonists (*Box 5.4*)**

3. **β-blockers with intrinsic sympathomimetic activity (ISA)**
    - Have agonist and antagonist activity
    - Include
      i. Oxprenolol
      ii. Pindolol

4. **α-antagonists**
    - Used in
      i. Benign prostatic hypertrophy (BPH)
      ii. Hypertension
    - α_1-antagonists include
      i. Tamsulosin
      ii. Prazosin
      iii. Phentolamine
      iv. Doxazosin

Box 5.3

Rhodopsin-like receptor family	Secretin receptor family	Metabotropic glutamate receptor family
• Chemokine receptors • Angiotensin II receptors • Bradykinin receptors • Bradykinin receptors • Somatostatin receptors • Leukotriene receptors • Vasopressin receptors • Relaxin receptors • Thyrotropin-releasing hormone receptors • Growth hormone receptors • Anaphylatoxin receptors • Melatonin receptors • Glycoprotein hormone receptors (LH, FSH, and thyrotropin) • Eicosanoid receptors • Adrenergic receptors • Muscarinic acetylcholine receptors • Dopamine receptors • Histamine receptors	• Secretin receptors • Calcitonin receptors • PTH receptors • VIP receptors • Glucagon receptors • CRH receptors	• Glutamate receptors

Table 5.1 Adrenergic receptors

Adrenergic receptors		Mechanism	Function
α	α_1	Activation of phospholipase C (thus increasing IP_3 and diacylglycerol leading to increased intracellular calcium)	Smooth muscle contraction (ureter, urethral sphincter, uterus, vas deferens, erector pili muscle) Smooth muscle relaxation of GIT Vasoconstriction of arteries and veins Glycogenolysis Gluconeogenesis
	α_2	Inactivation of adenylate cyclase leading to decreased intracellular cAMP	
β	β_1	Activation of adenylate cyclase, leading to increased intracellular cAMP, which in turn activates protein kinase A	Positive chronotropic effect on heart Positive inotropic effect on heart Increased conduction at atrioventricular node (AVN) Stimulates renin release Lipolysis in adipose tissue
	β_2		Smooth muscle relaxation (bronchi, uterus, detrusor muscle, GIT) Contracts anal sphincter Vasodilatory action Anabolism in skeletal muscle Stimulates renin release Inhibit histamine release from mast cells Reduces intraocular pressure
	β_3		Lipolysis in adipose tissue Thermogenesis in skeletal muscle

Box 5.4 Examples of β-antagonists

Non-selective	Cardioselective β₁	Mixed α₁β₁
• Proponolol	• Atenolol	• Carvedilol
• Timolol	• Metoprolol	• Labetalol
• Sotalol	• Bisoprolol	

- α₂-antagonists include
  - i. Yohimbine
  - ii. Phentolamine

5. **α- and β-agonists (Box 5.5)**

Box 5.5 Examples of α and β agonists

α₁-agonist	α₂-agonist	β₁-agonist	β₂-agonist
• Phenylephrine	• Clonidine	• Noradenaline	• Salbutamol
• Noradrenaline		• Isoprenaline	• Isoprenaline
		• Dobutamine	• Salmeterol
			• Terbutaline
			• Ritodrine

Acetylcholine receptors

1. **Acetylcholine**
   - Is a neurotransmitter found in the
     - i. Brain
     - ii. ANS
   - Is the only neurotransmitter used at the neuromuscular junction
   - Receptors include
     - i. Nicotinic receptors
     - ii. Muscarinic receptors
   - Both preganglionic sympathetic and parasympathetic fibres are cholinergic
   - All postganglionic parasympathetic fibres are cholinergic
   - All postganglionic sympathetic fibres are adrenergic

2. **Nicotinic receptors**
   - Belong to the ionotropic receptor superfamily
   - Form ligand-gated ion channels in the plasma membrane on the postsynaptic side of the neuromuscular junction
   - Do not make use of secondary messengers
   - Consist of 2 subtypes
     - i. Muscle-type
     - ii. Neuronal-type
   - Stimulation causes excitatory postsynaptic potential in neurones

3. **Muscarinic receptors**
   - Are members of the G protein-coupled receptor superfamily
   - Consist of 5 subtypes (**Box 5.6**)
   - Mechanism of action
     - i. M2 and M4 – act by decreasing intracellular cAMP

Box 5.6 Subtypes of muscarinic receptors

M1	M2	M3	M4
• Exocrine glands • CNS	• Heart	• Blood vessels • Lungs • Salivary glands	• CNS

M5

Box 5.7 Examples of nicotinic and muscarinic agonists and antagonists

Nicotinic agonist	Nicotinic antagonist	Muscarinic agonist	Muscarinic antagonist
• Acetylcholine • Choline • Nicotine • Suxamethonium	• Pancuronium • Tubocurarine • Atracurium	• Acetylcholine • Muscarine • Pilocarpine	• Atropine • Scopolamine • Ipratropium • Tolterodine • Oxybutinin • Darifenacin (M3) • Tiotropium (M3)

     ii. M1, M3 and M5 – act by upregulating phospholipase C and therefore inositol triphosphate and intracellular calcium
- Functions
  - i. Increase exocrine and endocrine secretions (e.g. salivary glands and stomach)
  - ii. Decrease HR
  - iii. Reduce cardiac contractility
  - iv. Smooth muscle contraction (e.g. bronchoconstriction)
  - v. Vasodilation
  - vi. Eye accommodation and pupillary constriction

4. **Non-depolarizing blocking agents (act by blocking the binding of ACh to its receptor)**
   - Tubocurarine
   - Vecuronium
   - Pancuronium

5. **Depolarizing blocking agents (act by depolarizing the plasma membrane of the skeletal muscle fibre)**
   - Suxamethonium

Intracellular receptors

1. **Intracellular receptors include**
   - Cytoplasmic receptors
   - Nuclear receptors

2. **Receptors that are exclusively intracellular include**
   - Steroid hormone receptors
   - Thyroid hormone receptors

- Retinoic acid receptors
- Vitamin D$_3$ receptors

Intracellular second messengers

1. **There are 3 main groups**
   - Ca^{2+}
   - Lipophilic messengers (e.g. diacylglycerol, inositol triphosphate (IP$_3$), eicosanoids)
   - NO
   - cAMP
     i. Synthesized from ATP by adenylate cyclase
     ii. Activation of protein kinase A
   - cGMP
     i. Synthesized from GTP by guanylate cyclase
     ii. Activates protein kinase G
     iii. Relaxes smooth muscle
     iv. Degraded by phosphodiesterases (sildenafil inhibits phosphodiesterase activity)

2. **NO**
   - Is also known as endothelium-derived relaxing factor
   - Is biosynthesized from L-arginine
     i. L-arginine → NO + L-citrulline
     ii. Catalyst enzyme = nitric oxide synthase (NOS)
   - Effects include
     i. Vasodilatation
     ii. Modulation of hair cycle
     iii. Penile erection
   - 3 types of NOS
     i. Endothelial (eNOS)
     ii. Inflammatory (iNOS)
     iii. Brain
   - eNOS
     i. Calcium-calmodulin dependent
     ii. Half life = 10 s
     iii. Acts on vascular smooth muscles
     iv. Expressed by syncytiotrophoblasts
   - iNOS
     i. Secreted by bacterial cell wall and neutrophils following activation by tumour necrosis factor (TNF) or interferon γ
     ii. Calmodulin independent
   - Mechanism of action (**Fig. 5.1**)

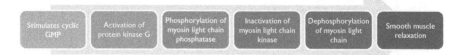

Figure 5.1 Mechanism of NO action

Carbohydrates

1. **General facts**
   - Consist of carbon, hydrogen, and oxygen only
   - Divided into
     - i.   Monosaccharides (e.g. glucose, fructose, galactose)
     - ii. Disaccharides (e.g. maltose, sucrose, lactose)
     - iii. Oligosaccharides (e.g. the ABO blood group classification)
     - iv. Polysaccharides (e.g. amylose, glycogen)
   - Carbohydrate **can** be converted to fat
   - Fat **cannot** be converted into glucose
   - ATP
     - i.   Stores energy
     - ii. Hydrolyses to release energy
   - Glucose
     - i.   Has a molecular formula of $C_6H_{12}O_6$
     - ii. Is the **only** substance that can undergo anaerobic metabolism
     - iii. Obligatory glucose requirement = 2 g/kg/day
     - iv. Physiological maximum amount of glucose that can be oxidized = 4 mg/kg/min
     - v.   Energy provided = 4.2 kcal/g
     - vi. Have a low Km value (Km is an indicator of the affinity of the transporter protein for glucose molecules; a low Km value suggest a high affinity)
   - The brain has an absolute requirement for glucose
     - i.   During normal food intake – needs 100 g/day
     - ii. During starvation – needs 25 g/day
   - Maltose is formed from 2 units of glucose
   - Lactose
     - i.   Is broken down to galactose and glucose by the enzyme lactase
     - ii. Deficiency of lactase produces lactose intolerance
   - Sucrose is broken down to glucose and fructose by the enzyme sucrase
   - Lactate is converted to glucose via the Cori cycle

2. **Glucose sources**
   - Glycogen
     - i.   Stored in muscle (cannot release glucose into circulation due to deficiency in glucose 6-phosphatase)
     - ii. Stored in liver
     - iii. Stores last 24 hours
   - Muscle protein conversion
   - Breakdown of other carbohydrates

3. **Glucose metabolism**
   - Anaerobic metabolism
     - i.   Follows the glycolytic pathway
     - ii. End-product is lactate (a 3-carbon atom)
     - iii. Produces 2 mol ATP per mol glucose
     - iv. Occurs in the cytosol
   - Aerobic metabolism
     - i.   Comprises of glycolysis, pyruvate oxidation, tricarboxylic acid cycle (TCA) pathway and oxidative phosphorylation
     - ii. Glucose is converted to pyruvate via glycolysis

iii. Pyruvate (a 3-carbon molecule) is converted to acetyl CoA (a 2-carbon molecule)
   - Enzyme = pyruvate dehydrogenase (which is membrane bound)
   - Irreversible reaction
iv. Acetyl-CoA enters TCA
v. TCA provides energy-rich molecules used in oxidative phosphorylation
vi. Yields 36–38 mol ATP per mol of glucose
vii. Occurs in the mitochondria

4. **Glycolysis pathway (*Fig. 5.2*)**
   - Converts glucose to pyruvate
   - Occurs in aerobic and anaerobic conditions
   - Undergoes double phosphorylation
   - Also known as Embden–Meyerhof pathway

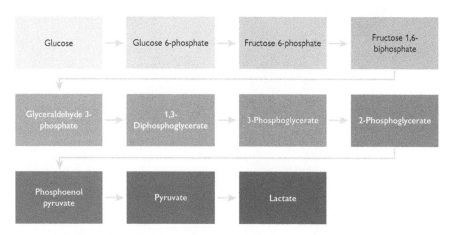

Figure 5.2 Glycolysis (Embden–Meyerhof) pathway

5. **TCA pathway**
   - Also known as
     i. Citric acid cycle
     ii. Kreb's cycle
   - Pathway (*Fig. 5.3*)
     i. Step 1: Acetyl CoA (2C) + oxaloacetate (4C) → citrate (6C); enzyme = citrate synthase
     ii. Step 2: Citrate (6C) → isocitrate (6C); enzyme = aconitase
     iii. Step 3: Isocitrate (6C) + NAD^+ → ketoglutarate (5C) + CO_2 + NADH + H^+; enzyme = isocitrate dehydrogenase
     iv. Step 4: Ketoglutarate (5C) + NAD^+ → succinyl CoA (4C) + CO_2 + NADH + H^+; enzyme = ketoglutarate dehydrogenase
     v. Step 5: Succinyl-CoA (4C) + GDP → succinate (4C) + GTP; enzyme = succinyl-CoA synthetase
     vi. Step 6: Succinate (4C) + FAD → fumarate (4C) + $FADH_2$; enzyme = succinate dehydrogenase
     vii. Step 7: Fumarate → malate; enzyme = fumarase
     viii. Step 8: Malate (4C) + NAD^+ → oxaloacetate (4C) + NADH + H^+; enzyme = malate dehydrogenase

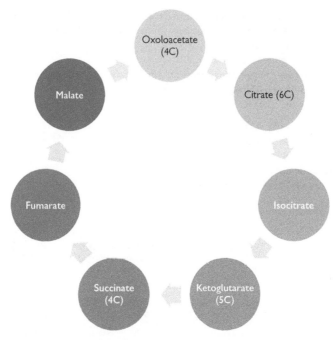

Figure 5.3 Kreb's cycle

6. **Tissues that can undergo ANAEROBIC metabolism**
   - RBC
     i.   Has no intracellular organelle
     ii. Entirely depends on glucose
     iii. **Cannot** use fat/ketones/amino acids
   - Retinal cells
   - Kidney medulla
   - Skeletal muscles

7. **Cori cycle**
   - Converts lactate (from anaerobic metabolism) back to glucose
   - Occurs in the liver
   - Importance
     i. Produces ATP
     ii. Prevents build up of lactic acid

8. **Blood glucose levels**
   - Normal = 4 mM
   - Postprandial = 8 mM
   - Pregnancy = 3.2 mM
   - Coma = <3 mM
   - Glycosuria >11 mM

9. **Features of gestational diabetes**
   - Loss of insulin sensitivity
   - Hyperglycaemia
   - Increased plasma fatty acids
   - Increased plasma ketone bodies

T. in
Obs
Gyn

Chpts 6.8
& 7.15

- Fetal macrosomia
- Increased risk of developing type 2 diabetes in later life

Fat

1. **General facts**
   - Energy provided = 9 kcal/g
   - Requirements = 200 g/week

2. **Triglycerides (TAGs, also known as triacylglycerol)**
   - Act as fuel store
   - Are dehydrated
   - Consist of
     i.   1 molecule of glycerol
     ii. 3 molecules of free fatty acid
   - Stored in adipocytes
   - Transported by chylomicrons

3. **Fatty acids**
   - Oxidation occurs in mitochondria
   - Undergo β oxidation
   - Metabolized to acetyl CoA
   - Essential fatty acids are
     i.   Linoleic acid
     ii. Linolenic acid
   - Unsaturated fatty acids
     i.   Linoleic acid (18 carbon atoms; double bond ×2)
     ii. Linolenic acid (18 carbon atoms; double bond ×3)
     iii. Arachidonic acid (20 carbon atoms; double bond ×4)

4. **Phospholipids**
   - Main component of cell membrane
   - 3 main groups
     i.   Lecithin
     ii. Sphingomyelin
     iii. Cephalins

5. **Ketone bodies**
   - Are by-products of fatty acid metabolism (fatty acid → acetyl CoA → ketone bodies)
   - Synthesized in the
     i.   Liver
     ii. Kidney
   - Consist of
     i.   β-hydroxybutyrate
     ii. Acetoacetic acid
     iii. Acetone (excreted in urine and lung)
   - Are fuel for intermediate or prolonged starvation
   - Ketone bodies (except for acetone) can be converted to acetyl CoA

6. **Limitations of fat**
   - Not metabolized by brain (except ketone bodies)
   - Not metabolized anaerobically
   - Cannot synthesize glucose

7. Adipose tissue
- There are 2 types
  - i. White adipose tissue
  - ii. Brown adipose tissue
- White adipose tissue stores energy
- Brown adipose tissue
  - i. Has large number of uncoupled mitochondria which do not produce ATP
  - ii. Produces heat

Proteins

1. Amino acids
- Molecules contain 2 functional groups
  - i. Amine
  - ii. Carboxyl
- Are both acid and base at the same time
- Zwitterions are neutral charged amino acid ions (i.e. at a certain isoelectric point the number of positive and negative charges are equal)
  - i. Positive charge is from protonated amine group
  - ii. Negative charge is from deprotonated carboxyl group
- Total number of amino acids in humans = 20
- Essential amino acids = 10
  - i. Lysine
  - ii. Leucine
  - iii. Isoleucine
  - iv. Valine
  - v. Methionine
  - vi. Phenylalanine
  - vii. Tryptophan
  - viii. Threonine
  - ix. Arginine*
  - x. Histidine*

  *Not strictly essential but depends on age and health status
- 7 subclasses (*Box 5.8*)

Box 5.8 Subclasses of amino acids

Acidic	Basic	Aromatic	Sulphydryl
• Glutamate • Aspartate	• Arginine • Histidine • Lysine	• Phenylalanine • Tryptophan • Tyrosine	• Methionine • Cysteine

Imino	Hydroxyl	Aliphatic
• Prolene	• Therionine • Serine	• Leucine • Isoleucine • Valine • Alanine • Glycine

- Amino acids as precursors
  i.   Tryptophan → serotonin
  ii. Glycine → porphyrins
  iii. Arginine → Nitric oxide
  iv. Tyrosine → L-DOPA → dopamine and noradrenaline

2. **Detoxification**
   - Begins before the urea cycle
     i.   Amino acid → glutamic acid → carbamyl phosphate
   - Urea cycle occurs in the liver
     i.   Liver mitochondria (*Fig. 5.4*)
     ii. Liver cytoplasm (*Fig. 5.5*)
   - Amino acid degradation can also produce uric acid and ammonia rather than urea

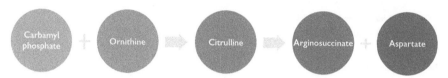

Figure 5.4 Urea cycle in liver mitochondria

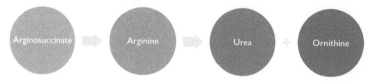

Figure 5.5 Urea cycle in liver cytoplasm

3. **Proteins**
   - Are made of polymerized amino acids
   - Peptide bonds link the amino acids in the polymer chain
   - Protein structure has 4 distinct aspects (*Box 5.9*)
   - Are divided into 3 classes
     i.   Globular proteins (are soluble and form enzymes)
     ii. Fibrous protein (often structural)
     iii. Membrane proteins (often serve as receptors)

Box 5.9 Protein structure

Primary structure	Secondary structure	Tertiary structure	Quaternary structure
• Is the amino acid sequence • Has peptide bonds	• 3-dimensional form of the primary structure • Held by hydrogen bonds	• Is the overall shape of a single protein molecule • Held by disulphide bonds • Controls the basic function of the protein	• Is the arrangement of multiple folded protein molecules

Chpt 1

Examples of proteins

1. **Haemoglobin**
   - Structure consist of
     i.   1 haem ring
     ii. 4 globin rings (i.e. 2 α and 2 β, γ, or δ subunits)
   - Gene location for subunits
     i.   α = chromosome 16 (short arm)
     ii. β = chromosome 11 (short arm)
   - Is synthesized in the mitochondria and cytosol of immature RBCs
   - Haem is metabolized to bilirubin and carbon monoxide by the liver
   - Haemoglobin is also found in non-erythroid cells
     i.   Dopaminergic neurones in substantia nigra
     ii. Macrophages
     iii. Alveolar cells
     iv. Kidney mesangial cells
   - Subtypes (*Box 5.10*)

Box 5.10 Haemoglobin subtypes

Embryo	Fetus	Adult	Variant
• Gower 1 ($\zeta_2\epsilon_2$) • Gower 2 ($\alpha_2\epsilon_2$) • Portland ($\zeta_2\gamma_2$)	• HbF ($\alpha_2\gamma_2$)	• HbA ($\alpha_2\beta_2$) • HbA$_2$ ($\alpha_2\delta_2$) • HbF ($\alpha_2\gamma_2$)	• HbS–sickle cell • HbC–variation in β chain • HbH (β_4) • Barts (γ_4) • HbE – variation in β chain

- HbA$_2$ makes up 3% of adult haemoglobin
- Fetal haemoglobin
  i.   Responsible for fetal oxygen transport from 12 weeks gestation
  ii. At birth makes up 50–95% of newborn's haemoglobin
  iii. Levels decline in newborn at 6 months of age

2. **Collagen**
   - Secreted by
     i.   Fibroblasts
     ii. Osteoblasts
   - Synthesized from pro-collagen
   - 4 subtypes
     i.   Type 1 (bone/dermis/tendon)
     ii. Type 2 (cartilage)
     iii. Type 3 (fetal/cardiac/scar/synovium)
     iv. Type 4 (basement membrane)
   - Type 1 collagen makes up 50% of total body protein

Hormones

1. **Hormones are divide into**
   - Endocrine
   - Exocrine

2. **Hormones fall into 3 chemical classes (*Box 5.11*)**

Box 5.11 Classes of hormones

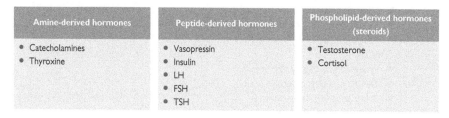

Amine-derived hormones	Peptide-derived hormones	Phospholipid-derived hormones (steroids)
• Catecholamines • Thyroxine	• Vasopressin • Insulin • LH • FSH • TSH	• Testosterone • Cortisol

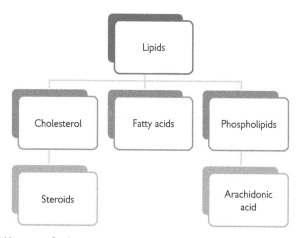

Figure 5.6 Lipid hormone family

Chpt 6

Steroids

1. **Cholesterol**
   - Ring-based structure
   - Contains 27 carbon atoms
   - Transported by lipoprotein
     i. LDL
     ii. HDL
   - Synthesized in the endoplasmic reticulum via HMG-CoA reductase pathway
   - Source
     i.   Acetyl-CoA
     ii. Plasma membrane cholesterol
     iii. Plasma lipoproteins
     iv. Intracellular lipid droplets (esterified cholesteryl oleate)

2. **General facts about steroids**
   - Have 4 rings
     i. 3 rings have 6 carbon atoms
     ii. 1 ring has 5 carbon atoms
   - Steroid receptors
     i. Are a subclass of nuclear receptors
     ii. Are associated with heat shock protein (HSP)

- Hydrophobic
- 5 groups
  i. Corticosteroids
      - Mineralocorticoids (aldosterone)
      - Glucocorticoids (cortisol)
      - Androgen (DHEA)
  ii. Gonadal
      - Progestogens (e.g. progesterone)
      - Oestrogens (e.g. oestradiol)
      - Androgens (e.g. testosterone)
- Act on nuclear receptors
- Increase gene transcription

3. **Steroid synthesis (*Fig. 5.7*)**
   - Cholesterol (C27) → progestin (C21) → androgen (C19) → oestrogen (C18)
   - Enzymes include
     i. Cytochrome P450 complex
     ii. Hydroxysteroid dehydrogenase (HSD)
   - Rate-limiting step is conversion of cholesterol to progestin, involving the enzyme cytochrome $P450_{CSCC}$ (cholesterol side chain cleavage)
   - Cytochrome $P450_{CSCC}$ resides in inner mitochondria
   - Cholesterol cannot transverse the aqueous space between the mitochondrial membranes unaided
     i. Intracellular membrane transport aided by STAR (steroidogenesis acute regulatory) protein and PBRs (peripheral benzodiazepine receptors)
   - STAR resides in
     i. Ovaries
     ii. Testes

4. **Cytochrome P450 complex**
   - Includes a variety of enzymes
     i. 17-hydroxylase
     ii. 21-hydroxylase
   - 17-hydroxylase catalyses the following reactions
     i.   Pregnenolone → 17α-hydroxy-pregnenolone
     ii. 17α-hydroxy-pregnenolone → DHEA
     iii. Progesterone → 17α-hydroxy-progesterone
     iv. 17α-hydroxy-progesterone → androstenedione
   - 21-hydroxylase catalyses the following reactions
     i. Progesterone → corticosterone
     ii. 17α-hydroxy-progesterone → cortisol

5. **HSD**
   - 2 types
     i. 3β
     ii. 17β
   - 3β-HSD
     i. Converts a weak steroid to a strong steroid
     ii. Catalyses the following reactions
         - Pregnenolone (C21) → pregnanedione (C21)
         - 17α-hydroxy-pregnenolone → 17α-hydroxy-progesterone
         - DHEA → androstenedione
   - 17β-HSD catalyses the following reactions

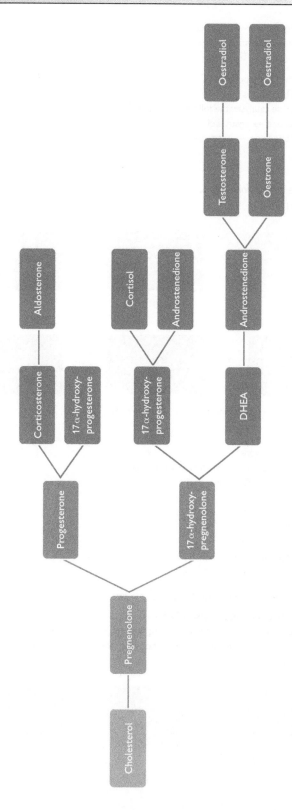

Figure 5.7 Overview of steroidogenesis

i. Androstenedione → testosterone

ii. Oestrone → oestradiol

6. Oestrogens

- Phenol aromatic compounds
- Have 18 carbon atoms
- P450 aromatase catalyses the following reaction
  i. Testosterone → oestradiol
  ii. Androstenedione → oestrone

7. Gonadal cells

- Leydig cells
  i. Produce testosterone (*Fig. 5.8*)
  ii. Have 17β-HSD

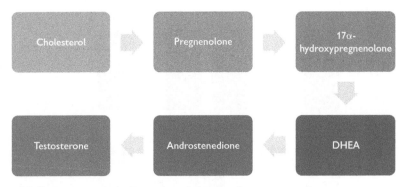

Figure 5.8 Testosterone production pathway in Leydig cells

- Theca cells
  i.   Produce androgens
  ii. Cannot produce testosterone and oestradiol
  iii. Does not have 17β-HSD
- Granulosa cells
  i. Produce oestradiol
  ii. Have 17β-HSD
- Luteal cells
  i. Produce progesterone
  ii. Produce oestradiol

Examples of abnormalities of steroidogenesis

1. Lipoid congenital adrenal hyperplasia (CAH)

- Is an autosomal recessive condition resulting from mutations of genes for enzymes mediating the biochemical steps of production of cortisol from cholesterol by the adrenal glands (*Fig. 5.9*)

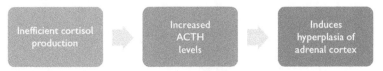

Figure 5.9 Pathogenesis of CAH

- Defect in
    i. STAR protein
    ii. Cytochrome P450$_{CSCC}$
    iii. 21-hydroxylase (accounts for 95% of CAH)
- Results in
    i. Failure of steroid production
    ii. Accumulation of large lipid droplets (cholesteryl ester) in adrenal cortex
- Depending on the type of CAH, it may be associated with
    i.   Ambiguous genitalia
    ii. Natriuresis (due to 21-hydroxylase deficiency)
    iii. Precocious puberty or failure of puberty
    iv. Infertility due to anovulation (due to 21-hydroxylase deficiency)
    v.   Virilization (due to 21-hydroxylase deficiency)
    vi. Hypertension (due to 11-hydroxylase deficiency)

Prostaglandins

1. **General facts**
    - Prostaglandins are
        i. Produced by all nucleated cells except lymphocytes
        ii. Hydrophilic
    - Vasomotor functions (*Box 5.12*)

Box 5.12 Vasomotor functions of prostaglandins

Vasoconstrictor	Vasodilator
- Thromboxane - Leukotriene	- PGD - PGE$_2$ - PGF$_2$ - Prostacyclin

- Other functions (*Box 5.13*)

Box 5.13 Non-vasomotor functions of prostaglandins

PGE$_2$	PGF$_2$	Prostacyclin
- Pyrogenic - Hyperalgesia - Uterine contraction - Increased gastric mucus secretion - GI smooth muscle contraction (receptor subtype 1 and 3) - GI smooth muscle relaxation (receptor subtype 2) - Bronchoconstriction (receptor subtype 1) - Bronchodilation (receptor subtype 2)	- Uterine contraction - Bronchoconstriction	- Inhibition of platelet aggregation - Bronchodilation

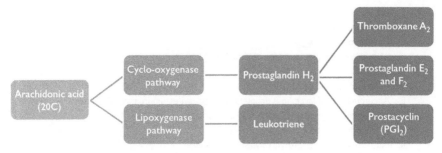

Figure 5.10 Prostaglandin synthesis pathway

2. **Synthesis pathway** (*Fig. 5.10*)

3. **Prostaglandin dehydrogenase (PGDH)**
   - Metabolizes prostaglandins
   - Found in
     - i.   Lungs
     - ii. Ovary
     - iii. Testes
     - iv. Placenta

4. **Prostaglandin receptors**
   - G-protein receptors
   - Seven-transmembrane domain
   - EP receptor = PGE_2
   - FP receptor = PGF_2

5. **Secondary messengers for**
   - $PGF_2 = IP_3$
   - $PGE_2 = cAMP$

6. **Clinical applications**
   - Induction of labour (PGE_2 and PGF_2)
   - To prevent closure of patent ductus arteriosus (PGE_2)
   - Treatment of
     - i.   Raynaud's phenomena
     - ii. Glaucoma
     - iii. Limb ischaemia
     - iv. Erectile dysfunction (alprostadil)
     - v.   Peptic ulcers (PGE_2)

7. **Prostaglandin antagonists include**
   - Non-steroidal anti-inflammatory drugs (inhibit cyclo-oxygenase)
   - Acetylsalicylic acid (irreversibly inhibits cyclo-oxygenase)
   - Corticosteroids (inhibit phospholipase A_2)
   - COX-2 selective inhibitors

Starvation

1. **General facts**
   - The brain has an absolute requirement for glucose
     - i.   During normal food intake – needs 100 g/day

    ii. During starvation – needs 25 g/day
- In starvation, the body is faced with an obligate need to generate glucose to sustain cerebral energy metabolism; achieved by
  i. Mobilizing glycogen stores
  ii. Hepatic gluconeogenesis
- 2 L intravenous 5% dextrose provides 100 g/day of glucose
- Death due to starvation occurs in 60 days

2. **Metabolic response to starvation (*Fig. 5.11*)**
   - Brain, RBCs, WBCs, and renal medulla can initially only use glucose for their metabolism
   - Starvation of 12 h or less leads to the following
     i. Fall in insulin levels
     ii. Rise in glucagon
     iii. Conversion of 200 g of liver glycogen to glucose (**glycogenolysis**)
     iv. Conversion of 500 g of muscle glycogen to lactate
     v. Lactate is exported to liver and converted to glucose via Cori's cycle
   - Starvation of >24 h
     i. Glycogen stores depleted
     ii. Glucose synthesis from alanine and glutamine (**gluconeogenesis**)
     iii. Protein catabolism of skeletal muscle up to 75 g/day
   - Starvation of >48 h
     i. Fat (TAG) oxidation to meet energy requirements (**lipolysis**)
     ii. TAG oxidation releases glycerol, which can be converted to glucose and fatty acids
     iii. Fatty acids are converted to ketones in the liver
   - Starvation of 2–3 weeks
     i. CNS adapts to using ketones as primary fuel source
     ii. This conversion to a 'fat fuel economy' reduces muscle breakdown by up to 55 g/day
   - Reduction in resting energy expenditure up to 20 kcal/kg/day
     i. Due to decline in conversion of T_4 to T_3

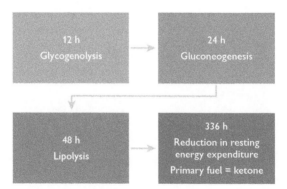

Figure 5.11 Evolution of metabolic response to starvation

Endocrinology

CONTENTS

Sex hormones

1. The ovary secretes 11 hormones (by definition a 'hormone' is a substance produced and secreted by a gland or from cell(s)/tissues) into the blood stream that circulates and acts at a target site remote from the source. Thus ovarian prostaglandins are strictly paracrine substances (*Fig. 6.1*)

2. Androgens in females are produced by
   - Ovary = 25%
   - Adrenal glands = 25%
   - Peripheral conversion of androstenedione = 50%

3. Markers of corpus luteum function are
   - 17-hydroxyprogesterone (**not** secreted by placenta)
   - Relaxin

4. Oestrogen
   - 3 naturally occurring oestrogens
     i. Oestrone (E1) – produced in menopause
     ii. Oestradiol (E2) – primary oestrogen in non-pregnant women
     iii. Oestriol (E3) – primary oestrogen in pregnancy
   - Oestradiol is the most active of the natural oestrogens
   - Produced by
     i. Developing follicles in ovary
     ii. Corpus luteum
     iii. Placenta
     iv. Liver
     v. Adrenal glands

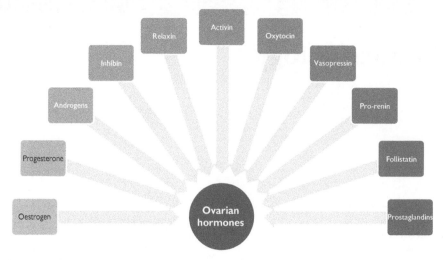

Figure 6.1 Ovarian hormones

    vi. Breast
    vii. Adipocytes
- In plasma binds to
  - i. Sex hormone-binding globulin (SHBG)
  - ii. Albumin
- Metabolized in the liver to oestrone and oestriol (*Fig. 6.2*)
- Excreted in the kidney as oestriol glucuronide
- Has 2 main receptors subtypes (other receptor subtypes exist)
  - i. α (found in endothelial cells)
  - ii. β
- Work by genomic expression

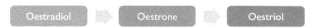

Figure 6.2 Metabolism of oestradiol

5. **Oestrogen functions**
   - Cardiovascular
     - i. Vasodilator (via an increase of NOS leading to an increase in NO)
     - ii. Prevents atherosclerosis
   - Bone
     - i. Maintenance of bone density – decreases resorption of bone by antagonizing PTH
     - ii. Fusion of epiphyseal plates
   - Increases clotting by
     - i. Increasing levels of factors II, VII, IX, X, and plasminogen
     - ii. Decreasing anti-thrombin 3
     - iii. Increase platelet adhesiveness
   - Gastrointestinal
     - i. Decrease motility of bowel
     - ii. Increases bile production
   - Metabolic changes
     - i. Increases high-density lipoprotein (HDL) levels

    ii. Decreases low-density lipoprotein (LDL) levels
    iii. Decreases cholesterol levels
    iv. Increases TAG synthesis
- Stimulates pigmentation of skin by increasing phaeomelanin
    i. Nipple
    ii. Areola
    iii. Genital regions
- Proliferation of endometrium
- Causes Na^+ and H_2O retention by kidney

6. **Progesterone**
- Sources
    i. *Dioscorea mexicana* (a type of plant)
    ii. Corpus luteum
    iii. Adrenal glands
    iv. Placenta
- Stored in adipose tissue
- In plasma binds to
    i. Corticosteroid-binding globulin (CBG)
    ii. Albumin
- Metabolized in liver to pregnanediol
- Excreted by kidney as pregnanediol glucuronide
- Levels
    i. Pre-ovulation = <2 ng/mL
    ii. Post-ovulation = 5 ng/mL
    iii. At term = 100–200 ng/mL
- At term placenta produces 250 mg/day progesterone

7. **Progesterone functions**
- Uterus, cervix, and vagina
    i. Converts proliferative to secretory endometrium
    ii. Withdrawal of progesterone causes menstruation
    iii. Thickens cervical mucus
    iv. Inhibits uterine contraction until term
- Increases core temperature following ovulation
- Smooth muscle relaxant
- Catabolic (thus causes an increase in appetite)
- Increases aldosterone production (leading to Na^+ and H_2O retention)
- Reduces pressor responsiveness to angiotensin-2
- Respiration
    i. Increased ventilator response to CO_2
    ii. Decreased arterial and alveolar pCO_2
- Inhibits lactation during pregnancy
- Neuroprotective (is being investigated in treatment of multiple sclerosis; demyelination halts during pregnancy)

8. **Inhibins**
- Are peptide members of transforming growth factor (TGF)-β family
- There are 2 forms of inhibin
    i. Inhibin A
    ii. Inhibin B
- Are secreted by ovarian granulosa cells
- Selectively inhibit FSH secretion but **not** LH secretion

- Produced in
  i. Gonads
  ii. Pituitary gland
  iii. Placenta
- Inhibin A is part of the quad screen test in the first trimester of pregnancy – elevated levels of inhibin A, elevated β-hCG, decreased α-fetoprotein (AFP), and decreased oestriol are suggestive of Down's syndrome

9. Activins
- Are peptide members of TGF-β family
- Are derived from
  i. Ovarian granulosa cells
  ii. Pituitary gonadotropes
- Functions
  i. Augment FSH action in the ovary
  ii. Stimulate FSH secretion in the pituitary
  iii. Inhibit prolactin, growth hormone, and ACTH responses

10. Relaxin
- Produced by
  i. Corpus luteum
  ii. Placenta
  iii. Breast
  iv. Prostate
- Relaxes pelvic ligaments in pregnancy
- Plays a role in cervical dilatation
- Inhibit contractility of myometrium

11. Testes secretes
- 3 main hormones
  i. Testosterone
  ii. DHT – strictly it is a paracrine hormone
  iii. Oestradiol
- Minor hormones
  i. DHEA
  ii. Androstenedione
  iii. Oestrone
  iv. Pregnenolone
  v. Progesterone
  vi. 17α-hydroxypregnenolone
  vii. 17α-hydroxyprogesterone

12. Testosterone
- Is an anabolic steroid
- Secreted by
  i. Testis (Leydig cells)
  ii. Ovary (theca cells)
  iii. Adrenals (zona reticularis)
  iv. Placenta (cyto or syncytiotrophoblastic cells)
- In serum exists
  i. Freely (2% of testosterone)
  ii. Bound to
    - SHBG (60% of testosterone)
    - Albumin (38% of testosterone)

- Effects of testosterone on tissue are via 2 mechanisms
  i. By activation of nuclear androgen receptors
  ii. By aromatization of testosterone to oestradiol (occurs in bone and brain)
- Is converted to DHT by 5α-reductase
- Excreted in urine as 17-ketosteroid

13. 5α-reductase
- Consist of 2 isoforms
- Is produced in
  i.   Skin
  ii. Seminal vesicles
  iii. Prostate
  iv. Epididymis
  v.   Brain
- Deficiency results in
  i.   Low DHT levels
  ii. Increased testosterone levels
  iii. Gynaecomastia
  iv. Ambiguous genitalia at birth (DHT is necessary for development of male genitalia *in utero*)

14. SHBG
- Is a glycosylated dimer protein
- Synthesized by liver
- Gene located on chromosome 17
- Levels are higher in females
- SHBG levels are influenced by the following (*Box 6.1*):

Box 6.1 Causes of altered SHBG levels

SHBG increased by	SHBG decreased by
• Oestrogen	• Exogenous androgens
• Tamoxifen	• Progestin
• Phenytoin	• Glucocorticoids
• Thyroid hormone	• Growth hormone
	• Hypothyroidism
	• Obesity

Hypothalamic hormones

1. Hypothalamic hormones (*Box 6.2*)

2. Paraventricular nucleus (PVN)
- Adjacent to 3rd ventricle
- Within blood–brain barrier
- Has 2 types of neurones
  i. Magnocellular
  ii. Parvocellular
- Magnocellular neurones produce
  i. Oxytocin
  ii. ADH

Box 6.2 Hypothalamic hormones

Paraventricular nucleus	Arcuate nucleus	Pre-optic nucleus	Peri-ventricular nucleus
• CRH • TRH	• Dopamine • GHRH	• GRH	• Somatostatin

Supraoptic and paraventricular nuclei
• ADH • Oxytocin

- Parvocellular neurones produce
  i. CRH
  ii. ADH
  iii. TRH

3. **Dopamine**
   - Is a prolactin-inhibitory hormone
   - Has 5 receptor types
   - Produced in
     i. Substantia nigra
     ii. Arcuate nucleus
     iii. Medulla of adrenal glands
   - Functions
     i. Plays an important role in behaviour, cognition, and voluntary movements
     ii. Inhibits prolactin
     iii. Inotropic
     iv. Chronotropic
     v. Induces vomiting via chemoreceptor trigger zone (metoclopramide is a dopamine receptor antagonist)
   - Does not cross blood–brain barrier
   - Is metabolized by
     i. Catechol-O-methyl transferase (COMT)
     ii. Monoamine oxidase (MAO)

4. **GnRH**
   - Release is pulsatile
     i. GnRH pulsatile frequency is high in follicular phase
     ii. GnRH pulsatile frequency slows in late luteal phase
   - Half life = 2–4 min
   - Gene is located on chromosome 8
   - Activity is low in childhood
   - Insulin increases GnRH activity
   - Prolactin decreases GnRH activity

5. **Somatostatin**
   - Is a GHRH inhibitor
   - Secreted by
     i. Stomach
     ii. Intestines
     iii. Pancreatic cells (D-cells)
     iv. Thyroid (parafollicular cells)
     v. Periventricular nucleus

- Functions are inhibitory
  i. Inhibits growth hormone (GH)
  ii. Inhibits TSH
  iii. Suppresses release of gastrointestinal hormones
     - Gastrin
     - CCK
     - Secretin
     - Vasoactive intestinal peptide (VIP)
     - Motilin
     - Insulin
     - Glucagon
  iv. Decreases gastric emptying, blood flow, and intestinal contractions
  v. Suppresses release of pancreatic hormones

6. **Thyrotrophin-releasing hormone (TRH)**
   - Stimulates release of
     i. Prolactin
     ii. TSH
   - Secreted by paraventricular nuclei

7. **Melatonin**
   - Is synthesized from serotonin
   - Is associated with biorhythms
   - Inhibits gonadotrophins
   - Diurnal
   - Produced in
     i. Pineal gland
     ii. Retina
     iii. Lens of eye
     iv. GIT
     v. Suprachiasmatic nucleus
   - Melatonin secretion increases in response to
     i. Hypoglycaemia
     ii. Darkness

Pituitary gland hormones

1. **The 6 anterior pituitary hormones can be classified into 3 groups (Box 6.3)**

Box 6.3 Classification of anterior pituitary hormones

Corticotrophin-related peptides	Somatomammotrophin peptides	Glycoproteins (have 2 subunits α and β)
• ACTH	• Growth hormone	• TSH
• MSH	• Prolactin	• Gonadotrophin (LH & FSH)

2. **FSH**
   - Is a glycoprotein
   - Released in response to GnRH

- Structure has 2 subunits
  i. α (gene located on chromosome 6)
  ii. β (gene located on chromosome 11)
- Functions
  i. Stimulates maturation of germ cells
  ii. In females – stimulates ovary to produce Graafian follicle
  iii. In males – induces Sertoli cells to synthesize and secrete inhibin
- High levels of FSH are due to
  i. Premature menopause
  ii. Reduced ovarian reserve
  iii. Gonadal dysgenesis
  iv. Castration
  v. Swyer's syndrome
  vi. CAH
- Half life = 3–4 hours
- Receptors are **only** in granulosa cells

3. **LH**
   - Is a heterodimeric glycoprotein
   - Structure has 2 subunits
     i. α (gene located on chromosome 6)
     ii. β (gene located on chromosome 19)
   - α-subunit has 92 amino acids and is identical to the α-subunit of
     i. TSH
     ii. FSH
     iii. hCG
   - In females
     i. Triggers ovulation
     ii. Prevents apoptosis of corpus luteum
     iii. Stimulates oestrogen and progesterone production
   - In males – stimulates Leydig cells to produce testosterone
   - Low LH levels are due to
     i. Kallmann's syndrome
     ii. Hypothalamic suppression
     iii. Hypopituitarism
     iv. Hyperprolactinaemia
   - High levels of LH are due to
     i. Premature menopause
     ii. Gonadal dysgenesis
     iii. Castration
     iv. Polycystic ovary syndrome (PCOS)
     v. Swyer's syndrome
     vi. CAH
   - Surge
     i. Is biphasic
     ii. Ovulation occurs
        - 36 h after LH surge
        - 16–26 h after peak of LH
     iii. Causes
        - Prostaglandin production
        - Progesterone secretion from corpus luteum
        - Resumption of meiosis by oocyte

- Half life = 20 min
- Gonadotrophins reach 2 peaks at
  i. 20 weeks in fetal life
  ii. 1–2 months in infancy
- LH and testosterone increases in the first 3–6 months of life
- Receptors are found in
  i. Granulosa cells
  ii. Theca cells

4. **Prolactin**
   - Is a peptide hormone
   - Has a molecular weight of 24 000 Daltons
   - Consists of 199 amino acids
   - Structure is similar to
     i. GH
     ii. Placental lactogen
   - Gene located on chromosome 6
   - Cycle is
     i. Diurnal
     ii. Ovulatory
   - Functions
     i. Lactogenesis
     ii. Promotes breast development
   - Is also responsible for decreasing serum levels of
     i. Oestrogen
     ii. Testosterone
   - Also produced by
     i.   Decidua
     ii. Breast
     iii. Brain
     iv. Immune system
   - Factors affecting prolactin secretion (**Table 6.1**)

5. **GH**
   - Most of GH effects are mediated by IGF
   - Gene located on chromosome 17
   - Consists of 191 amino acids
   - Functions are
     i. Mainly anabolic
         - Increases protein synthesis
         - Decreases protein catabolism
     ii. Lipolysis
     iii. Anti-insulin actions
   - Factors affecting GH secretion (**Table 6.2**)

6. **ACTH**
   - Released in response to CRH from hypothalamus
   - Can be produced by cells of the immune system
     i.   T-cell
     ii. B-cell
     iii. Macrophage
   - Stimulates production of steroids from the adrenals

Table 6.1 Factors affecting prolactin secretion

Hyperprolactinaemia		
Physiological	**Pharmacological**	**Pathological**
Pregnancy	TRH	Pituitary tumour
Lactation	Oestrogen	Chest wall lesions
Exercise	Dopamine antagonists	Spinal cord lesions
Stress	MAOI	Hypothyroidism
Sleep	Cimetidine	Chronic renal failure
Hypoglycaemia	Verapamil	Liver failure
		Stalk syndrome
Hypoprolactinaemia		
Pharmacological		**Pathological**
Dopamine agonists		Sheehan's syndrome
		Hypopituitarism
		Bulimia

Table 6.2 Factors affecting GH secretion

Raised serum GH		
Physiological	**Pharmacological**	**Pathological**
Sleep	GHRH	Chronic renal failure
Stress	Oestrogen	Anorexia nervosa
Exercise	Adrenergic agonist	
Hypoglycaemia	Dopamine agonist	
Decreased serum GH		
Physiological	**Pharmacological**	**Pathological**
Hyperglycaemia	Somatostatin	Obesity
Elevated free fatty acids	Progesterone	
	Glucocorticoids	

- Released in circadian rhythm – highest in the morning
- Derived from pro-opiomelanocortin (POMC)
- By-products are
  i. melanocyte-stimulating hormone (MSH)
  ii. Endorphins

7. **Oxytocin**
   - Is a nanopeptide (consists of 9 amino acids)

- Produced in supra-optic and paraventricular nucleus of hypothalamus
- Stored in posterior pituitary
- Involved in smooth muscle contraction of
  i. Uterine muscle
  ii. Myoepithelial cells surrounding breast alveoli (letdown reflex)
- Oxytocin receptor
  i. Is a G-protein-coupled receptor which requires Mg^{2+} and cholesterol
  ii. Also found in brain and spinal cord

8. **ADH**
   - Is a nanopeptide
   - Also known as vasopressin
   - Is derived from pre-pro-hormone precursors synthesized in the hypothalamus
   - Released when body fluid volume decreases
   - Functions
     i. Vasoconstrictor
     ii. Increases urine osmolarity
     iii. Increases reabsorption of H_2O at DCT and collecting duct
     iv. Na^+ reabsorption in ascending loop of Henle
     v. Implicated in memory formation

Thyroid gland hormones

1. **Action of thyroid hormone**
   - Increases activity of Na^+-K^+ ATPase (in all tissue except brain, spleen, and testis) causing
     i. Increased O_2 consumption
     ii. Heat production
   - Decreases superoxide dismutase levels
   - Increases β-adrenergic receptors in
     i. Myocardium (leading to positive ionotropic and chronotropic effects)
     ii. Skeletal muscles
     iii. Adipose tissue
     iv. Lymphocytes
   - Blood
     i. Increases EPO
     ii. Increases erythropoiesis
     iii. Increases DPG content of erythrocyte
   - Bone
     i. Increases bone turnover
     ii. Increases bone resorption, leading to osteopenia
   - Metabolism
     i. Increases hepatic gluconeogenesis
     ii. Increases glycogenolysis
     iii. Increases lipolysis

2. **Thyroid hormone production**
   - I_2 absorbed from bloodstream via iodide trapping
   - Thyroglobulin synthesis
   - Iodination (I_2 binds to tyrosine contained in thyroglobulin)
     i. I_2 + tyrosine = monoiodotyrosine (MIT)
     ii. I_2 + MIT = diiodotyrosine (DIT)

- Coupling of iodinated residues
    i.   MIT + DIT = T_3
    ii. DIT + DIT = T_4
- Stored in colloid of the follicular cells

3. **Thyroid hormones**
- Bound to
    i.   Thyroid-binding globulin (TBG) = 70%
    ii. Albumin = 15%
    iii. Pre-albumin (transthyretin) = 15%
- T_4
    i.   Amount is approximately 20 times more than T_3
    ii. Half-life = 7 days
- T_3 is
    i.   The active component
    ii. Half-life = 1 day
- rT_3
    i.   Is inactive
    ii. Half life = 4 h

4. **Changes in pregnancy (*Fig. 6.3*)**

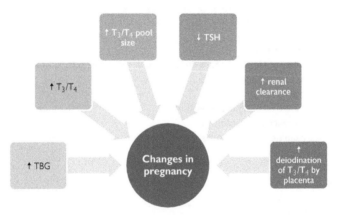

Figure 6.3 Thyroid changes in pregnancy

Adrenal hormones

1. **Adrenal hormones are derived from the**
- Adrenal cortex and
- Adrenal medulla

Adrenal cortex

1. **Mediates the stress response via the production of**
- Mineralocorticoids
- Glucocorticoids

2. **Consists of 3 layers**
- Zona glomerulosa (produces mineralocorticoids)

- Zona fasciculata (produces glucocorticoids)
- Zona reticularis (produces weak androgens)

3. **All adrenocortical hormones are synthesized from cholesterol**

4. **Glucocorticoids include**
   - Cortisol
   - Corticosterone

5. **Glucocorticoid actions**
   - Protein catabolism
     i.   Inhibit DNA synthesis
     ii. Inhibit RNA and protein synthesis (except in the liver)
   - Formation of ATP
   - Metabolism
     i.   Increases gluconeogenesis
     ii. Inhibits peripheral glucose usage
     iii. Increases lipolysis
   - Connective tissue and bone
     i.   Inhibits fibroblasts
     ii. Loss of collagen
     iii. Increases bone resorption
   - Renal
     i.   Increases excretion of Na^+ and water
     ii. Increases GFR
   - Increases secretion of stomach acid
   - Blood
     i.   Increases neutrophil count
     ii. Decreases lymphocyte count

6. **Aldosterone**
   - Is a mineralocorticoid
   - Has 21 carbon atoms
   - Is part of the renin–angiotensin system
   - Functions
     i.   Reabsorption of Na^+ from DCT and collecting ducts
     ii. Excretion of H^+ and K^+ via kidneys
     iii. Acts on posterior pituitary to release ADH
   - Secretion is regulated by
     i.   Renin–angiotensin system
     ii. Sympathetic nerves
     iii. Juxtaglomerular apparatus
     iv. Carotid artery baroreceptors
     v.   Plasma concentration of K^+
     vi. Plasma concentration of Na^+

7. **During adrenarche**
   - Adrenal androgen production starts at
     i.   Males = 7–9 years old
     ii. Females = 6–7 years old
   - The adrenal cortex secretes weak androgens
     i.   DHEA
     ii. Dehydroepiandrosterone sulphate (DHEAS)
     iii. Androstenedione

Adrenal medulla

1. Is composed mainly of chromaffin cells

2. Adrenal medulla cells are modified neural crest cells which did not complete their development to postganglionic neurones, but retain the same functions

3. Synthesizes
   - Adrenaline
   - Noradrenaline
   - Dopamine

4. Adrenaline
   - Synthesis: Tyrosine → L-DOPA → dopamine → noradrenaline → adrenaline
   - Actions
     i. Lipolysis
     ii. Glycogenolysis
     iii. Salt and water balance
     iv. Vasoconstriction
     v. GIT – relaxes smooth muscle
     vi. Increases plasma levels of
       ▪ Insulin
       ▪ Renin–angiotensin system
   - Adrenaline acts on α and β receptors
   - Noradrenaline acts **only** on α receptors
   - The dominant fetal catecholamine is L-DOPA
   - Metabolized by
     i. MAO
     ii. COMT

Renin–angiotensin system

1. Juxtaglomerular apparatus in kidney
   - Composed of
     i. Juxtaglomerular cells of afferent arterioles
     ii. Macula densa (cells on ascending loop of Henle)
   - Regulates renin secretion

2. Renin
   - Also known as angiotensinogenase
   - Secreted by juxtaglomerular cells in response to
     i. Decreased arterial blood pressure
     ii. Decrease Na^+ levels in plasma
   - Renin cleaves angiotensinogen to form angiotensin 1
   - Renin inhibitors are used to treat hypertension
   - Synthesis (*Fig. 6.4*)

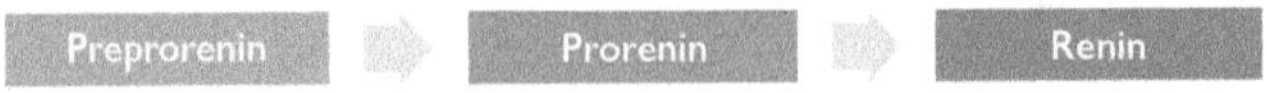

| Preprorenin | ⇨ | Prorenin | ⇨ | Renin |

Figure 6.4 Renin synthesis

3. Angiotensinogen
   - Secreted by liver

- Production is increased by
  i. Oestrogen
  ii. Glucocorticoids

4. **Angiotensin**
   - Synthesis
     i. Angiotensinogen → angiotensin 1 (catalyst = renin)
     ii. Angiotensin 1 → angiotensin 2 (catalyst = ACE)
   - Function
     i. Vasoconstriction
     ii. Stimulates aldosterone secretion

5. **ACE**
   - Found in
     i. Endothelial cells of the pulmonary capillaries
     ii. Brain
     iii. Glomeruli
   - Also catalyses
     i. Bradykinin breakdown
     ii. Enkephalin breakdown
     iii. Substance P breakdown

Pancreatic hormones

1. **Insulin actions**
   - Anabolic effects
     i. Glycogen synthesis
     ii. TAG synthesis
   - Inhibits catabolism
     i. Inhibits glycogenolysis
     ii. Inhibits ketogenesis
     iii. Inhibits gluconeogenesis
   - Stimulates glucose uptake into
     i. Muscle
     ii. Adipose tissue

2. **Insulin antagonists**
   - Glucagon
   - Cortisol
   - Growth hormone
   - Adrenaline
   - Oestrogen
   - Thyroid hormone
   - Prolactin
   - Human placental lactogen (responsible for the insulin resistance of pregnancy)

3. **Glucagon**
   - Main target tissue = liver
   - Actions
     i. Glycogenolysis
     ii. Inhibits glycogen synthesis
     iii. Gluconeogenesis

    iv. Lipolysis

    v. Ionotropic

    vi. Causes release of

        ■ Insulin

        ■ Catecholamines

Endocrine diseases

1. **Syndrome of inappropriate antidiuretic hormone hypersecretion (SIADH)**
   - Clinical features
     i. Hyponatraemia
     ii. Hypo-osmolality of plasma (<280 mOsm/kg)
     iii. Excessive renal excretion of Na^+ (>20 mEq/L)
     iv. Hypervolaemia
     v. Absence of oedema
     vi. Normal renal function
     vii. Normal adrenal function
   - Aetiology
     i. Tumour – oat cell carcinoma
     ii. CNS disease
     iii. Respiratory disease
     iv. Myxoedema
     v. Porphyria
     vi. Drugs
        ■ Vinblastine
        ■ SSRIs
        ■ Thiazide
        ■ Carbamazepine
     vii. Trauma
     viii. Infection
     ix. Surgery
   - Treatment
     i. Fluid restriction (1 L/day)
     ii. Diuretics
     iii. Demeclocycline (is a tetracycline which induces nephrogenic diabetes insipidus)
     iv. Conivaptan (is an ADH inhibitor)
     v. Hyponatraemia can be corrected by using hypertonic saline 5% (rapid rise in sodium levels may cause central pontine myelinolysis; aim for maximum increase of 12 mEq/L/day of Na^+)

2. **Diabetes insipidus (DI)**
   - Is a disorder resulting from deficient ADH action
   - Treatment = desmopressin
   - Classification of DI (*Box 6.4*)
   - Also associated with pregnancy-related diseases such as
     i. Pre-eclampsia
     ii. HELLP syndrome
     iii. Acute fatty liver of pregnancy (due to activation of hepatic vasopressinase)

3. **Hypothyroidism**
   - Can result in congenital hypothyroidism in the fetus, known as cretinism
   - Aetiology (*Box 6.5*)

Box 6.4 Classification of diabetes insipidus

Neurogenic	Nephrogenic	Gestational
• Idiopathic	• Chronic renal disease	• Vasopressinase is produced in the placenta, which breaks down ADH
• Familial	• Hypokalaemia	
• Syphilis	• Hypercalcaemia	
• Tuberculosis (TB)	• Sickle cell disease	
• Tumour	• Sjogren's syndrome	
• Autoimmune	• Lithium	

Box 6.5 Aetiology of hypothyroidism

Primary	Secondary	Tertiary
• Hashimoto's	• Hypopituitarism	• Hypothalamic dysfunction
• Iatrogenic		
• Iodide deficiency		

- Associated with
  i. Pernicious anaemia
  ii. Sjogren's syndrome
  iii. Rheumatoid arthritis
  iv. Systemic lupus erythematosus (SLE)
  v. Diabetes
- Clinical features
  i. Cardiomegaly
  ii. Decreased intestinal peristalsis
  iii. Renal
     ▪ Decreased GFR
     ▪ Myxoedematous facies
  iv. Anaemia
  v. Amenorrhoea/menorrhagia
  vi. Overweight
  vii. Hands
     ▪ Dry
     ▪ Cool
     ▪ Rough
     ▪ Inelastic skin
     ▪ Non-pitting oedema
     ▪ Carpal tunnel syndrome
  viii. Face
     ▪ Thin, dry and brittle hair
     ▪ Loss of outer 1/3 of eyebrow
     ▪ Yellowish complexion
  ix. Reflex – slow relaxing reflex
- Complication = myxoedema coma
- Tested for by Guthrie's test

4. **Hyperthyroidism**
   - Aetiology (*Fig. 6.5*)
   - Treatment
     i. Carbimazole and propylthiouracil (PTU)

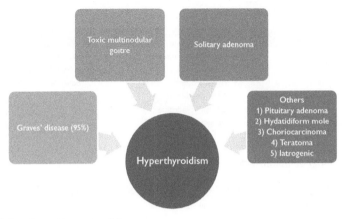

Figure 6.5 Aetiology of hyperthyroidism

  ii. Surgery

  iii. Radioactive iodine

- Clinical features
  - i. Hands
    - Pulse suggestive of atrial fibrillation
    - Excessive sweating
    - Tremor
  - ii. Weight loss
  - iii. Muscular weakness
  - iv. Heat intolerance
  - v. Insomnia
  - vi. Eyelid retraction
  - vii. Lid-lag
  - viii. Exophthalmos
  - ix. Thyroid acropachy
- Complication = thyroid crisis

5. **Exophthalmos**
   - Is due to
     - i. Cross-reaction of autoimmune antibodies to intraorbital muscle
     - ii. Increased retro-orbital fat
     - iii. Intraorbital muscle infiltrated with lymphocytes
   - Complications of exophthalmos include
     - i. Chemosis
     - ii. Ophthalmoplegia
     - iii. Diplopia

6. **Addison's disease**
   - Is due to decreased levels of cortisol
   - Is primary adrenocortical insufficiency
   - Clinical features
     - i. Hypotension
     - ii. Hyponatraemia
     - iii. Hypoglycaemia
     - iv. Hyperkalaemia
     - v. Hyperpigmentation (due to increased ACTH)

- Aetiology
  i. CAH
  ii. Infection
     - TB
     - CMV
  iii. Autoimmune
  iv. Adrenal haemorrhage
  v. Infiltrative disorder
     - Amyloidosis
     - Haemochromatosis
  vi. Rapid removal of exogenous hormone
  vii. Drugs
     - Ketoconazole
     - Etomidate

7. **Cushing's syndrome**
   - Is chronic glucocorticoid excess
   - Aetiology (**Box 6.6**)

Box 6.6 Causes of Cushing's syndrome

ACTH dependent	ACTH independent
• Pituitary adenoma (Cushing's disease) • Ectopic ACTH	• Iatrogenic • Adrenal neoplasm

- Clinical features
  i. Hypertension
  ii. Hyperglycaemia
  iii. Hyperlipidaemia
  iv. Hypokalaemia
  v. Amenorrhoea
  vi. Osteoporosis
  vii. Obesity
- Tumours causing ectopic ACTH secretion
  i. Small cell carcinoma of lung
  ii. Pancreatic cancer
  iii. Carcinoid
  iv. Medullary carcinoma of thyroid
  v. Phaeochromocytoma

8. **Conn's disease**
   - Is primary hyperaldosteronism
   - Aetiology = adrenal adenoma
   - Shows low renin : aldosterone ratio
   - Clinical features
     i. Hypokalaemia
     ii. Hypernatraemia
     iii. Hypertension
   - Treatment = spironolactone

9. **Phaeochromocytoma**
   - Are tumours arising from chromaffin cells
   - Secretes

   i.   Adrenaline
   ii. Noradrenaline
   iii. Dopamine
- Associated with
   i.   MEN type 2 syndrome
   ii. Neurofibromatosis
- Can be caused by *RET* proto-oncogene mutations
- Clinical features
   i.   Hypertension
   ii. Hyperglycaemia
   iii. Headache
   iv. Sweating
- Diagnosis is achieved by measuring urinary levels of vanillylmandelic acid (VMA) and metanephrine
- Untreated phaeochromocytoma leads to inhibition of renin–angiotensin system
- Treatment
   i.   Surgery
   ii. Preoperative salt loading
   iii. Intraoperative α-blocker (e.g. phenoxybenzamine)
   iv. Avoid pure β-blockers (e.g. atenolol)

10. Prolactinoma
- Is a benign tumour of the pituitary gland
- Results in hyperprolactinaemia
- Classification
   i.   Macroprolactinoma (i.e. tumour size >10 mm)
   ii. Microprolactinoma (i.e. tumour size <10 mm)
- Features
   i.   Headache
   ii. Bitemporal hemianopia (due to pressure on optic chiasm)
   iii. Galactorrhoea
   iv. Hypogonadism (resulting in amenorrhoea)
   v.   Erectile dysfunction
- Treatment
   i.   Dopamine agonist (shrinks tumour in 80% of patients)
   ii. Trans-sphenoidal surgery
   iii. Radiotherapy
- May result in osteoporosis due to reduced oestrogen and testosterone

Puberty

1. Sex determination
- Default phenotype *in utero* = female
- Male phenotype determined by
   i.   SRY
   ii. Testosterone (promotes Wolffian ducts)
   iii. Mullerian inhibiting substance (MIS) – secreted by Sertoli cells

2. Physical changes in puberty
- Stages of development described by Tanner (5 stages in total) (*Fig. 6.6*)

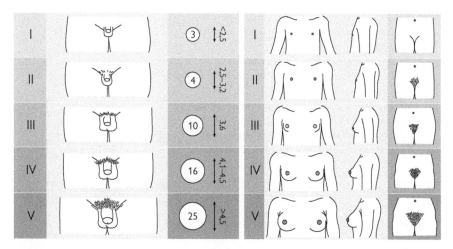

Figure 6.6 Tanner's stages for male (circled numbers represent testicular volume in ml, numbers next to arrows represent testicular length in cm) and female

Reproduced from the *Oxford Handbook of Reproductive Medicine and Family Planning*, by McVeigh, Homburg and Guillebaud, © Oxford University Press (2008). Original data from Marshall WA and Tanner JM. *Archives of Disease in Childhood* 1969; 44:291–303.

- Male development
  i. Chronologically: testes → scrotum → penis → pubic hair
  ii. Seminiferous tubule is solid until the age of 5
- Female development
  i. Chronologically: increased growth velocity → breast (thelarche) → pubic hair (adrenarche) → axillary hair → menarche
  ii. Breast development is determined by ovarian oestrogen
  iii. Pubic hair development is determined by adrenal and ovarian androgens
  iv. Average age of menarche is 12.3 years in African girls and 12.8 in Western Caucasians

3. **Growth spurt in puberty**
   - Is under endocrine control
     i. GH
     ii. IGF
   - Oestrogen is important for epiphyseal fusion
   - Begins in males 2 years later than females
   - Bone mineralization peak
     i. Girls at the age of 14–16 years old
     ii. Boys at the age of 17.5 years old

4. **GnRH and gonadotropin changes up to puberty**
   - GnRH
     i. Is secreted in a pulsatile manner (every 90–120 min)
     ii. Increased GnRH pulse frequency increases LH : FSH ratio
     iii. Continuous GnRH secretion causes suppression of gonadotrophins
     iv. Increased LH : FSH ratio is characteristic of midcycle dynamics
   - Fetal life
     i. Fetal LH and FSH peak at mid-gestation then decline until term
     ii. Fetal GnRH increases until mid-gestation

- Age 2–9
  i. Gonadotrophin level is low (juvenile pause)
- Peripubertal
  i. Gonadotrophin release is circadian
  ii. GnRH secretions increase in frequency and amplitude during early sleep
- Early puberty
  i. The peak of LH and FSH occurs during the day
- Late puberty
  i. The peak of LH and FSH occurs all the time
  ii. Gonadotrophin diurnal rhythm is eliminated

Endocrine changes in pregnancy

1. **Maternal hormonal changes in pregnancy include (*Fig. 6.7*)**
   - LH and FSH levels are minimal
   - Cortisol and corticosteroids – increase in 2nd trimester
   - T_3 and T_4 – peak at 10–15 weeks gestation
   - Relaxin – highest in the first trimester

2. **Proteins associated with pregnancy (*Box 6.7*)**

Placental hormones

1. **Placenta produces 9 hormones during pregnancy (*Fig. 6.8*)**

2. **hCG**
   - Is a peptide hormone (glycoprotein)
   - Is composed of 244 amino acids
   - Is secreted by the syncytiotrophoblast
   - Functions
     i. Prevents degradation of corpus luteum
     ii. Induces ovulation
     iii. Stimulates Leydig cells to produce testosterone
   - Is heterodimeric
   - Structure has 2 subunits
     i. α – identical to LH/FSH/TSH
     ii. β – unique to hCG
   - Peaks at 9–12 weeks to 290 000 mIU/mL
   - Secreted by some types of tumour
     i. Choriocarcinoma
     ii. Germ cell tumour
     iii. Hydatidiform mole

3. **hPL**
   - Consists of 190 amino acids linked by disulphide bonds
   - Is an anti-insulin (i.e. is diabetogenic)
   - Is secreted by the syncytiotrophoblast
   - Gene located on chromosome 17
   - Belongs to the same family as
     i. GH
     ii. Prolactin

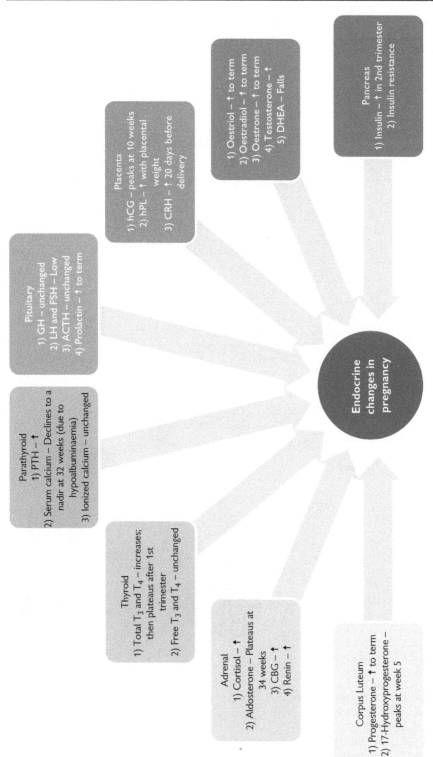

Figure 6.7 Maternal endocrine changes in pregnancy

Box 6.7 Proteins associated with pregnancy

Fetal compartment	Placental compartment	Maternal compartment

• α-fetoprotein	• GnRH
	• CRH
	• TRH
	• Somatostatin
	• GHRH
	• hCG
	• hPL
	• hGH
	• hCT
	• ACTH
	• Oxytocin
	• IGF-1 and IGF-2
	• Epidermal growth factor
	• Platelet-derived growth factor
	• Fibroblast growth factor
	• Transforming growth factor
	• Inhibin
	• Activin
	• Follistatin
	• Cytokines
	• Opiates
	• Pregnancy-associated plasma protein A
		• Prorenin
		• Decidual proteins, which include
		  • Prolactin
		  • Progesterone-associated endometrial protein
		  • Interleukin-1
		  • Colony-stimulating factor-1

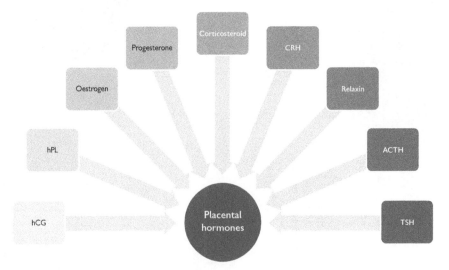

Figure 6.8 Placental hormones

- Peaks at 35 weeks gestation (5–7 mg/mL)
- Half-life = 15 min
- Functions
  i. Induces lipolysis – raises maternal free fatty acids (FFAs)
  ii. Decreases maternal insulin sensitivity

Labour

1. **Initiation of labour involves 2 endocrine systems**
   - Fetal
   - Maternal

2. **Labour is characterized by**
   - Uterine contractions
   - Cervical effacement and dilatation

3. **Cervical ripening (obvious in the last 5 weeks of pregnancy) has much in common with an inflammatory process involving**
   - Prostaglandin E_2
   - Cytokines (especially interleukin (IL)-8)
   - Recruitment of neutrophils
   - Synthesis of metalloproteinases (including collagenases and elastase)
   - Increased cervical tissue water content
   - Reduction in cervical tissue collagen concentration, and rearrangement and realignment of collagen

4. **The fetus is thought to trigger parturition**
   - Fetal pituitary releases corticotrophin, which acts on the fetal adrenals
   - Fetal adrenals release
     - i. Cortisol
     - ii. DHEAS

5. **Hormonal changes leading to labour**
   - Fetal adrenal cortisol rises towards the end of term causing
     - i. Increased oestrogen production
     - ii. Formation of oxytocin receptors
   - Fetal adrenal DHEAS is metabolized in the placenta leading to increased oestrogen levels, which provoke the release of prostaglandin $F_{2\alpha}$ from the decidua, causing myometrial contractions
   - Rise in placental CRH, causing augmentation of levels of
     - i. Oxytocin
     - ii. Prostaglandin $F_{2\alpha}$

6. **Other factors initiating labour**
   - NO withdrawal
   - Progesterone
     - i. Withdrawal
     - ii. Switch from type 1 to type 2 progesterone receptors
   - Increased placental release of
     - i. CRH
     - ii. Oestrogen
   - Upregulation of oxytocin receptors
   - Increased prostaglandin synthesis in
     - i. Uterus
     - ii. Fetal membranes
   - Increased IL
     - i. IL-1
     - ii. IL-8

- Fetal release of
  i. Cortisol
  ii. Platelet-activating factor
- Catecholamines
  i. β_2-adrenergic receptor agonists inhibit labour
  ii. α_2-adrenergic receptor agonists cause uterine contractions
- Fetal posterior pituitary (umbilical artery oxytocin > umbilical vein oxytocin)
- Increased myometrial gap junctions during labour

7. **Ferguson reflex**
   - Is a neuronal reflex triggered by pressure application to the
     i. Cervix
     ii. Vagina
   - Causes spurts of oxytocin release
   - Occurs during the following labour phases
     i. Active
     ii. Expulsive

Puerperium and lactation

Puerperium

1. **Most hormone levels drop dramatically except for the rise in**
   - Prolactin (only in breast-feeding women)
   - Oxytocin

2. **The following hormone levels decline in the puerperium**
   - Oestrogen
   - Progesterone
   - Thyroid
   - Most hormones takes 6 weeks to return to normal

3. **Menses returns in**
   - Breastfeeding women at 28 weeks post partum
   - Non-breast feeding women at 9 weeks post partum

4. **Prolactin levels drop 2 weeks post partum in non-breast feeding women, resulting in cessation of lactation**

Breastfeeding

1. **Lactation**
   - Maternal breast changes occur from 7 weeks gestation onwards
   - Influenced by
     i. Oestrogen
     ii. hPL
     iii. Prolactin
     iv. Decreased serum progesterone levels
     v. Oxytocin
     vi. LH
     vii. FSH

2. **Lactational amenorrhoea is a reliable form of contraception (98% effective according to the World Health Organization (WHO)) if the following criteria are met**
   - The baby is exclusively breastfed (intervals between breastfeeding are no longer than 5 h)
   - Amenorrhoea (less than 6 months postpartum)

3. **Breast milk**
   - Composition (*Box 6.8*)

Box 6.8 Composition of breast milk

Carbohydrate	Fat	Protein	Vitamin
• Lactose • Oligosaccharides	• Polyunsaturated fatty acid • Palmitic acid • Oleic acid • Vaccenic acid • Conjugated linoleic acid	• Casein • Lactoferrin • Immunoglobulin (A, G, M, and D) • Lysozymes • Albumin	• A • B_1 • B_2 • C

Cells
• Macrophage • Lymphocyte

   - Also contains
     i.   2-arachidonoyl glycerol (a type of endocannabinoid)
     ii. Growth factors (e.g. epidermal growth factor (EGF), IGF)
     iii. Digestive enzymes (e.g. bile acid-stimulating lipase, amylase)
     iv. Hormones (e.g. feedback inhibitor of lactation (FIL), prolactin, insulin, ACTH)
   - Benefits (*Box 6.9*)

Box 6.9 Benefits of breastfeeding

Maternal	Neonatal
• Weight loss (breastfeeding uses 500 kcal/day) • Strengthens maternal bonding • Helps uterus contract post delivery and reduces risk of postpartum bleeding • Reduces risk of breast cancer • Reduces risk of ovarian cancer • Reduces risk of endometrial cancer	• Decreases sudden infant death syndrome (SIDS) • Protects against diabetes mellitus • Reduce risk of obesity • Reduces atopy • Reduces risk of necrotizing enterocolitis (NEC) • Confers passive immunity • Lower the risk of infection (e.g. otitis media, upper respiratory tract infection, urinary tract infection) • Acts as a mild laxative

- Typical breast milk volume at day 5 post partum is 500 mL/day
- Colostrum
  i. Secreted for the first 3–5 days after delivery
  ii. Typical volume = 100 mL/day
  iii. Rich in the following (compared with mature breast milk)
     - Vitamin A
     - Lactoferrin
     - Ig A
     - Sodium

Fetal and neonatal endocrine system

1. Fetal endocrine system is largely functional by term

2. Surfactant production is controlled by
   - Cortisol
   - Oestrogen
   - Adrenaline
   - Thyroid hormone

3. Development of gonads and adrenals in the 1st trimester is directed by hCG

4. Fetal endocrine development (*Box 6.10*)

Box 6.10 Fetal endocrine development

Thyroid	Parathyroid	Adrenal	Gonad
• Hormone synthesis begins at 12 weeks • T₄ is predominant	• Hormone synthesized in 1st trimester • Fetal PTH levels are low • Fetal calcitonin is elevated • Fetus is hypercalcaemic	• Cortex identifiable at 4 weeks • Steroidogenesis starts at 7 weeks • Fetal zone involution complete 1 month post delivery	• Testes seen at 6 weeks • Ovaries seen at 7–8 weeks • Testosterone production starts at 10 weeks • Oestrogen production starts at 20 weeks

Pituitary
• Oxytocin and Vasopressin present at 12 weeks • Anterior pituitary hormone levels are significant in fetal circulation at 20 weeks

Pathology

CONTENTS

Inflammation

1. **The inflammatory response consists of 2 main components**
   - Vascular response
   - Cellular response

2. **Vascular response**
   - Chronology of vascular response (*Fig. 7.1*)

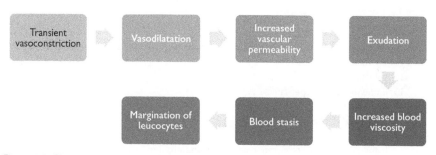

Figure 7.1 Chronology of vascular response

   - Vasodilation
     i. Is the earliest manifestation of acute inflammation
     ii. Involves arterioles first
     iii. Is induced by the action of
        - Histamine
        - NO
     iv. Results in increased blood flow
     v. Results in increased hydrostatic pressure

- Exudation results in
  - i.   Reduced intravascular osmotic pressure
  - ii. Increased interstitial osmotic pressure
  - iii. Oedema
- Exudate is an inflammatory extravascular fluid that has a high protein concentration and a specific gravity >1.02
- Increased vascular permeability occurs in distinct phases
  - i.   Phase 1 – immediate transient response
    - Is mediated by histamine, leukotrienes, neuropeptide substance P, and bradykinin in venules
    - Is short lived (less than 30 minutes)
    - Is reversible
  - ii. Phase 2 – delayed response
    - Is mediated by kinin and complement products
    - Is long lived
    - Involves venules and capillaries
    - Onset is delayed for 2–12 h
  - iii. Phase 3 – prolonged response after direct endothelial injury, which affects all levels of microcirculation

3. **Cellular response**
   - Involves 2 events
     - i. Leucocyte extravasation
     - ii. Phagocytosis
   - Extravasation is the sequence of events in the movement of leucocytes from the vessel lumen to the interstitial tissue (**Fig. 7.2**)

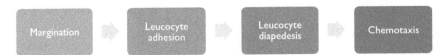

Figure 7.2 Extravasation sequence

- Leucocyte adhesion to the endothelium is regulated via endothelial binding receptors that belong to 4 main groups
  - i.   Selectins
  - ii. Immunoglobulin super-family
  - iii. Integrins
  - iv. Mucin-like glycoproteins
- Diapedesis
  - i. Is the process of transmigration across the endothelium
  - ii. Occurs predominantly in the venules
- Chemotaxis is elicited by
  - i. Exogenous agents (e.g. bacterial products)
  - ii. Endogenous agents
    - Components of the complement system
    - Leukotriene
    - Cytokines
- Microbicidal substances
  - i. Are released into the extracellular space and phagolysosomes during phagocytosis by leucocytes

Chpt 8

ii. Include
- Lysosomal enzymes
- Reactive oxygen intermediates (e.g. H_2O_2)
- Products of arachidonic acid metabolism (e.g. leukotrienes and prostaglandins)

     iii. Are capable of causing endothelial and tissue damage (leucocyte-induced injury) including
- Acute respiratory distress syndrome
- Acute transplant rejection
- Asthma
- Reperfusion injury

4. **Chemical mediators of inflammation include**
   - Hageman factor activation
     - i. Source = liver and plasma
     - ii. Also known as factor 12
     - iii. Functions
       - Activates kinin system
       - Activates clotting system
       - Activates fibrinolytic system
       - Activates complement system
   - Complement system
     - i. Source = liver and plasma
   - Cytokines and NO
     - i. Source = endothelium and macrophage
   - Platelet-activating factor
     - i. Source = endothelium and leucocytes
   - Serotonin
     - i. Source = platelets and mast cells
     - ii. Increases vascular permeability
   - Histamine
     - i. Source = platelets and mast cells
     - ii. Associated with IgE
   - Bradykinin
     - i. The kinin system is triggered by the activation of the Hageman factor
     - ii. Functions
       - Increased vascular permeability
       - Vasodilation
       - Smooth muscle contraction
       - Chemotaxis
       - Activates Hageman factor
     - iii. Is formed by the action of kallikrein (converts kininogen → bradykinin)
     - iv. Is inactivated in the lungs by ACE
     - v. ACE inhibitor (ACEi) prevents inactivation of kinin in the lungs
   - Prostaglandins
   - Leukotrienes
   - Platelet-activating factor
   - Lysosomal enzymes

5. **Signs of inflammation**
   - Raised ESR (due to RBC clumping)
   - Leucocytosis – increased number of immature neutrophils
   - 4 cardinal signs

  i.   Rubor (redness)
  ii. Tumour (swelling)
  iii. Calor (heat)
  iv. Dolor (pain)
- Virchow sign (loss of function)

6. **Systemic acute phase response is predominantly induced by**
   - Interleukin-1
   - TNF

7. **There are 2 patterns of inflammation**
   - Acute
   - Chronic

Acute inflammation

1. **Characteristics**
   - Rapid onset
   - Short duration

2. **Vascular and cellular changes**
   - Alteration in vascular calibre
     i.   Initial vasoconstriction followed by vasodilation
     ii. Slowing of circulation (stasis)
     iii. Margination of leucocytes
     iv. Central sludging of RBCs
   - Increased vascular permeability
   - Exudation of fluid
     - Serous
     - Fibrinous
     - Purulent
   - Emigration of leucocytes (predominantly neutrophils)

3. **Outcomes**
   - Complete resolution
   - Fibrosis
   - Abscess formation
   - Chronic inflammation

4. **Morphological patterns of acute inflammation**
   - Serous inflammation
   - Fibrinous inflammation
   - Suppurative inflammation
   - Ulcers

Chronic inflammation

1. **Chronic inflammation is caused by**
   - Persistent infection (e.g. *Mycobacterium*)
   - Prolonged exposure to foreign agents (e.g. silica)
   - Immune reaction to own tissue (e.g. autoimmune disease)

2. **Can start de novo without acute inflammation**

3. **Features**
   - Long duration

- Associated histologically with the presence of
  i. Lymphocytes
  ii. Macrophages

4. **Characterized by**
   - Infiltration by mononuclear cells (macrophages) – predominant by 48 h
   - Tissue destruction
   - Attempted repair by proliferation of new blood vessels
   - Fibrosis

5. **Granulomatous inflammation**
   - Is a distinctive pattern of chronic inflammation characterized by
     i. Granulomas (focal area)
     ii. Epithelioid cells (activated macrophages)
   - Epithelioid cells are surrounded by mononuclear leucocytes
   - E.g.
     i. TB
         - Caseating granuloma
         - Langhans giant cell
         - Mantoux test can be positive/negative
     ii. Cat-scratch disease
         - Stellate granuloma
         - Contains neutrophils
     iii. Schistosomiasis (contains eosinophils)
     iv. Sarcoidosis
         - Non-caseating granuloma
         - Schaumann's body
         - Raised ACE levels
         - Kveim's test can be positive/negative
     v. Temporal arteritis
   - Any granulomatous lesion can contain giant cells

Cellular adaptation

1. **Cellular adaptation**
   - Cellular changes that occur in response to a persistent physiological or pathological stress
   - There are 5 major forms of adaptation (*Box 7.1*)

2. **Causes of atrophy**
   - Decreased workload
   - Loss of innervation
   - Diminished blood supply
   - Inadequate nutrition
   - Loss of endocrine stimulation (e.g. loss of oestrogen during menopause)
   - Senile atrophy
   - Pressure

3. **Hyperplasia**
   - Is a result of increased cell mitosis
   - Can be divided into
     i. Physiological
     ii. Pathological

Box 7.1 Forms of adaptation

Atrophy	Hypertrophy	Hyperplasia	Metaplasia
• Decrease in cell size	• Increase in cell size	• Increase in number of cells	• Occurs when a cell is replaced by another cell type • Reversible • If stimuli persist can induce cancer

Dysplasia
• Abnormal changes in cellular shape and size • Also known as atypical hyperplasia

- Physiological hyperplasia is further divided into
  i. Hormonal
  ii. Compensatory
- Endometriosis is a form of pathological hyperplasia

T. in
Obs
Gyn
Chpt 13.2

Cell injury

1. **Cell injury**
   - Occurs when limits of adaptive responses are exceeded
   - It may be reversible or irreversible
   - Hallmarks include
     i. Decreased oxidative phosphorylation
     ii. Depleted ATP
     iii. Cellular swelling
   - Cellular swelling is also known as
     i. Hydropic degeneration
     ii. Vacuolar degeneration

2. **Cell death**
   - Results from irreversible cell injury
   - Hallmarks include
     i. Mitochondrial damage
     ii. Loss of membrane permeability
   - Characterized by
     i. Pyknosis (condensation of chromatin)
     ii. Karyorrhexis (fragmentation of nuclear material)
     iii. Karyolysis (dissolution of nucleus)
   - There are 3 types
     i. Necrosis (traumatic cell death)
     ii. Apoptosis (programmed cell death, follows a characteristic pattern)
     iii. Autolysis (non-traumatic cell death occurring through the action of its own enzymes)

3. **Mechanisms of cell injury**
   - Depletion of ATP
   - Influx of Ca^{2+}
   - Oxygen-derived free radicals

4. **Depletion of ATP leads to**
   - Anaerobic glycolysis – leading to
     i. Decreased pH
     ii. Clumping of nuclear chromatin
   - Decreased protein synthesis – leading to lipid deposition
   - Failure of membrane Na^+-K^+ pump – leading to
     i. Influx of Ca^{2+}
     ii. Influx of Na^+
     iii. Loss of K^+
     iv. ER swelling
     v. Cellular swelling
     vi. Loss of microvilli
     vii. Bleb formation

5. **Influx of Ca^{2+} leads to**
   - Increased cytosol Ca^{2+}
   - Activation of
     i. Endonuclease $\rightarrow$ DNA damage
     ii. ATPase $\rightarrow$ decreased ATP
     iii. Phospholipase $\rightarrow$ decreased phospholipids $\rightarrow$ membrane damage
     iv. Protease $\rightarrow$ disruption of cell membrane

6. **Oxygen-derived free radicals**
   - Cause
     i. DNA lesions
     ii. Protein fragmentation
     iii. Membrane lipid peroxidation
   - Can be neutralized by antioxidants, which include
     i. Vitamin A, C, and E
     ii. Glutathione
     iii. Superoxidase dismutase (SOD)
     iv. Iron and copper transport proteins (ferritin/transferritin/ lactoferritin/ ceruloplasmin)

7. **Apoptosis**
   - Programmed cell death
   - Characterized by
     i. Intact cell membrane
     ii. Degradation of nuclear DNA
   - Can be physiological or pathological (*Box 7.2*)

Box 7.2 Causes of apoptosis

Physiological	Pathological
• During embryogenesis	• Cell death in tumours
• Hormone-dependent involution	• Atrophy after obstruction
• Elimination of harmful self-reactive lymphocytes	• Cytotoxic drugs and radiation
• Cell death induced by cytotoxic T-cells	• Cell injury in viral disease

- Does not release proinflammatory markers
- Morphology
    i.   Cell shrinkage
    ii. Chromatin condensation
    iii. Formation of
        ▪ Cytoplasmic blebs
        ▪ Apoptotic bodies
    iv. Phagocytosis
- There are 2 pathways
    i.   Extrinsic (death-receptor initiated)
        ▪ TNF receptor
        ▪ Fas
    ii. Intrinsic (mitochondrial) – involves release of pro-apoptotic molecules into the cytoplasm through the loss of the action of the Bcl-2 anti-apoptotic gene

8. **B-cell lymphoma 2 (*Bcl-2*) gene family is**
    - A family of oncogenes
    - Can be both anti-apoptotic (e.g. Bcl-2 proper gene) and pro-apoptotic (e.g. *BAD* gene) in function
    - Reside in mitochondria

9. **Necrosis**
    - Cell death in living tissues by enzymatic degradation
    - Characterised by
        i.   Loss of membrane integrity
        ii. Enzymatic digestion of cells
        iii. Host reaction
    - Occurs within 4–12 h of insult
    - Types of necrosis (**Box 7.3**)
    - Gangrene is a term used to describe black necrotic tissue
        i.   Wet gangrene – tissues undergo colliquative necrosis
        ii. Dry gangrene – tissues undergo coagulative necrosis
        iii. Gas gangrene – tissues accumulate gas (evident as crepitation) due to exotoxin-producing clostridial species (usually *Clostridium perfringens*)
    - Patterns of necrosis are also determined by the blood supply to the organ
    - Necrosis of striated muscle is called rhabdomyolysis

10. **Cell injury can be mediated via intracellular accumulation of metabolites or pigments, e.g.**
    - Lipids
        i.   TAG causing steatosis ('fatty changes'). Observed in
            ▪ Heart
            ▪ Liver
            ▪ Kidney
        ii. Cholesterol leading to
            ▪ Arthrosclerosis
            ▪ Xanthoma
            ▪ Foamy macrophages
            ▪ Niemann–Pick disease
            ▪ Cholesterolosis (in the gall bladder)
    - Protein
    - Hyaline changes (giving rise to Russell bodies)
    - Glycogen

Box 7.3 Types of necrosis

Colliquative necrosis (liquefaction)	Coagulative necrosis	Caseous necrosis	Fibrinoid necrosis
• Due to action of tissue digestive enzymes • Seen mainly in CNS, kidney, and pancreas • Caused by focal bacterial/fungal infections	• Occurs in hypoxic cell injury • Due to protein denaturation • Intracellular organelles are disrupted but the shape of tissues is maintained because the proteins stick together	• Features between colliquative and coagulative necrosis • Tissues become semi-solid/liquid	• Due to immune-mediated vascular injury causing fibrin-like protein deposits in arterial walls

Fat necrosis
• Due to action of lipase • Tissues aquire a chalky appearance • Seen in breast, pancreas, omentum, and skin

- Pigments such as
  - i. Lipofuscin
    - It is the end product of free radical injury
    - Brown in colour
  - ii. Melanin (derived from tyrosine)
  - iii. Haemosiderin

11. Cellular ageing process
- Replicative senescence
  - i. Is the concept that cells have a limited capability for replication
  - ii. After a fixed number of divisions all cells become arrested in a terminally non-dividing state
  - iii. Caused by telomere (short repeated sequences of DNA present at the ends of chromosome) shortening
- Telomerase
  - i. Is a specialized enzyme composed of both RNA and protein that uses RNA as a template for adding nucleotides to the end of chromosomes
  - ii. Maintains length of telomere
  - iii. Prevents replicative senescence
  - iv. Its activity is
    - High in germ cells
    - Low in stem cells
    - Absent in somatic cells
    - Reactivated in cancer cells

- Free radical oxidative damage
- Genetic influence

Response to cell injury

1. **Physiological response to injury**
   - Immobility/rest
   - Loss of appetite
   - Catabolism

2. **Metabolic and systemic response to injury**
   - Is graded into
     i.   Minor – Increased HR/RR/temperature/WBC count
     ii. Major – SIRS/hypermetabolism/catabolism/multiorgan dysfunction syndrome (MODS)
   - Divided into ebb and flow phases (the 'ebb and flow model')
   - Ebb phase (shock phase)
     i.   Begins at the time of injury
     ii.   Lasts for 24–48 h
     iii. Characterized by hypovolaemia; reduced CO; decreased basal metabolic rate; hypothermia; lactic acidosis
     iv.   Predominant hormones are catecholamines; cortisol; aldosterone
     v.   It functions to conserve circulating volume and energy stores
   - Flow phase
     i.   It is a predominantly hypermetabolic phase
     ii.   Corresponds to SIRS
     iii. Divided in an initial catabolic phase (lasting 3–4 days) aimed at mobilizing energy stores and a later anabolic phase (lasting for weeks)
     iv.   Characterized by tissue oedema (vasodilation); increased CO; hypermetabolism; increased temperature; leucocytosis; increased oxygen consumption; increased gluconeogenesis
   - In the catabolic phase there is
     i.   Weight loss (muscle wasting approximately 500 g/day)
     ii.   Increased urinary nitrogen excretion (up to 20 g/day)
     iii. Once the body protein mass loss has reached 30–40% of the total, survival is unlikely
   - Consists of
     i.   An immunological response
     ii.   A neuroendocrine response

3. **The immunological response in injury evolves from a proinflammatory to a compensatory anti-inflammatory response (CARS)**
   - The proinflammatory response is mediated by the innate immune system
   - The innate immune system interacts with the adaptive immune system (T- and B-cells)
   - Proinflammatory cytokines (IL-1, TNF; IL-6; IL-8)
     i.   Produced in first 24 h
     ii.   Act directly on hypothalamus causing pyrexia (IL-6 mediated)
     iii. Act directly on skeletal muscles to induce proteolysis
     iv.   Induce acute phase proteins production in liver (IL-6 mediated)
     v.   Cause peripheral insulin resistance (can last for 2 weeks)
   - Proinflammatory response is followed rapidly by an increase in levels of cytokine antagonists (IL-1 receptor antagonist; TNF-soluble receptors I and II), leading to CARS

4. **Neuroendocrine response to injury**
   - Is biphasic

     i. Acute phase – active secretion of pituitary and counter-regulatory hormones (glucagon; cortisol; adrenaline)

    ii. Chronic phase – hypothalamic suppression and low serum levels of respective target organ hormones. Contributes to chronic wasting.

- Hormonal flow
  - i. Increased CRH from hypothalamus causes increased secretion of ACTH from anterior pituitary
  - ii. ACTH causes release of cortisol from adrenal glands
- Counter-regulatory hormones function to
  - i. Reduce insulin levels
  - ii. Increase metabolism
  - iii. Promote hepatic gluconeogenesis
  - iv. Promote adipocyte lipolysis
  - v. Promote skeletal muscle protein catabolism
  - vi. Inactivate peripheral thyroid hormone (T_3)
  - vii. Reduce testosterone levels
  - viii. Increase prolactin and GH in response to low levels of circulating IGF

5. **Energy expenditure is increased in trauma by 25% due to**
- Central thermo-dysregulation
- Increased sympathetic activity
- Abnormalities in wound circulation
  - i. Ischaemic areas produce lactate that is metabolized in Cori's cycle
  - ii. Hyperaemic areas cause increased CO
- Increased protein turnover

6. **Skeletal muscle protein metabolism in response to injury**
- Protein degradation occurs in peripheral tissues (skin, skeletal muscle, adipose tissue)
- Major site of protein loss is peripheral skeletal muscle, respiratory muscle, and GIT
- Muscle catabolism cannot be inhibited fully
- Muscle protein turnover rate = 1–2%/day

7. **Hepatic protein metabolism in injury**
- Liver protein turnover rate = 20%/day
- Hepatic protein synthesis is divided roughly 50 : 50 between renewal of structural protein and synthesis of export protein (albumin)
- During inflammation
  - i. Hepatic synthesis of positive acute phase protein (fibrinogen and C-reactive protein (CRP)) is increased
  - ii. Serum albumin levels are decreased due to transcapillary escape

Wound healing

1. **Wound healing has 3 phases**
- Inflammatory
  - i. Starts immediately
  - ii. Last 2–3 days
  - iii. Local vasoconstriction
  - iv. Thrombus formation and fibrin mesh
  - v. Platelets line the damaged endothelium and release ADP/platelet-derived growth factor (PDGF)/cytokines/histamine/serotonin/prostaglandins

      vi. ADP causes thrombus aggregation

      vii. Cytokines attract lymphocytes and macrophages

      viii. Histamine causes increased capillary permeability

- Proliferative
  - i.   Lasts from day 3 to week 3
  - ii. Increased fibroblast activity producing collagen type 3 and ground substance (requires vitamin C)
  - iii. Angiogenesis
  - iv. Re-epithelialization of wound surface
  - v. Formation of granulation tissue
- Remodelling
  - i.   Maturation of collagen (type 1 replaces type 3)
  - ii. Decrease in wound vascularity
  - iii. Wound contraction

2. **Classification of wound closure**
   - Primary intention
   - Secondary intention
   - Tertiary intention (also known as delayed primary intention)

3. **Primary intention healing**
   - Is **not** an acute inflammatory reaction
   - Process
     - i.   A fibrin-rich haematoma develops first
     - ii. Neutrophils appear at the margin of the wound within 24 h and move towards the fibrin clot
     - iii. Movement of epithelial cells from the wound edge deposit a basement membrane in 24–48 h
     - iv. Macrophages replace the neutrophils at day 3
     - v. Granulation tissue invasion takes place
     - vi. Neovascularization occurs and is maximal at day 5
     - vii. Fibroblast proliferation at week 2
     - viii. Scar is devoid of inflammatory cells by week 4

4. **Secondary intention healing**
   - Heals by granulation, contraction, and epithelialization
   - Is marked by wound contraction (5–10% reduction in size)
   - Requires action of myofibroblast

5. **Wound strength (skin)**
   - At week 1 strength is at 10% that of un-wounded skin
   - At 3 months it is 80% that of un-wounded skin

6. **Growth factors involved in healing**
   - EGF
   - TGF
   - VEGF (vascular endothelial growth factor)
   - PDGF
   - FGF (fibroblast growth factor)
   - IGF

7. **Wound healing is**
   - Promoted by
     - i.   Good blood supply
     - ii. Vitamin C

    iii. Zinc
    iv. Protein
    v. Insulin
    vi. UV light
- Inhibited by
    i. Glucocorticoids
    ii. Infection
    iii. Extreme temperatures

Chpt 9

8. **Scar**
- Matures over 2 years
- Immature scar is
    i. Pink
    ii. Hard
    iii. Raised
    iv. Itchy
- Types of mature scar
    i. Atrophic
    ii. Hypertrophic (defined as excessive scar tissue that does not extend beyond the boundaries of the original wound) – due to the excessive production of granulation tissue
    iii. Keloid (defined as excessive scar tissue that extends beyond the boundaries of the original wound) due to the persistence of type 3 collagen
- Treatment of keloid/hypertrophic scar is by
    i. Excision of scar
    ii. Laser
    iii. Intralesion steroid injection
    iv. Pressure
    v. Silicone gel sheeting
    vi. Postoperative radiation
    vii. Vitamin E
- Surgical scarring can be reduced by
    i. Use of monofilament sutures
    ii. Removal of sutures at day 3–5
    iii. Tensionless suturing
    iv. Use of fine sutures and using Steri-Strips to strengthen the wound
    v. Subcuticular suturing technique

Neoplasia

1. **Neoplasia**
- Means 'new growth'
- Characterized by
    i. Abnormal growth
    ii. Uncontrolled growth
    iii. Uncoordinated growth
- Growth persists after cessation of stimuli

2. **Malignant neoplasia characterized by**
- Invasion
- Rapid growth
- Metastases
- Poor differentiation

3. **Definitions**
   - Carcinoma is malignancy of **epithelial** origin
   - Sarcoma is malignancy of **mesenchymal** origin
   - Teratoma is a neoplasm containing more than one germ cell layer
     i.   Ovarian teratoma is benign
     ii. Testicular teratoma is malignant
   - Choristoma is a non-malignant mass of normal tissue in an ectopic location
   - Hamartoma is a non-malignant mass of disorganized but mature tissue indigenous to the site

4. **Growth of a tumour**
   - Is gompertzian (i.e. in early stages growth is exponential but as the tumour grows the growth rate slows)
   - Majority occurs before it is clinically detectable
   - A radiologically detectable tumour is
     i.   10 mm in size
     ii. Has 10^9 cells
   - 2^n describes the number of cells produced after 'n' generations of division
     i.   E.g. $10^9 = 2^{30}$ since after the 30th division there will be 10^9 cells
   - Tumour size that is usually fatal = 2^{45} (i.e. after 45 generations)
     i.   However, there is also concurrent tumour loss, which reduces the number of tumour cells

5. **Features of malignant transformation**
   - Establishment of an autonomous lineage
     i.   Resisting signals that inhibit growth
     ii. Acquisition of independence from signal-stimulating growth
     iii. Oncogenes are a key factor in this process
   - Obtaining immortality
     i.   Normal cells undergo a finite number of division (i.e. between 40 and 60)
     ii. This limitation is imposed by the progressive shortening of the end of the chromosomes (the telomere)
     iii. Cancer cells do not undergo telomeric shortening
   - Evasion of apoptosis (p53 is responsible for apoptosis)
   - Acquisition of angiogenic competence
   - Acquisition of ability to invade (invasion)
   - Acquisition of ability to disseminate and implant
   - Evading detection and elimination
   - Genomic instability

6. **Differentiation**
   - It refers to the extent to which neoplastic cells resemble normal cells
   - Benign tumours are well differentiated (i.e. morphologically and functionally similar to mature normal cells)
   - Anaplasia is lack of differentiation
   - A high-grade tumour is one that is poorly differentiated

7. **Metastasis**
   - All cancers can metastasize except for basal cell carcinoma and gliomas
   - Occurs via (*Box 7.4*)

8. **Inherited genetic predisposition to cancer includes**
   - Inherited cancer syndromes (are autosomal dominant)
     i.   Retinoblastoma
     ii. Adenomatous polyposis coli
     iii. MEN

Box 7.4 Routes of metastasis

Lymphatic	Blood	Body cavity
• Typical of carcinoma	Typical of • Sarcoma • Renal cell carcinoma • Osteosarcoma • Choriocarcinoma	Typical of • Ovarian cancer • Breast cancer • Pseudomyxoma peritonei

    iv. Neurofibromatosis 1 and 2
    v. von Hippel–Lindau syndrome
- Inherited autosomal recessive syndromes of defective DNA repair
    i. Xeroderma pigmentosum
    ii. Ataxia-telangiectasia
    iii. Bloom's syndrome
    iv. Fanconi's anaemia
- Familial cancers
    i. Breast cancer
    ii. Ovarian cancer
    iii. Hereditary non-polyposis colonic cancer (HNPCC)

9. Cancer genes include
- BRCA genes
- *HNPCC*
- *RB* gene (retinoblastoma)
- *p16* (melanoma)

10. *BRCA* genes
- *BRCA*-1 gene
    i. Located on the long arm of chromosome 17
    ii. Predisposes to
      ■ Breast cancer
      ■ Ovarian cancer
- *BRCA*-2 gene
    i. Located on the long arm of chromosome 13
    ii. Predisposes to
      ■ Breast cancer
      ■ Male breast cancer
      ■ Ovarian
      ■ Prostate cancer
      ■ Pancreatic cancer
- 85% lifetime risk of developing breast cancer
- Lifetime risk of ovarian cancer is
    i. 55% with *BRCA-1*
    ii. 25% with *BRCA-2*

11. HNPCC
- Also known as Lynch's syndrome
- Has an autosomal dominant inheritance
- Has 5 genes
- Has 80% lifetime risk of colonic cancer
- Has 30–50% lifetime risk of endometrial cancer
- Has 10% lifetime risk of ovarian cancer

12. Non-genetic predisposing factors to cancer include
- Chronic inflammation
  - i. Crohn's disease
  - ii. Ulcerative colitis
- Pre-cancerous conditions
  - i. Leukoplakia
  - ii. Solar keratosis
  - iii. Pernicious anaemia
  - iv. Cervical dysplasia
- Carcinogenic agents (*Table 7.1*)

Table 7.1 Carcinogenic agents

Carcinogen	Neoplasm
Wood dust	Adenocarcinoma of nose and nasal sinuses
Aflatoxin B1	Hepatocellular carcinoma
Asbestos	Mesothelioma GIT cancers Bronchogenic carcinoma
Vinyl chloride	Haemangiosarcoma of liver
Chromium and nickel	Lung cancer
Arsenic	Skin cancer
Diethylstilbestrol	Vaginal clear cell carcinoma
High fat/low fibre	Colonic carcinoma
Alkylating agents	Lymphoma Leukaemia
Aniline dye β-naphthylamine	Bladder cancer
Polycyclic aromatic hydrocarbon	Lung cancer
Anabolic steroids	Hepatocellular carcinoma
Human papillomavirus (HPV) 16 and 18	Cervical cancer
Epstein–Barr virus	Burkitt's lymphoma Nasopharyngeal carcinoma
Hepatitis B virus	Hepatocellular carcinoma
Human T-cell lymphotrophic virus (HTLV)-1	T-cell leukaemia Lymphoma

13. Tumour markers (*Table 7.2*)

14. Paraneoplastic syndromes (*Table 7.3*)
- Are symptom complexes in cancer patients
- Are not due to the spread of cancer but due to their endocrine function or immunological response

15. p53
- Is a transcription factor that regulates cell cycle

Table 7.2 Tumour markers

Marker	Neoplasm
hCG	Trophoblastic tumour (choriocarcinoma) Non-seminomatous germ cell tumour
Calcitonin	Medullary carcinoma of thyroid
Catecholamines	Phaeochromocytoma
AFP	Hepatocellular carcinoma Non-seminomatous germ cell tumour (YST)
Carcinoembryonic antigen (CEA)	Colonic carcinoma Pancreatic carcinoma Gastric carcinoma Lung cancer
PSA/PAP	Prostatic neoplasm
Immunoglobulins	Multiple myeloma
CA 125	Ovarian carcinoma Primary peritoneal carcinoma
CA 19-9	Colonic carcinoma Pancreatic carcinoma
CA 15-3	Breast carcinoma

Table 7.3 Paraneoplastic syndromes

Paraneoplastic syndrome	Neoplasm
Cushing's syndrome	Small cell lung cancer Pancreatic carcinoma
SIADH	Small cell lung cancer Intracranial neoplasm
Carcinoid syndrome	Bronchial adenoma Pancreatic carcinoma Gastric carcinoma
Polycythaemia	Renal cell carcinoma Cerebellar haemangioma Hepatocellular carcinoma Fibroid (leiomyoma)
Myasthenia	Bronchogenic carcinoma
Acanthosis nigrans	Lung carcinoma Uterine carcinoma
Dermatomyositis	Bronchogenic carcinoma Breast carcinoma
Venous thrombosis Trousseau's phenomenon	Bronchogenic carcinoma Pancreatic carcinoma

- Is a tumour suppressor
- Gene located on chromosome 17
- Functions
  i. Activates DNA repair
  ii. Initiates apoptosis
- Li-Fraumeni syndrome
  i. Is an autosomal dominant disorder
  ii. Linked to mutation of *p53* gene
  iii. Has a 25-fold greater chance of developing malignancy by the age of 50 compared to the general population

Coagulation

Coagulation system

1. **The endothelium has both anti-thrombotic and pro-thrombotic properties** (*Fig. 7.3*)
   - Anti-thrombotic agents (*Box 7.5*)
   - Pro-thrombotic agents (*Box 7.6*)

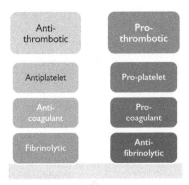

Figure 7.3 Anti-thrombotic and pro-thrombotic properties of endothelium

Box 7.5 Types of anti-thrombotic agents

Anti platelet	Anti coagulant	Fibrinolytic
• Prostacyclin • NO • ADPase	• Thrombomodulin • Anti-thrombin III • Tissue factor pathway inhibitor	• Tissue-type plasminogen activator (t-PA)

Box 7.6 Types of pro-thrombotic agents

Pro-platelet	Pro-coagulant	Anti-fibrinolytic
• von Willebrand Factor (vWF)	• Thromboplastin	• Plasminogen activator inhibitor

2. **Tissue factor pathway inhibitor – inhibits activated factor VIIa and Xa**

3. Platelets
- Contain
  - i.   Fibrinogen
  - ii. Fibronectin
  - iii. PDGF
  - iv. Histamine
  - v.   Serotonin
  - vi. Factor V and VIII
- Platelet aggregation induced by
  - i.   vWF
  - ii. ADP
  - iii. Thromboxane A_2
- Form part of the haemostatic plug formation process (**Box 7.7**)

Box 7.7 Haemostatic plug formation process

Primary haemostatic plug	Secondary haemostatic plug	Fibrin binds to plug
• Platelet aggregation • Reversible	• Thrombin binds to platelets • Irreversible	• ADP mediated activation of platelets causes changes to the platelet surface Gp2b-3a receptor for fibrinogen, causing fibrin to form and bind to the plug

4. Coagulation cascade
- Intrinsic pathway (**Fig. 7.4**)
- Extrinsic pathway (**Fig. 7.5**)
- Both the extrinsic and intrinsic pathways act on the common pathway via activation of factor IX (**Fig. 7.6**)
- Common pathway (**Fig. 7.7**)
- Final pathway (Fig. 7.8)

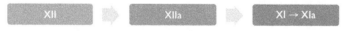

Figure 7.4 Coagulation cascade (Step 1)

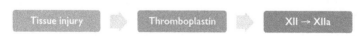

Figure 7.5 Coagulation cascade (Step 2)

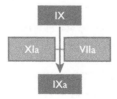

Figure 7.6 Coagulation cascade (Step 3)

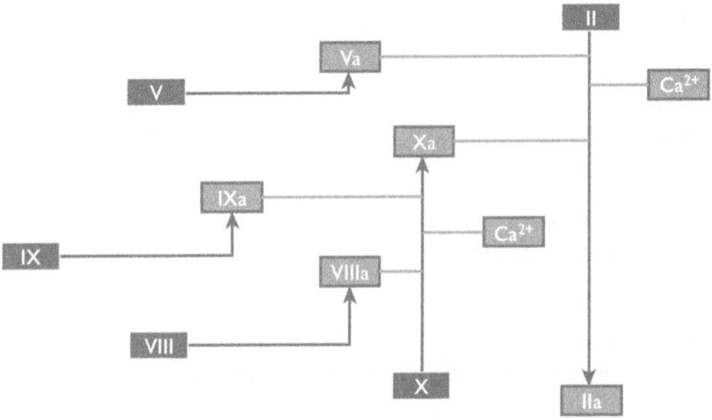

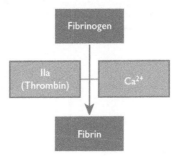

Figure 7.7 Coagulation cascade (Step 4)

Figure 7.8 Coagulation cascade (Step 5)

5. **Protein C**
   - Is a physiological anticoagulant
   - Degrades factor Va and VIIIa
   - Activated by thrombin

6. **Protein S**
   - Cofactor with activated protein C for the degradation of factor Va and VIIIa
   - Is an anticoagulant
   - Binds to complement factors

7. **Factor V Leiden**
   - Is a variant of factor V that cannot be inactivated by protein C
   - Causes a hypercoagulant state
   - An autosomal dominant condition
   - Prevalence in Caucasians is 5%
   - Is present in 30% of patients with deep vein thrombosis (DVT) and pulmonary embolism (PE)

8. **Fibrinolytic cascade**
   - Accomplished by generation of plasmin
   - Plasminogen conversion to plasmin is via
      i. Hageman dependent pathway

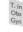

ii. Plasminogen activators (PA)
  - Urokinase-like PA
  - Tissue-type PA (t-PA)

T. in Obs Gyn Chpt 6.2

9. **Changes in pregnancy**
   - Physiological drop of platelet levels (due to haemodilution despite increased platelet production)
   - Hypercoagulant state – caused by increased levels of coagulant factors (all except factors XI and XIII)
   - Increased fibrinogen levels
   - Increased ESR
   - Fibrinolytic system
     i. Placenta secretes PAI-2, which inhibits fibrinolytic system
     ii. Increased anti-thrombin III levels
     iii. Increased FDPs
     iv. Activity remains low in labour
     v. Returns to normal 1 h after delivery of placenta

Coagulation abnormalities

1. **Thrombosis**
   - Pathogenesis is based on Virchow's triad
     i. Endothelial injury
     ii. Stasis
     iii. Hypercoagulability
   - Hypercoagulability states are due to
     i. Primary (genetic) disorders
       - Protein C deficiency
       - Protein S deficiency
       - Anti-thrombin III deficiency
       - Factor V Leiden
     ii. Secondary (acquired)
       - Pregnancy
       - Combined contraceptive pill
       - Antiphospholipid antibodies
       - Nephrotic syndrome
       - Trousseau's syndrome
       - Heparin-induced thrombocytopenia syndrome
   - Fate of thrombus
     i. Propagation
     ii. Embolization
     iii. Dissolution
     iv. Organization and recanalization
   - Types of thrombosis
     i. Venous
     ii. Arterial
     iii. Cardiac

T. in Obs Gyn Chpt 7.27

2. **Antiphospholipid syndrome (APS)**
   - Also known as Hughes' syndrome
   - Is characterized by a triad of
     i. Thrombosis (arterial and venous)
     ii. Recurrent miscarriage

      iii. Presence of antiphospholipid antibody
- Is an autoimmune disease
- Clinical features
  - i. Recurrent venous or arterial thrombi
  - ii. Recurrent miscarriages (i.e. >3 consecutive miscarriages <10 weeks gestation)
  - iii. Pre-eclampsia
  - iv. Preterm deliveries
  - v. Fetal death
  - vi. Thrombocytopenia
  - vii. Cardiac valvular vegetations
  - viii. Livido reticularis
- Types
  - i. Primary (when not associated with any other autoimmune conditions)
  - ii. Secondary (associated with other autoimmune conditions, e.g. SLE)
- Fetal loss in women with APS is due to
  - i. Pro-coagulant state caused by antiphospholipid antibody
  - ii. Decreased levels of annexin-V (an anticoagulant on normal placental villi)
- Treatment is
  - i. Aspirin
  - ii. Anticoagulants (low molecular weight heparin (LMWH))

3. **Antiphospholipid antibodies**
   - Are a group of heterogeneous antibodies directed against anionic phospholipids or their binding proteins which include
     - i. Prothrombin
     - ii. Factor V
     - iii. Protein C and S
     - iv. Annexin-V
   - Consist of
     - i. Lupus anticoagulant
     - ii. Anticardiolipin antibodies
   - Prevalence in
     - i. Normal obstetric population = 2–5 %
     - ii. Patients with recurrent miscarriage = 15%
     - iii. SLE women = 30%

4. **Trousseau's syndrome**
   - Is also known as migratory thrombophlebitis
   - Associated with underlying malignancy

5. **Heparin-induced thrombocytopenia syndrome**
   - Is caused by the formation of antibodies that bind to the heparin–platelet complex
   - Activates platelets
   - Clinical features
     - i. Low platelet count
     - ii. Thrombosis
   - Treatment is with lepirudin

6. **Disseminated intravascular coagulation (DIC)**
   - Is also known as consumptive coagulopathy
   - Aetiology
     - i. Cancer
     - ii. Massive tissue injury

     iii. Massive haemorrhage

     iv. Infection

     v. Liver disease

     vi. Placental abruption

     vii. Pre-eclampsia

     viii. Amniotic fluid embolism

- Clinical features and lab findings
  i. Prolonged clotting time (increased prothrombin time (PT) and activated partial thromboplastin time (APTT))
  ii. High levels of FDPs
  iii. Increased soluble fibrin complex
  iv. Decreased levels of fibrinogen
  v. High levels of D-dimers
  vi. Thrombocytopenia
  vii. Fragmented RBCs (schistocytes) on blood film

7. Embolism

- Types include
  i. Pulmonary thromboembolism
  ii. Systemic thromboembolism
  iii. Fat embolism
  iv. Air embolism (symptoms seen only in an embolus >100 mL of air)
  v. Amniotic fluid embolism
- PE
  i. 60% are silent
  ii. Results in cor pulmonale
- Clinical features of fat embolism
  i. Neurological symptoms
  ii. Pulmonary insufficiency
  iii. Anaemia
  iv. Thrombocytopenia
- Decompression sickness
  i. Is a form of air embolism
  ii. Is also known as Bends' or Caisson's disease
- Amniotic fluid embolism
  i. Incidence is 1 : 8000–80 000 deliveries
  ii. Mortality rate of up to 60%

T. in
Obs
Gyn

Chpt 10.1

T. in
Obs
Gyn

*Chpts 8.14
& 8.15*

8. Thrombocytopenia

- Aetiology (**Fig. 7.9**)
- Is prevalent in 5–10% of pregnancies at term
- Gestational thrombocytopenia
  i. Is a benign condition
  ii. Does not require treatment
  iii. Maternal platelets return to normal post delivery
- TTP/HUS
  i. Characterized by thrombocytopenia, microangiopathic haemolytic anaemia, and renal impairment
  ii. TTP is also associated with CNS involvement
  iii. Is a platelet consumption disorder leading to thrombocytopenia
  iv. Treatment = plasma exchange (platelet transfusion is contraindicated)

- Platelet count
  i.   >80 = regional anaesthesia is safe
  ii. >50 = LMWH thromboprophylaxis is safe

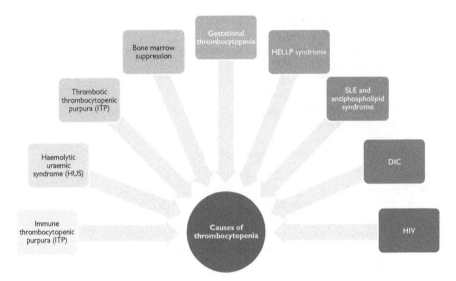

Figure 7.9 Causes of thrombocytopenia

9. ITP
- Is due to autoantibodies against platelet surface glycoproteins
- Incidence = 1–2 : 10 000 pregnancies
- Antiplatelet IgG
  i.   Can cross placenta
  ii. Can cause fetal thrombocytopenia (risk is 5–10%)
- Treatment of ITP
  i.   Corticosteroids (first-line therapy)
  ii. Immunoglobulins (in resistant cases)
  iii. Splenectomy
  iv. Azathioprine
  v.   Platelet transfusion

10. Infarction
- Is an area of ischaemic necrosis caused by occlusion of either the arterial supply or venous drainage to a tissue
- Aetiology
  i.   Thrombosis
  ii. Embolism
  iii. Vasospasm
  iv. Expansion of atheroma
  v.   Extrinsic compression of vessel
- Classification of infarcts (based on the colour; reflecting the amount of haemorrhage)
  i.   Red (haemorrhagic) – due to venous obstruction
  ii. White (anaemic) – due to arterial obstruction

Sepsis

1. Protective mechanisms against infection

- Mechanical
- Chemical – low pH
- Humoral – antibodies/complement
- Cellular – natural killer (NK) cells/macrophages

2. Septic ladder

- SIRS is defined as 2 of the following
  i.   Temp <36 °C or >38 °C
  ii. Tachycardia >90 bpm
  iii. Tachypnoea >20/ min
  iv. WBC <4 or >12
- Sepsis is defined as SIRS if it is a result of infection
- Severe sepsis is sepsis with evidence of failure of more than 1 organ system
- MODS leads to multiple organ system failure (MOSF)
- MODS
  i.   Is defined as 2 or more failed organ systems
  ii. Carries a 60% mortality rate

3. Abscess

- Is a collection of pus surrounded by an acute inflammatory response and a pyogenic membrane
- Contains hyperosmolar material that draws fluid in and increases the pressure causing pain
- Clinical features
  i.   Calor
  ii. Rubor
  iii. Dolor
  iv. Tumour
- Pus is composed of dead and dying WBCs
- Most abscesses relating to surgical wounds take 7–10 days to form
- Outcomes
  i.   Resolution via incision and drainage
  ii. Antibioma – if treated with antibiotics
  iii. Chronic abscess (contains plasma cells/lymphocytes)
  iv. Fistula
  v.   Sinus

4. Determinants of wound infection

- Host response
- Virulence and inoculums of infective agent
- Vascularity and tissue health
- Presence of foreign body
- Presence of antibiotics during the decisive period (decisive period is the 4 h taken to mobilize host defences)

5. Categories of surgery according to infection risk

- Clean (infection rate with antibiotic prophylaxis is 2%)
- Clean-contaminated (infection rate with antibiotic prophylaxis is 10%)
- Contaminated (infection rate with antibiotic prophylaxis is 20%)
- Dirty (infection rate with antibiotic prophylaxis is <40%)

Shock

1. Shock is a systemic state of low tissue perfusion, which is inadequate for normal cellular respiration

2. Shock pathogenesis
   - Lack of oxygen leads to metabolic acidosis (*Fig. 7.10*)
   - Consumption of cellular glucose stores leads to cessation of anaerobic respiration causing cell lysis (*Fig. 7.11*)
   - Microvascular – hypoxia and acidosis activate the immune and coagulation systems, leading to increased capillary permeability (*Fig. 7.12*)

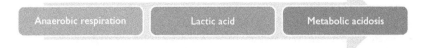

Figure 7.10 Shock pathogenesis 1

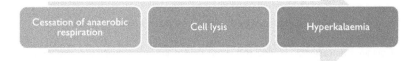

Figure 7.11 Shock pathogenesis 2

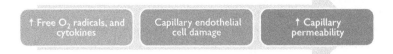

Figure 7.12 Shock pathogenesis 3

- Cardiovascular
  i. Decreased pre-load and after-load cause reflex tachycardia and vasoconstriction
  ii. Reduced perfusion leads to reduced heat generation (causing hypothermia)
- Respiration
  i. Metabolic acidosis causes an increased respiratory rate and minute ventilation (in an attempt to excrete CO_2)
  ii. A compensatory respiratory alkalosis results
- Renal
  i. Decreased filtration at glomeruli
  ii. Oliguria
  iii. Activation of renin–angiotensin system, leading to vasoconstriction
- Hormonal – release of
  i. ADH
  ii. Cortisol
- Acidosis leads to coagulopathy

3. **Ischaemia-reperfusion syndrome**
   - Metabolites (H^+ and K^+) that build up during tissue hypoperfusion are flushed back into the systemic circulation
   - This leads to
     i. Acute lung injury
     ii. Acute renal injury
     iii. MODS

4. **Classification of causes of shock (*Box 7.8*)**

Box 7.8 Causes of shock

Hypovolaemic	Cardiogenic	Obstructive	Distributive
• Haemorrhagic	• Myocardial infarction	• Tamponade	• Septic
• Non-haemorrhagic	• Arrhythmias without	• PE	• Anaphylactic
• 3rd spacing	output	• Pneumothorax	• Neurogenic

Endocrine
• Adrenal insufficiency
• Hypothyroidism
• Hyperthyroidism

5. **Characteristics of different types of shock**
   - Mixed venous saturation – only high in distributive shock
   - Venous pressure – high in obstructive and cardiogenic shock
   - CO – only high in distributive shock
   - Vascular resistance – only low in distributive shock
   - Base deficit – high in all types of shock

6. **Occult hypoperfusion**
   - Is a state characterized by normal vital signs but where there is continued tissue hypoperfusion
   - Manifests only by
     i. Low mixed venous oxygen saturation
     ii. Persistent lactic acidosis

7. **Dynamic fluid response**
   - Patients can be divided into 3 groups based on their response to a 250–500 mL of intravenous fluid challenge over 10 min
     i. Responders – show a sustained improvement (no active bleeding or fluid loss)
     ii. Transient responders – improve but revert back to their previous state over 20 min (have moderate ongoing fluid losses)
     iii. Non-responders – show no improvement (persistent uncontrolled haemorrhage or fluid loss)

8. **Central venous pressure (CVP)**
   - Normal CVP value = 5–15 cmH$_2$O
   - After an intravenous fluid challenge of 250–500 mL over 10 min
     i. The normal CVP response is a rise of 2–5 cmH$_2$O which gradually drifts back to the original level over 20 min
     ii. No CVP change indicates an underfilled patient
     iii. Large sustained CVP change indicates an overfilled patient

9. **Markers of global hypoperfusion**
   - Base deficit
   - Lactate (when >6 mmol/L patients have higher morbidity and mortality rates than those with no metabolic acidosis)

10. **Mixed venous oxygen saturation**
    - Is obtained from the right atrium
    - Is a measure of O_2 delivery and extraction by tissues
    - Normal value = 50–70%
    - Levels < 50% indicate
      i.   Inadequate oxygen delivery
      ii. Increased oxygen extraction
    - Levels >70% is seen in sepsis due to decreased utilization of O_2 at the cellular level

11. **Haemorrhage**
    - Leads to
      i.   Acidosis
      ii. Hypothermia
      iii. Coagulopathy
    - Degree of haemorrhage
      i.   <15% is within the limits of compensatory mechanisms (compensation is at the expense of GIT, muscle, and skin)
      ii. 15–30% (decompensation starts)
      iii. 30–40% (fall in BP detected)
      iv. >40%
    - 3 types of haemorrhage (**Box 7.9**)

Box 7.9 Types of haemorrhage

Primary	Reactionary	Secondary
• Occurs immediately	• Delayed haemorrhage within 24 h of primary event • Can be due to dislodgement of clot/vasodilation/normalization of BP	• Occurs within 7–14 days of primary event • Caused by sloughing of vessel wall

12. **Blood transfusion**
    - Packed red cells
      i.   Each unit has 330 mL red blood cells (RBC)
      ii. Each unit has 250 mg iron
      iii. Stored at 2–6 °C
      iv. Shelf life is 5 weeks
    - Fresh frozen plasma (FFP)
      i.   Stored at −40 °C
      ii. Shelf-life is 2 years
    - Cryoprecipitate (is rich in factor VIII and fibrinogen)
    - Platelets
      i.   Each pool contains 250×10^9 cells/L
      ii. Stored at 20–24 °C
      iii. Shelf-life is 5 days

13. Complications of transfusion can be divided into 2 groups

- Single transfusion
  i. Haemolytic transfusion reaction (due to ABO incompatibility)
  ii. Febrile transfusion reaction (non-haemolytic and due to graft versus host response from residual leucocytes in blood)
  iii. Allergic reaction
  iv. Infections
  v. Air embolism
  vi. Thrombophlebitis
  vii. Transfusion-related acute lung injury (from FFP)
- Massive transfusion
  i. Coagulopathy
  ii. Hypocalcaemia
  iii. Hyperkalaemia
  iv. Hypokalaemia
  v. Hypothermia
  vi. Iron overload

14. Management of transfusion induced coagulopathy

- FFP if PT >1.5 × normal
- Cryoprecipitate if fibrinogen <0.8 g/L
- Platelets if platelets <50 × 10^9/mL
- Tranexamic acid
- Aprotinin
- Recombinant factor VIIa (NovoSeven®)

15. Blood substitutes

- Biomimetics
  i. Mimic the standard oxygen-carrying capacity of blood
  ii. Haemoglobin based
- Abiotics
  i. Synthetic oxygen carriers
  ii. Perfluorocarbon based

Disorders of the genital tract

T. in
Obs
Gyn

Chpts
15.2–15.4

Cervical pathology

1. Cervical screening in the UK

- Routine age range of 20–64 (25–60 in England)
- Every
  i. 3 years in 25–49 year olds
  ii. 5 years in 50–65 year olds
- Statistics
  i. Screening false negative is 10%
  ii. Pap-smear false negative is 50%
- Incidence of
  i. Borderline and mild dyskaryosis is 10%
  ii. Moderate and severe dyskaryosis is 1–2%
  iii. Inadequate smears is 10%

2. **Cervical intraepithelial neoplasia (CIN)**
   - Is a
     i. Form of cervical dysplasia
     ii. A premalignant condition
   - Major aetiology is HPV 16 and 18
   - Most CINs spontaneously regress (50% of CIN 2 will regress within 2 years without treatment)
   - Progression to cancer takes about 15 years
   - Cytological characteristics include
     i. Nuclear enlargement
     ii. Increased nuclear : cytoplasmic ratio
     iii. Nuclear pleomorphism
     iv. Hypochromasia
     v. Increased mitotic activity
   - Evolution over 5 years
     i. CIN 3
        - 32% regress
        - 55% remains persistent
        - 12% progress to invasive cancer
     ii. CIN 2
        - 43% regress
        - 35% remain persistent
        - 5% progress to invasive cancer

3. **Cervical glandular intraepithelial neoplasia (CGIN)**
   - Usually coexists with squamous disease
   - Is multifocal in 15%
   - Incidence of smears showing CGIN is 1 : 2000
   - Ratio of CGIN : CIN is 1 : 50
   - Risk of recurrence following treatment is 15%

4. **Cervical cancer**
   - Incidence is 9 : 100 000
   - Is the commonest gynaecological cancer worldwide
   - Mean age of presentation = 52 years old
   - Distribution is bimodal with peaks at
     i. 35–39 years old
     ii. 60–64 years old
   - Lifetime risk in
     i. Europe = 1%
     ii. Asia/Africa = 5%
   - 99.7% of cervical cancers are due to all types of HPV
   - 70% of cervical cancers are due to HPV 16 and HPV 18
   - Types
     i. Squamous cell carcinoma (80%)
     ii. Adenocarcinoma (15%)
     iii. Adenosquamous carcinoma
     iv. Rare (< 1%)
        - Small cell carcinoma (is a type of neuroendocrine tumour that carries a poor prognosis due to early lymphatic and systemic spread; may present with carcinoid syndrome)
        - Clear cell carcinoma

- ▪ Glassy cell carcinoma
- ▪ Sarcoma Botryoides (i.e. a type of embryonal rhabdomyosarcoma)
- Staging (*Table 7.4*)

Table 7.4 FIGO 2010 classification of cervical cancer

FIGO classification of cervical cancer		Treatment
Stage 0	Carcinoma *in situ*	
Stage 1	Limited to cervix: micro-invasive lesion	Hysterectomy or
	$1A_1$ Depth <3 mm Length <7 mm	Large loop excision of the transformation zone (LLETZ) or
	$1A_2$ Depth 3–5 mm Length <7 mm	trachelectomy
	Limited to cervix: visible lesion	Radical hysterectomy
	$1B_1$ Lesion <4 cm	and
	$1B_2$ Lesion >4 cm	lymphadenectomy
Stage 2	Invades beyond uterus but not to pelvic wall or lower 1/3 of vagina	Radiation therapy and cisplatin-based chemotherapy and
	2A Without parametrial invasion	hysterectomy
	2B With parametrial invasion	
Stage 3	Extends to pelvic side wall or lower 1/3 of vagina or hydronephrosis	Radiation therapy and cisplatin-based chemotherapy
	3A No pelvic side wall involvement	
	3B Pelvic side wall involvement or hydronephrosis	
Stage 4	Extends beyond true pelvis	Radiation therapy and cisplatin-based chemotherapy
	4A Invades mucosa of bladder and rectum	
	4B Distant metastasis	

- Risk of lymph node involvement
  - i. In stage $1A_1$ is 1 in 3000
  - ii. In stage $1A_2$ is 5%
  - iii. In stage 2A is 25%
  - iv. In stage 3 is 45%
  - v. In stage 4a is 55%

Uterine pathology

Chpts 12.5 & 12.6

1. Uterine fibroids (also known as uterine leiomyomas)
- Affects 20–40% of women in the reproductive age
- Oestrogen-dependent benign tumours
- Arise from uterine smooth muscle
- Well circumscribed
- There is no conclusive evidence that benign fibroids can become malignant
- The risk of malignant transformation to leiomyosarcoma in rapidly growing fibroids is 0.25%
- Intravenous leiomyomatosis
  - i. Is a variant fibroid

ii.   Can metastasize via haematological spread

iii. Can occur in any organ

Chpt 13.2

2. **Endometriosis**
   - Disease characterized by the occurrence of ectopic endometrium
   - Frequent sites
     i.   Pouch of Douglas
     ii. Ovaries
   - Occurs in women of fertile age
   - Prevalence is 1–2%
   - Aetiology is unknown
   - Theories
     i.   Oestrogen dependent
     ii.   Genetic
     iii. Transplantation
     iv.   Retrograde implantation of endometrium from menstruation
     v.   Coelomic epithelium metaplasia
   - Endometriotic tissue consists of
     i.   Endometrial stroma
     ii. Glands
   - Can be associated with cancers (clear cell carcinoma)
   - Symptoms include
     i.   Dysmenorrhoea
     ii.   Dyspareunia
     iii. Dyschezia
     iv.   Dysuria
     v.   Chronic pelvic pain
     vi.   Infertility in 40% of patients with endometriosis
   - CA-125 is elevated in endometriosis
   - Staging is based on the revised classification of the American Society of Reproductive Medicine
     i.   Stage 1 – superficial lesions and filmy adhesions
     ii.   Stage 2 – deep lesions at cul-de-sac
     iii. Stage 3 – all the above and endometriomas on ovaries
     iv.   Stage 4 – all the above and extensive adhesions

3. **Adenomyosis**
   - Is defined as presence of endometrial glands in the myometrium
   - Prevalence is 20%

4. **Endometrial hyperplasia**
   - Is related to prolonged oestrogen stimulation of the endometrium
   - Consists of 3 groups
     i.   Simple hyperplasia
     ii.   Complex hyperplasia
     iii. Atypical hyperplasia
   - Atypical hyperplasia has the highest rate of progression to malignancy (25%–50%)
   - Treatment is
     i.   Progestogens (for simple and complex hyperplasia)
     ii. Total abdominal hysterectomy and bilateral salpingo-oophorectomy (for atypical hyperplasia)

Chpts 15.5
& 15.6

5. **Endometrial cancer**
   - Risk factors (**Fig. 7.13**)

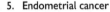

- Types (*Fig. 7.14*)
  - i.   Uterine adenocarcinoma
  - ii. Uterine carcinosarcoma
- Non-endometrioid carcinoma
  - i.   Is a poorly differentiated carcinoma

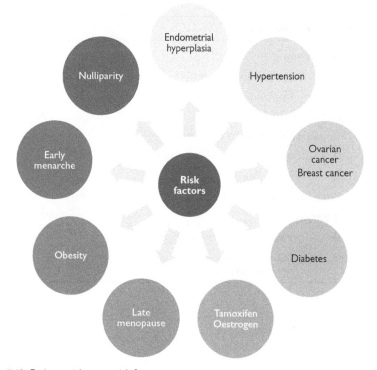

Figure 7.13 Endometrial cancer risk factors

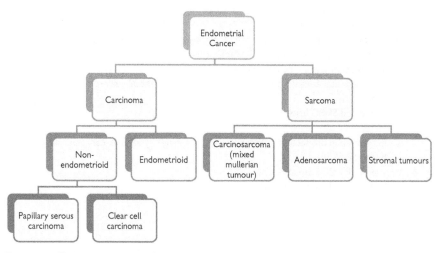

Figure 7.14 Endometrial cancer subtypes

ii. Resembles serous ovarian carcinoma

iii. Has a poorer prognosis

iv. Is managed the same as a grade 3 endometrial carcinomas

- Staging (*Table 7.5*)
- Carcinosarcomas have a 5-year survival of 25–30 %

Table 7.5 FIGO 2010 classification of uterine cancer

FIGO classification of uterine cancer			5-year survival
Stage 1	Limited to uterus		85–90%
	1A	Invasion <1/2 of myometrium	
	1B	Invasion >1/2 of myometrium	
Stage 2	Cervical stromal invasion		65%
Stage 3	Extension beyond uterus but confined to pelvis		45–60%
	3A	Invasion of uterine serosa, adnexa and peritoneal fluid	
	3B	Vaginal invasion	
	3C	Nodal involvement (C1 = pelvic and C2 = para-aortic)	
Stage 4	Distant metastasis		15%
	4A	Invasion of mucosa of rectum and bladder	
	4B	Distant metastases including abdominal metastases and/or inguinal lymph nodes	

T. in Obs Gyn

Chpt 12.11

PCOS

1. PCOS

- Prevalence is 5%
- Also known as Stein–Leventhal syndrome
- Diagnosis based on Rotterdam criteria (2 out of 3 to be met)
  i. Oligo-ovulation
  ii. Excess androgen activity
  iii. Polycystic ovaries on imaging (i.e. >12 follicles in each ovary measuring 2–9 mm in diameter or an ovarian volume >10 mL)
- High androgen levels are possibly due to
  i. Increased luteinizing hormone levels (cause increased thecal cell production of androgens)
  ii. Decreased SHBG levels
  iii. Increased insulin levels
  iv. Extra-ovarian production of androgens (e.g. Cushing's syndrome, congenital adrenal hyperplasia)
- Women with PCOS are at risk of
  i. Endometrial hyperplasia/neoplasia
  ii. Insulin resistance
  iii. Dyslipidaemia

Ovarian tumours

1. Primary ovarian cancer types are divided into 3 groups (*Box 7.10*)

Box 7.10 Types of primary ovarian cancer

Epithelial (85%)	Stromal (5%)	Germ cell (5%)

• Serous (75%)
• Mucinous
• Brenner's
• Clear cell
• Differentiated
• Endometrioid
• Fibroma
	• Sertoli–Leydig (testosterone-
	  secreting)
	• Thecofibroma
	• Granulosa (oestrogen-secreting)
		• Germinoma
		• Endodermal sinus tumour
		  (secretes AFP and α-antitrypsin)
		• Choriocarcinoma
		  (secretes hCG)
		• Teratoma
		• Embryonal (secretes LDH)

2. **Secondary ovarian cancer arise from**
   - Primary peritoneal cancer
   - Breast cancer
   - GIT cancer

3. **Germ cell tumour accounts for 70% of ovarian tumours in the under 20 age group**

4. **Krukenberg cancer**
   - Is secondary ovarian cancer from a gastrointestinal primary cancer
   - Characterized by appearance of mucin-secreting signet-ring cells
   - Usually affects both ovaries

5. **Teratomas**
   - Include
     i. Dermoid cysts (derived from all 3 germ cell layers)
     ii. Mature teratomas
     iii. Struma ovarii (contains mostly thyroid tissue) – only 5% are malignant
     iv. Carcinoid component
   - Benign teratomas
     i. Are the commonest ovarian tumour (accounts for 40% of all ovarian tumours)
     ii. Are bilateral in 10–15%
     iii. 1% undergo malignant transformation
   - Struma ovarii may cause hyperthyroidism

6. **5-year survival rate for all stages of ovarian cancer is 45.5%**

7. **30% of ovarian adenocarcinomas express *HER2* oncogenes**

8. **Ovarian endometrioid carcinoma**
   - 15% coexist with endometriosis
   - 15–30% are associated with uterine endometrial carcinoma

9. **Brenner's tumour**
   - Is composed of transitional cells
   - Secretes oestrogen
   - Mostly benign
   - 15% are bilateral

10. **Dysgerminomas**
    - Are the commonest malignant germ cell tumours
    - Are female equivalent to a seminoma
    - Bilateral in 20%
    - Are extremely radiosensitive

11. Fibroma-thecomas

- Pure thecomas are rare
- Associated with
  i. Meigs' syndrome (ovarian tumour, hydrothorax (more common on the right side), and ascites)
  ii. Basal cell nevus syndrome

12. Granulosa-theca cell tumour

- Secretes oestrogen
- May produce
  i. Endometrial hyperplasia
  ii. Precocious sexual development
- Risk of endometrial carcinoma in 10–15% of patients

13. Leydig cell tumour

- Also known as hilus cell tumour
- Derived from theca cells
- Reinke crystalloids are present in the cytoplasm of the Leydig cell
- Are unilateral
- Associated with elevated levels of 17-ketosteroid
- Almost always benign

14. Tumour markers

- Biochemical
  i. CA 125 (elevated in 50% with early disease & 80% in late disease)
  ii. CA 119 (elevated in mucinous epithelial ovarian cancer)
  iii. CEA
  iv. AFP
  v. β-HCG
  vi. Lactate dehydrogenase (LDH)
- Cytokeratins
  i. CK 7 positive
  ii. CK 20 negative
- Risk of malignancy index (RMI) = CA 125 × menopausal status × ultrasound features
  i. Premenopausal score = 1
  ii. Postmenopausal score = 3
  iii. >1 ultrasound feature seen = 3
  iv. RMI >200 is highly indicative of malignancy

14. Staging (*Table 7.6*)

Chpts 13.9, 15.11, & 15.12 *Vulval and vaginal pathology*

1. Lichen sclerosis

- Also known as chronic atrophic vulvitis
- Affects women of all ages
- Common after menopause
- Clinical features
  i. Narrowed introitus
  ii. Labial atrophy
- Cardinal histological features
  i. Epidermal atrophy
  ii. Hydropic degeneration of the basal layer
  iii. Dermal inflammation

iv. Sclerotic stroma
- May be associated with squamous vulval carcinoma in 5%

Table 7.6 FIGO 2010 classification of ovarian carcinoma

FIGO classification of ovarian carcinoma		
Stage 1	Limited to 1 or both ovaries	
	1A	Involves 1 ovary Peritoneal washing's negative
	1B	Involves both ovaries Peritoneal washing's negative
	1C	Capsule ruptures Peritoneal washing's positive
Stage 2	Pelvic extensions	
	2A	Implants on uterus
	2B	Implants on pelvic structure
	2C	Peritoneal washing's positive
Stage 3	Peritoneal implants beyond pelvis or with extension to small bowel/omentum	
	3A	Microscopic implants
	3B	Macroscopic implants <2 cm
	3C	Macroscopic implants >2 cm
Stage 4	Distant metastasis	

2. **Lichen simplex chronicus**
   - Also known as hyperplastic dystrophy
   - Is secondary to pruritus
   - Clinical features
     i. Acanthosis of vulval squamous epithelium
     ii. Hyperkeratosis
   - Histological features
     i. Thickened epithelium
     ii. Increased mitotic activity in basal and prickle cell layer

3. **Vulval intraepithelial neoplasia (VIN)**
   - Characterized by
     i. Epithelial nuclear atypia
     ii. Increased mitosis
     iii. Lack of surface differentiation
   - 90% of VIN is associated with HPV
   - 10–30% is associated with another primary squamous neoplasm in the vagina or cervix

4. **Extramammary Paget's disease**
   - Is a non-invasive intraepithelial adenocarcinoma
   - Not usually associated with underlying invasive malignancy
   - Can be associated with adenocarcinoma arising from
     i. Urethra

      ii. Rectum

      iii. Bartholin's gland

  • Clinical features of the lesion

      i.   Sharp demarcation

      ii. Erythematous

      iii. Pruritic

5. **Vulval cancer**
   - Incidence in UK = 3 : 100 000 women
   - Accounts for 4% of all gynaecological cancers
   - Median age of presentation = 74
   - Commonest symptom = itching (75%)
   - 10% of vulval cancer patients are under 40 years old
   - Types
     i.   Squamous cell carcinoma (85%)
     ii. Melanoma (5%)
     iii. Basal cell carcinoma (1%)
     iv. Adenocarcinoma
     v.   Sarcoma

6. **Vulval cancer staging (*Table 7.7*)**

Table 7.7 FIGO 2010 classification of vulval carcinoma

FIGO classification of vulval carcinoma		
Stage 1	Confined to vulva	
	1A	Lesions <2 cm in size with stromal invasion <1 mm
	1B	Lesions >2 cm in size with stromal invasion >1 mm
Stage 2	Extension to adjacent perineal structures	1/3 lower vagina
		1/3 lower urethra
		Anus
Stage 3	Positive inguino-femoral nodes	
	3A	<2 lymph node metastases
	3B	>2 lymph node metastases
	3C	With extracapsular spread
Stage 4	Extension to upper urethra and vagina	
	4A	Upper vagina
		Upper urethra
		Bladder
		Rectum
	4B	Distant metastases including pelvic lymph nodes

7. **Vaginal cancer**
   - Accounts for 1% of gynaecological malignancies
   - Primary carcinoma of the vagina is uncommon
   - Associated with HPV
   - Types
     i.   Squamous cell carcinoma (90%)
     ii. Adenocarcinoma (clear cell)
     iii. Germ cell tumours
     iv. Sarcoma Botryoides

Disorders in pregnancy

T. in
Obs
Gyn

Chpts
8.11–8.13

1. Pre-eclampsia

- Definition is blood pressure >140/90 with proteinuria after 20 weeks gestation (**Fig. 7.15**)

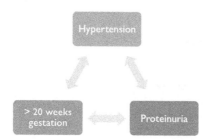

Figure 7.15 Triad of pre-eclampsia

- Prevalence of
  i. Hypertension is 10–15% of pregnancies
  ii. Pre-eclampsia is 2–3%
  iii. Eclampsia is 0.05% in the UK
  iv. Eclampsia in pre-eclamptic women is 2%
- Aetiology is unknown
- Pathophysiology is thought to be due to poor placentation causing
  i. Utero-placental resistance
  ii. Abnormal placental function
- Pre-eclampsia is a
  i. Vasoconstricted state
  ii. Plasma contracted state
- Associated with intravascular coagulation
- Associated with endothelial dysfunction
  i. Increased capillary permeability
  ii. Increased vascular tone
  iii. Increased fibronectin
  iv. Platelet thrombosis
- Biochemical changes
  i. Decreased nitric oxide by increasing ADMA
  ii. Increased thromboxane A_2, angiotensin, and endothelin
  iii. Decreased prostacyclin
- Classification (**Box 7.11**)

Box 7.11 Classification of pre-eclampsia

Mild	Severe
• BP > 140/90	• BP > 160/110
• Proteinuria 300 mg/24 h	• Proteinuria > 5 g/24 h

- Clinical features
  i. Symptoms
     - Headache
     - Visual disturbance
     - Epigastric/right upper quadrant pain

- Vomiting
- Ankle swelling
- Seizures

ii. Signs
- Hyper-reflexia
- Clonus
- Oliguria

iii. Investigations can show
- Deranged liver enzymes
- Low platelets
- Abnormal renal function
- Deranged clotting
- Elevated urinary protein

- Risk factors
  i.   Age >40 years old (doubles the risk of pre-eclampsia)
  ii. Body mass index (BMI) >30
  iii. Family history of pre-eclampsia (4 fold increase in pre-eclampsia risk)
  iv. Primiparity
  v.   Multiple pregnancy
  vi. Previous pre-eclampsia (7 fold increase in pre-eclampsia risk)
  vii. Hydatidiform mole
  viii. Triploidy
  ix. Pre-existing hypertension
  x.   Renal disease
  xi. Diabetes
  xii. Antiphospholipid syndrome

- Complications
  i.   Haemolysis, elevated liver enzymes, and low platelets (HELLP) syndrome
  ii. Placental abruption
  iii. FGR
  iv. Eclampsia
  v.   Pulmonary oedema
  vi. DIC
  vii. Commonest causes of death in pre-eclampsia are
    - Cerebral haemorrhage
    - ARDS

2. **Obstetric cholestasis**
   - Prevalence varies geographically. It is higher in
     i.   Scandinavia
     ii. Chile
     iii. Bolivia
     iv. China
   - Clinical features
     i.   Pruritus of limbs and trunk (mainly palms and soles)
     ii. No rash
     iii. Abnormal liver function tests
     iv. Jaundice is rare
   - Pathogenesis is multifactorial (genetic, environmental, endocrine) and is not well understood
   - Complications
     i.   Vitamin K deficiency
     ii. Postpartum haemorrhage

iii. Pre-term delivery

iv. Intrapartum fetal distress in 22%

v. Meconium-stained amniotic fluid in 25–45%

vi. Intrauterine fetal death (is 1–4% but with active management is comparable to the general population)

vii. Fetal intracranial haemorrhage

- Risk of recurrence is 90% in future pregnancies
- Affects 0.7% of pregnancies

3. **Acute fatty liver of pregnancy**

Chpt 8.14

- Prevalence is 1 : 9000–13 000 pregnancies
- Usually presents after 30 week gestation
- Risk factors
  i. Primigravida
  ii. Obesity
  iii. Male fetus (ratio 3 : 1)
  iv. Multiple pregnancy
- Maternal mortality is 10–20%
- Perinatal mortality is 20–30%
- Clinical features
  i. Vomiting
  ii. Abdominal pain
  iii. Jaundice
  iv. Abnormal liver function
  v. Profound hypoglycaemia
  vi. Marked hyperuricaemia
  vii. Coagulopathy
- Complications are
  i. Fulminant hepatic failure
  ii. Encephalopathy

4. **HELLP syndrome**

Chpt 8.14

- Incidence is 20% in women with severe pre-eclampsia
- Pathogenesis involves
  i. Endothelial cell injury
  ii. Microangiopathic platelet activation and consumption
- Effects on pregnancy
  i. Abruption
  ii. Acute renal failure
  iii. Hepatic necrosis
  iv. Liver rupture
  v. Subcapsular liver haematoma
  vi. Perinatal mortality = 10–60%
  vii. Maternal mortality = 1%
- Risk of recurrence in future pregnancies is 3–5%
- Risk of pre-eclampsia in future pregnancies is 75%

5. **Peripartum cardiomyopathy**
- Is a form of dilated cardiomyopathy
- Occurs between 8 months gestation to 5 months post partum
- Associated with
  i. Congestive heart failure
  ii. Decreased left ventricular ejection fraction

iii. Cardiac arrhythmias
iv. Thromboembolism
v. Sudden death
- The cause is unknown
- It is a diagnosis of exclusion
- Maternal mortality = 25–50%
- Management
  i. Diuretics
  ii. β-blockers
  iii. ACEi
  iv. Anticoagulation
  v. In refractory cases
    ■ Left ventricular assist device
    ■ Heart transplant

Pathology – specific blood tests

1. **Coombs' test**
   - 2 types
     i. Direct
     ii. Indirect
   - Is positive if agglutination occurs
   - Indirect Coombs' test
     i. Detects antibodies against RBCs present in patient's serum
     ii. Used for antibody screening (both for cross-matching and for antenatal screening)
   - Direct Coombs' test (*Box 7.12*)

Box 7.12 Diseases that give a positive direct Coombs test

Alloimmune haemolysis	Autoimmune haemolysis	Drug-induced immune-mediated haemolysis
- Haemolytic disease of newborn	- SLE - Idiopathic (primary cold haemagglutinin syndrome) - Secondary due to a lymphoproliferative disease or an infection such as infective mononucleosis (secondary cold haemagglutinin syndrome)	- Methyldopa - Penicillin - Quinidine

   i. Detects antibodies bound to RBC surface antigens
   ii. Indicates immune-mediated attack on RBCs

2. **Kleihauer's test**
   - Is used to measure the fetal RBCs in the maternal circulation
   - Normally fetal maternal haemorrhage is <4 mL at delivery
   - Anti-D immunoglobulin
     i. 500IU neutralizes 4mL of Rhesus positive RBC
     ii. Should be given within 72 h of sensitisation in non-sensitised Rhesus negative women
     iii. Provides protection for 6 weeks

CHAPTER 8

Immunology

CONTENTS

General immunology

1. **The immune system is divided into 2 functional units**
   - Innate
   - Adaptive

2. **Innate immune system**
   - Is the first line of defence
   - Also known as the non-specific immune system (i.e. its response is non-specific and antigen independent)
   - Is unchanged over time (i.e. has no memory)
   - Is fast to develop (within hours)
   - Consists of soluble and cellular mediators (*Box 8.1*)
   - Also includes anatomical barriers (e.g. skin and epithelial layers)

Box 8.1 Mediators of the innate immune system

Soluble mediators	Cellular mediators
• Complement system components	• Monocyte
• Coagulation system components	• Dendritic cells
• Lactoferrin and transferrin	• Neutrophil
• Interferon	• Eosinophil
• Cytokines and chemokines (e.g. interleukins)	• Mast cells
• Acute phase proteins (e.g. CRP)	• Basophil
	• Natural killer (NK) cells

3. **Adaptive immune system**
   - Is responsible for specific lymphocytic activity
   - Is slow to development (within days)
   - Has memory
   - Augments with time
   - Has immune tolerance to self (i.e. no immune response to self-antigens)

- Has diversity
- Has 2 arms
  i. Humoral immunity (antibody production)
  ii. Cellular immunity
- Consists of soluble and cellular mediators (*Box 8.2*)

Box 8.2 Mediators of the adaptive immune system

Soluble mediators	Cellular mediators
• Complement system components	• T-cell
• Antibodies	• B-cell
• Cytokines	• Antigen-pesenting cells

4. **Immune tolerance**
   - Is the process through which immune response to self-antigens is prevented
   - There are 3 forms
     i.   Central tolerance
     ii. Peripheral tolerance
     iii. Acquired tolerance
   - Prevents the development of autoimmunity
   - Central tolerance
     i. Occurs in the thymus and bone marrow
     ii. Begins in fetal life
   - Acquired tolerance includes the immune tolerance that occurs in pregnancy

5. **Hypersensitivity – there are 4 types (Box 8.3)**

Box 8.3 Types of hypersensitivity

Type 1 Mast cell mediated	Type 2 Complement mediated	Type 3 Antibody–antigen complex mediated	Type 4 T-cell mediated

• Mast cell degranulation
• Associated with IgE
• E.g.
  • Hay fever
  • Allergy
	• Antibody dependent
	• Activation of complement via classical pathway by IgM and IgG
	• E.g.
	  • Haemolytic disease of newborn
	  • Pernicious anaemia
	  • Transfusion
	  • Graves' disease
	  • Myasthenia gravis
	  • Autoimmune disease
	  • Food allergies
		• Immune complex deposition
		• Develops in ≈ 10 days
		• E.g.
		  • Rheumatoid arthritis
		  • SLE
		  • Glomerulonephritis
		  • Serum sickness
			• Cell-mediated reaction
			• Delayed reaction (takes ≈ 48 hrs to develop)
			• Involves T-cells
			• E.g.
			  • Graft rejection
			  • Contact sensitivity
			  • Symptom of TB
			  • Symptom of leprosy

6. **Transplantation**
   - Graft classifications
     i.   Autograft = from the same person
     ii. Allograft = from a different individual of the same species
     iii. Xenograft = from a different species

- Types of rejection
  - i. Hyperacute rejection = a severe immunological response to the graft that occurs within minutes to hours of transplantation (due to pre-formed host antibodies)
  - ii. Acute rejection = a primary immune response to the graft that occurs within days to weeks (due to the presence of donor leucocytes)
  - iii. Chronic rejection (occurs months to years after transplantation)

7. **There are 3 types of vaccine**
   - Attenuated (MMRBOYV), which are live organisms
     - i. Mumps
     - ii. Measles
     - iii. Rubella
     - iv. Bacille Calmette Guérin (BCG)
     - v. Polio (Sabin, which is oral)
     - vi. Yellow fever
     - vii. Varicella zoster
   - Killed
     - i. Cholera
     - ii. Polio (Salk, which is i.m.)
     - iii. Rabies
     - iv. Hepatitis A
   - Acellular – toxoid
     - i. Tetanus
     - ii. Diphtheria
   - Acellular – organism subunits
     - i. Pertussis (whooping cough)
     - ii. Hepatitis B
     - iii. Influenza
     - iv. *Neisseria meningitidis*

Soluble mediators

1. **Complement system**
   - Consists of approximately 30 proteins
   - Are a part of both the innate and adaptive immune systems
   - Synthesized in the liver
   - Present in inactive form in plasma
   - Constitutes 10% of total body protein
   - Activity is analogous to the coagulation cascade
   - Complement activation has 3 pathways
     - i. Classical
       - Requires antibody as a trigger
       - Fixation of C1 to IgG/M
     - ii. Alternative
       - Requires antigen as a trigger (e.g. lipopolysaccharides (LPS)/endotoxin)
     - iii. Mannose-binding lectin pathway
     - iv. All 3 pathways
       - Produce protease C3 convertase
       - Cleave C3 to C3a and C3b
   - Complement system functions
     - i. Opsonization (via C3b)
     - ii. Leucocyte adhesion, chemotaxis, and activation (via C5a)

iii. Cell lysis via membrane attack complex (MAC)
iv. Inflammatory mediator (via activation of lipoxygenase pathway of arachidonic acid metabolism by C5a)
v. Increase in vascular permeability (via C3a and C5a)
- Specific complement component functions
  i. C3b – opsonization
  ii. C3a and C5a
   - Have anaphylatoxin activity
   - Stimulate histamine release
  iii. C5a
   - Chemotaxis
   - Activates lipoxygenase pathway
  iv. C5b and C6-9 – cell lysis via MAC

2. **Interferons (IFN)**
 - Are glycoproteins
 - Are a class of cytokines
 - Functions
   i. Antiviral – inhibit viral replication within cells
   ii. Anti-oncogenic
   iii. Activate
    - NK cells
    - Macrophages
   iv. Upregulation of major histocompatibility complex (MHC) class 1
   v. Increased p53 activity (p53 promotes apoptosis)
 - Production of IFNs is induced by
   i. Microorganisms (via infected host cells)
   ii. Cytokines
 - 3 major classes of IFN
   i. IFN-1 (α)
   ii. IFN-2 (β and γ)
   iii. IFN-3

3. **CRP**
 - Is an acute phase serum protein
 - Coats pathogens to promote opsonization
 - Is produced by the liver
 - Gene is located on chromosome 1

4. **ESR (Box 8.4)**
 - Is a non-specific measure of inflammation
 - Basal ESR is higher in females
 - ESR (mm/H) = (Age (years) + 10 (if female))/2

Box 8.4 Causes of altered ESR level

ESR decreased in	ESR increased in
• Sickle cell	• Inflammation
• Polycythaemia	
• Heart failure	

5. **Cytokines**
   - Are group of proteins responsible for cellular signalling
   - Are produced by leucocytes and other body cells
   - Are water soluble
   - Are glycoproteins
   - Bind to cell surface receptors
   - Classification of cytokines
     i. Promoters of Th-1 helper cells
         - IFN-γ
         - IL-2
     ii. Promoters of Th-2 helper cells
         - IL-4/5/6
         - TGF-β
     iii. Non-immunological cytokines
         - EPO
         - Thrombopoietin
     iv. Chemokines
     v. Colony-stimulating factor

6. **IL-1 and TNF**
   - Are 2 major cytokines that mediate inflammation
   - They act on
     i.   Endothelium
     ii. Leucocytes
     iii. Fibroblasts
   - They induce systemic acute phase reactions, which include
     i.   Fever
     ii. Increased sleep
     iii. Decreased appetite
     iv. Increased acute phase proteins
     v.   Neutrophilia
     vi. Shock
   - Effects on endothelium include
     i.   Increased leucocyte adherence
     ii. Increased prostacyclin synthesis
     iii. Increased procoagulant activity
     iv. Increased anticoagulant activity
     v.   Increased levels of
          - IL-1, 6, and 8
          - PDGF
     vi. Induce synthesis of nitric oxide
   - Effects on fibroblasts include
     i.   Increased proliferation
     ii. Increased collagen synthesis
     iii. Increased collagenase secretion
     iv. Increased protease secretion
     v.   Increased prostaglandin E synthesis

7. **EPO**
   - Is a glycoprotein
   - Produced by the kidney
   - Regulates RBC production

8. **Thrombopoietin**
   - Is a glycoprotein
   - Produced by
     - i.   Kidney
     - ii. Liver
     - iii. Striated muscle
     - iv. Stromal cells in bone marrow
   - Regulates production of platelets (megakaryocytes)

Cellular mediators

1. **Cellular mediators**
   - Originate from the bone marrow
   - Include
     - i. Myeloid cells (e.g. leucocytes)
     - ii. Lymphoid cells (e.g. B-cells, T-cells, and NK cells)
   - Myeloid progenitor cells give rise to
     - i.   Erythrocytes
     - ii. Platelets
     - iii. Leucocytes
     - iv. Dendritic cells

2. **Leucocytes**
   - Are divided into 2 groups (**Box 8.5**)

Box 8.5 Groups of leukocytes

Granulocytes	Agranulocytes
• Neutrophil (65%) • Eosinophil • Basophil	• Monocyte (half-life = 1 day) • Macrophage = Monocyte outside blood vessels (half-life = months) • Lymphocyte (25%)

   - Granules
     - i. Store antibiotic compounds and enzymes
     - ii. Utilized in the digestion of endocytosed particles
   - Neutrophils are incapable of replication
   - Eosinophils
     - i.   Combat parasitic infections
     - ii. Associated with atopy and allergy
     - iii. Stain pink with eosin which is a red dye (acid-loving)
     - iv. Induce mast cell degranulation
     - v.   Contain
       - ▪ Histamine
       - ▪ Plasminogen
       - ▪ Lipase
       - ▪ Major basic protein
   - Only macrophages can form giant cells
   - Hofbauer cells are phagocytic cells present in the placenta

3. **Lymphocytes consist of 3 cell types**
   - T-cells (80%)
   - B-cells (15%)

- NK cells (10%)
  i. Specific for MHC class 1 and have CD16 receptors
  ii. Decidual NK cells (present in pregnancy) stain positive for CD56 but are negative for CD16

4. T-cells

- Are part (principal mediators) of the adaptive immune system
- Are divided into
  i. T-cells expressing the surface protein CD4 (i.e. Th-1 and -2 cells)
    - MHC class 2 restricted
    - Express α or β T-cell receptors
  ii. T-cells expressing the surface protein CD8 (i.e. T cytotoxic and suppressor)
    - Specific for MHC class 1
    - Express α or β T-cell receptors
  iii. T-cells expressing both surface proteins CD4 and CD8
    - Are MHC-unrestricted
    - Express γ or δ T-cell receptors
- T-cell development
  i. Originates in the bone marrow
  ii. Cells mature in the thymus
  iii. Undergo clonal deletion (i.e. a process by which T- and B-cells expressing receptors for self-antigens are deactivated)
- Do not recognize free antigens
- Recognize antigens bound to MHC molecules (MHC dependent)
- Th-1 cells
  i. Mediate cellular response
  ii. Interact with monocytes, macrophages, and CD8-positive T-cells
  iii. Produce IFN-γ and IL-2
- Th-2 cells
  i. Mediate humoral response
  ii. Interact with B cells
  iii. Produce IL-4 and -5

5. B-cells

- Development
  i. Originate in the bone marrow
  ii. Differentiation induced by
    - Th cells
    - Antigens
- Differentiate into
  i. Plasma cells – secrete antibodies
  ii. Memory cells
- Contain on their surface
  i. Fc receptors
  ii. Complement receptors
  iii. MHC class 2
- Produce immunoglobulins (Ig G, A, M, E, and D)

6. Lymph nodes

- Are divided anatomically into
  i. Cortex
  ii. Medulla

- Cortex is divided into 2 regions
  - i. Outer (nodular) – contains B-cells
  - ii. Inner (juxtamedullary) – contains T-cells
- Medulla has 2 parts
  - i. Medullary cord – contains plasma and T-cells
  - ii. Medullary sinuses – contains histiocytes (immobile macrophages) and reticular cells

7. **MHC**
   - Encodes for cell-surface antigen-presenting proteins
   - Gene is located on short arm of chromosome 6
   - There are 2 classes
     - i. MHC class 1
       - Expressed on all nucleated cells
       - Has 3 major sub-loci genes (A, B, and C)
       - Has 3 minor sub-loci genes (E, F, and G)
       - Presents intracellular antigens
     - ii. MHC class 2
       - Has 3 major sub-loci genes (DP, DQ, and DR)
       - Has 2 minor sub-loci genes (DM and DO)
       - Expressed on antigen-presenting cells
       - Presents extracellular antigens to T-lymphocytes

8. **Antigen-presenting cells include**
   - B-cells
   - Dendritic cells
   - Macrophages

9. **Immunoglobulins**
   - Structure (**Fig. 8.1**)
     - i. 2 heavy chains
     - ii. 2 light chains
     - iii. Bound by disulfide bonds
     - iv. There is a variable region
       - Forms the antigen-binding site

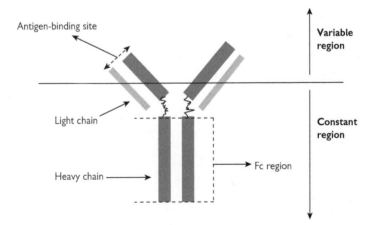

Figure 8.1 Immunoglobulin structure

- Also known as Fab (fragment antigen binding) region
- Consists of portions of a light and a heavy chain
v. There is a constant region
  - Fc (fragment crystallizable region) receptor binding site
  - Made up of 2 heavy chains only
- Consist of 5 classes (Ig G, A, M, E, and D) (*Box 8.6*)

Box 8.6 Classes of immunoglobulin

IgG	IgA	IgM	IgE
• 75% of total Ig pool • Monomer • Has 4 subtypes (IgG1, IgG2, IgG3, IgG4)	• 20% of total Ig pool • Dimer • Has 2 isoforms • Found in mucosal epithelium (GIT; respiratory tract; urogenital tract)	• 5% of total Ig pool • 1st Ig produced in infection • Pentamer • Confined to intravascular pool	• Binds to basophil and mast cells • Monomer • Involed in allergy and parasitic infections

IgD
• <1% of total Ig pool • Monomer

Immunohistochemistry (IHC)

1. **IHC is the process of identifying antigens in cells by using antibodies**

2. **Widely used in diagnosis of abnormal cells**

3. **2 methods used in IHC detection of antigens**
   - Direct (where only one antibody is used)
   - Indirect (where two antibodies are used)

4. **Diagnostic IHC markers (*Table 8.1*)**

T. in
Obs
Gyn

Chpts 7.24
& 7.25

Immunological disorders

1. **SLE**
   - Prevalence
     i. 1 : 1000 women
     ii. Women are affected more than men with a ratio of 9 : 1
   - Clinical features
     i. Joint involvement – arthritis
     ii. Skin involvement
         - Malar rash
         - Photosensitivity
         - Raynaud's phenomenon
     iii. Haematological manifestations
         - Haemolytic anaemia
         - Thrombocytopenia
         - Leucopenia

Table 8.1 Diagnostic IHC markers

Marker	Positive in	Negative in
CK 7	Lung adenocarcinoma Breast adenocarcinoma Ovarian adenocarcinoma (serous and endometrioid) Cervical adenocarcinoma Bladder adenocarcinoma	Squamous cell carcinoma Colonic carcinoma Mucinous adenocarcinoma of ovary Hepatocellular carcinoma Prostatic adenocarcinoma Renal epithelial tumour
CK 20	Gastrointestinal epithelium Urothelium Colorectal carcinoma Rectal carcinoma Pancreatic duct adenocarcinoma Mucinous ovarian adenocarcinoma	
CA 19.9	GIT carcinomas Pancreaticobiliary carcinomas Mucinous ovarian tumour	
CA 125	Ovary adenocarcinoma Cervical adenocarcinoma Endometrial adenocarcinoma GIT adenocarcinoma Breast adenocarcinoma Thyroid adenocarcinoma	
CA 15.3	Recurrent breast carcinoma	
Calretinin	Ovarian sex cord stromal tumour	
CEA (is an oncofetal glycoprotein)	GIT adenocarcinoma Lung adenocarcinoma Medullary carcinoma of thyroid	
Epithelial membrane antigen (found in human milk fat globule membranes)	Mesotheliomas	
Inhibin	Ovarian sex cord stromal tumour	

    iv. Renal involvement
    v. Neurological involvement
- SLE autoantibodies include
    i. Antinuclear antibodies (ANA)
    ii. Antibodies to double-stranded DNA
    iii. Extractable nuclear antigens (ENA)
       ■ Anti-Ro antibodies
       ■ Anti-La antibodies
    iv. Anticardiolipin antibodies
- Pregnancy increases the risk of SLE relapses
- Complications of SLE during pregnancy include
    i. Miscarriage
    ii. Pre-eclampsia

    iii. FGR

    iv. Fetal death

    v. Pre-term delivery

    vi. Congenital heart block

    vii. Cutaneous neonatal lupus

- Complications during pregnancy are decreased if
    i.   SLE in remission around the time of conception
    ii. There is no of renal disease
- Cutaneous neonatal lupus
    i.   Is transient
    ii. Occurs in 5% of infants born to anti-Ro/La positive mothers
- Congenital heart block
    i.   Is permanent
    ii. Occurs in 2% of infants born to anti-Ro/La positive mothers
    iii. Perinatal mortality rate is 19%
    iv. Fetal heart rate responses during labour unreliable

2. Multiple sclerosis (MS)

- Is an autoimmune disorder of the CNS due to auto antibodies directed against myelin-producing oligodendrocytes
- Destruction of myelin is due to cell-mediated immunity by Th-1 cells
- Diagnosis is based on 2 demyelinating lesions in the brain or spinal cord disseminated in time and space
- There are 2 forms of MS
    i.   Relapsing-remitting (85% of patients)
    ii. Primary progressive MS
- Prevalence in UK is 0.1%
- Lifetime risk of developing MS if
    i.   One parent affected = 2%
    ii. One sibling affected = 3%
    iii. Two parent affected = 20%
    iv. Dizygotic twin affected = 7%
    v.   Monozygotic twin affected = 30%
- Relapse rate
    i.   Decreases in pregnancy due to decreased cell-mediated immunity and increase in humoral immunity associated with pregnancy
    ii. Increases by 50% during the first 3 months after delivery
- Investigations include
    i.   Magnetic resonance imaging (MRI)
    ii. CSF – raised IgG in 70% of patients and oligoclonal bands on CSF electrophoresis
    iii. Visual evoked potential
- Treatments include
    i.   Corticosteroid
    ii. IFN beta
    iii. Plasma exchange
    iv. Glatiramer acetate

3. Myasthenia gravis

- Prevalence is between 1 : 10 000 and 1 : 50 000
- Is due to IgG antibodies against the nicotinic acetylcholine receptor on the motor endplate
- Only affects skeletal muscles
- Diagnosis is via the Tensilon test

- Complications in pregnancy
    i.   Arthrogryposis multiplex congenital (development of fetal contractures due to lack of movement caused by transplacental passage of myasthenic antibodies) in 20%
    ii. Pre-term delivery
    iii. Intrauterine FGR
- In pregnancy
    i.   40% have exacerbation
    ii. 30% have remission
    iii. 30% have no change in disease progress

Immunology – pregnancy

1. **The fetus**
    - Is a semi-allograft
    - Is antigenically competent
        i.   Produces IgM at 11 weeks
        ii. T-cell development is slow
        iii. NK cell activity is 50% that of adults
        iv. Cytotoxic T cell function is 1/3 that of adults
    - Maternal Ig transfer to the fetus
        i.   Only IgG can cross the placenta
        ii. Starts at 12 weeks
        iii. Peaks at 32 weeks (although significant protection is provided ≥36 weeks)
        iv. Is passive

2. **Uterine immune system cells**
    - Lymphocytes
        i.   B-cells (virtually none)
        ii. T-cells (10%)
        iii. NK cells (70%)
    - Uterine large granulolymphocytes (ULGLs)
    - Macrophages (20%)
    - Dendritic cells (2%)
    - Ratio of T-cells : B-cells = 1 : 1
    - CD 8$^+$ T-cells >CD 4$^+$ T-cells

3. **Maternal immunology**
    - Humoral and cellular response remain about the same with mild discrepancies
        i.   Humoral immunity tends to dominate (Th-2 cell mediated) hence SLE (Th-2 dependent) worsens in pregnancy
        ii. Progesterone suppresses Th-1 cell hence rheumatoid arthritis (Th-1 dependent) improves in pregnancy
    - Increased complement activation
    - Increased acute phase protein levels
    - Decreased NK cell activity
    - Increased endothelial cell activation mediated via
        i.   VEGF
        ii. PAI-1
    - Decreased immunoglobulin levels of
        i.   Ig G
        ii. Ig A
        iii. Ig M

4. **Fetal cells**
   - Syncytiotrophoblast
     i.   Is in direct contact with maternal cells
     ii. Does not express class 1 and 2 MHC antigens
     iii. Does not stimulate cytotoxic activity
     iv. Inhibits NK cell activity
   - There are 2 immunological interfaces in human pregnancy
     i.   Extra-villous cytotrophoblast/decidua (early pregnancy)
     ii. Syncytiotrophoblast/maternal blood (late pregnancy)
   - Extra-villous trophoblast
     i.   Expresses class 1 MHC antigens (e.g. HLA-C, HLA-E, HLA-G)
     ii. Does not express class 2 MHC antigens
   - Blastocyst develops MHC class 1 and 2 at 4 weeks

5. **Immuno-contraception**
   - Is a birth control method using the body's immune response to avert pregnancy
   - Not used in humans but utilized in animals (e.g. for controlling the numbers of some species of wild deer)
   - Antibodies can act on 3 potential antigen sites
     i.   Sperm surface
     ii. Zona pellucida
     iii. Implantation-associated antigens (e.g. hCG)

CHAPTER 9

Microbiology

CONTENTS

Bacteria

1. **Bacteria**
   - Are prokaryotic (i.e. have no membrane-bound organelles)
   - Can be classified into 3 main groups (**Box 9.1**)

Box 9.1 Bacterial groups

Gram stainable	Acid-fast bacilli	Unusual
• Gram positive • Gram negative • Gram variable (*Gardenella vaginalis, Mobiluncus*)	• Cell wall has high lipid content - hence difficult to stain (e.g. *Mycobacteria, Norcardia*)	• Have no peptidoglycans (e.g. *Chlamydia, Mycoplasma*)

   - Are visible by light microscopy (average diameter ≈ 1 μm)
   - Have a cell wall which is made up of
     - i. *N*-acetyl glucosamine/muramic acid
     - ii. Peptidoglycans
       - Have penicillin-binding sites
       - Are the target for β-lactams
     - iii. Polypeptides
     - iv. Polysaccharides

2. **Taxonomy**
   - By shape
     - i. Bacilli (rods)
     - ii. Cocci (grains)
   - By O_2 requirement
     - i. Aerobes
     - ii. Anaerobes

- By spore forming
- By staining

3. **Anaerobe organisms can be classified into 2 types**
   - Facultative anaerobes, which are capable of aerobic respiration if O_2 is present
   - Obligate anaerobes, which die in the presence of O_2

4. **Gram stain**
   - Process involves
     i. Staining with crystal violet
     ii. Then staining with Gram's Iodine
     iii. Decolourizing with acetone
     iv. Counter-stain with methyl red
   - Gram-positive bacteria
     i. Stain blue – retain crystal violet stain
     ii. Stain due to peptidoglycan – a thick polysaccharide coat that loses stain very slowly once taken up
     iii. Include (**Box 9.2**)

Box 9.2 Examples of gram positive bacteria

Cocci	Bacilli
• *Staphylococcus* (form chains) • *Streptococcus* (form grape-like clusters)	• *Clostridium* • *Corynebacterium* • *Listeria* • *Bacillus* • *Actinomycetes*

- Gram-negative bacteria (**Fig. 9.1**)
  i. Stain pink because the cell wall is thinner and does not retain the crystal violet dye, so it takes up the methyl red stain
  ii. Cell wall consists of
     - Outer layer of LPS
     - Periplasmic layer containing β-lactamase

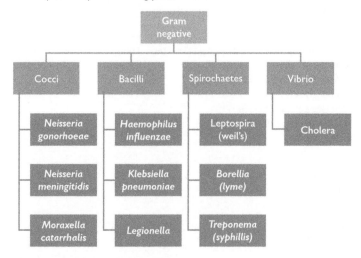

Figure 9.1 Gram-negative bacteria nomenclature

- ▪ Inner peptidoglycan layer
iii. Gram-negative bacilli include
  - ▪ *Haemophilus influenzae*
  - ▪ *Klebsiella pneumonia*
  - ▪ *Legionella*
  - ▪ *Pseudomonas aeruginosa*
  - ▪ *Escherichia coli*
  - ▪ *Proteus mirabilis*
  - ▪ *Helicobacter pylori*
  - ▪ *Salmonella typhi*
  - ▪ *Campylobacter*
iv. Can also be divided based on lactose fermentation (**Box 9.3**)

Box 9.3 Gram negative bacteria classification according to lactose fermentation

Lactose fermenters (orange on McConkey agar)	Lactose non-fermenters (pink on McConkey agar)
• Klebsiella	• *Pseudomonas*
• *Escherichia coli*	• *Salmonella*
• Enterobacter	• *Shigella*
• Citrobacter	• *Yersinia*
	• *Salmonella*
	• *Helicobacter pylori*
	• *Proteus*

5. **Bacterial toxins consist of 2 types**
   - Exotoxins
     i. Secreted by organisms
     ii. A feature of Gram-positive and Gram-negative bacteria
     iii. Form toxoids
   - Endotoxin
     i. Released on cell death and lysis
     ii. A feature of Gram-negative bacteria
     iii. The main forms is lipid A from LPS

6. **Bacterial antimicrobial resistance occurs via**
   - Bacterial mechanisms of antimicrobial resistance
     i. Drug inactivation (e.g. production of β-lactamases)
     ii. Alteration of drug target site (e.g. alteration of penicillin-binding sites)
     iii. Bacterium metabolic pathway alteration
     iv. Fibronectin coat
     v. IgA cleaving protease
   - Mechanisms of transfer of antimicrobial resistance
     i. Horizontal gene transfer
     ii. Vertical gene transfer
   - Mechanisms of horizontal gene transfer
     i. Plasmid DNA transfer
     ii. Chromosomal mediated resistance
     iii. Bacterial conjugation

7. **Vaginal flora is influenced by oestrogen levels contributing to**
   - Increased vaginal glycogen concentration
   - pH 3.5–4.5 due to conversion of glycogen to lactic acid by lactobacilli

8. **Clinical isolation of bacteria**
   - Use of specific microbiological swabs
   - Storage at 4 °C
   - Preliminary laboratory report takes 18 h
   - Identification is via detection of
     i. Antigens
     ii. Antibodies
     iii. Nucleic acids

Examples of Gram-positive organisms

1. *Streptococcus* – **general facts**
   - Many are facultative anaerobes
   - They can be
     i. Catalase negative
     ii. Oxidase negative
   - Form chains
   - Divided into 3 groups based on levels of haemolysis when cultured on horse blood agar (*Box 9.4*)

Box 9.4 Streptococci classification according to haemolysis when cultured on horse blood agar

Non-haemolytic	Partial haemolytic (α)	Complete haemolytic (β)
• *E. faecalis*	• *S. viridans* • Enterococcus • Pneumococcus	• Group A, C, and G • Group B • Group F

2. **β-haemolytic streptococci are subdivided by Lancefield grouping (A–O)**
   - Groups A, C, and G are associated with
     i. Toxic shock syndrome
     ii. Necrotizing fasciitis
     iii. Vaginitis
   - Group B is associated with
     i. Chorioamnionitis
     ii. Neonatal sepsis
     iii. Endometritis
   - Group F – can cause abscesses

3. **Group A streptococcus**
   - Also known as *Streptococcus pyogenes*
   - Virulence factor is determined by the presence of
     i. M protein
     ii. Hyaluronidase
     iii. Streptokinase
     iv. DNAse
     v. Superantigens
   - M-protein is
     i. A fimbrial protein
     ii. Involved in capsule formation
     iii. Is anti-phagocytic
     iv. Involved in destroying C3 convertase and preventing opsonization by C3b
     v. Responsible for organism adhesion and invasion

- Causes
  - i. Scarlet fever
  - ii. Toxic shock
  - iii. Rheumatic fever
  - iv. Glomerulonephritis
  - v. Necrotizing fasciitis

4. **Group B streptococcus (GBS)**

Chpt 6.6

  - Also known as *Streptococcus agalactia*
  - Maternal carriage
    - i. 20–35% carry GBS
    - ii. Intermittent carriage
  - Fetal
    - i. Maternal to fetal colonization rate = 80%
    - ii. Invasive neonatal disease occurs in 0.5 : 1000 births
    - iii. Neonatal mortality from early-onset GBS disease in UK is 6%
  - Indications for antibiotic prophylaxis during labour (following a risk-based approach)
    - i. Early-onset GBS disease in a previous baby
    - ii. GBS found in vagina/urine during index pregnancy
    - iii. Prolonged rupture of membranes at term (>18 h)
    - iv. Preterm labour <37 completed weeks of gestation
    - v. Preterm rupture of membranes with known GBS
    - vi. Intrapartum pyrexia
  - Antibiotic regimens
    - i. Benzylpenicillin
      - 3 g i.v. loading dose followed by
      - Benzylpenicillin 1.5 g i.v. 4 hourly until delivery
    - ii. Clindamycin 900 mg i.v. 8 hourly until delivery
    - iii. Erythromycin 500 mg 6 hourly until delivery
    - iv. Vancomycin as a very last resort

5. *Streptococcus pneumoniae*
  - Is a diplococcus (forms pairs)
  - Forms draughtsman-shaped colonies
  - Is optochin sensitive
  - Is bile soluble
  - Causes
    - i. Meningitis
    - ii. Pneumonia
    - iii. Primary bacterial peritonitis (in prepubertal girls)

6. *Enterococcus* **genus**
  - Consists of 2 species
    - i. *Enterococcus faecalis*
    - ii. *Enterococcus faecium*
  - Are gastrointestinal commensal organisms
  - Are resistant to many antimicrobials
  - Causes
    - i. Endocarditis
    - ii. Proctitis
  - Can be haemolytic or non-haemolytic – used to be classified as group D

7. *Listeria monocytogenes*
   - Affects 1 : 10 000 pregnant women
   - Some strains are β-haemolytic
   - Produces flagella at room temperature but not at 37 °C
   - Causes – listeriosis
     i.   Meningitis
     ii. Hepatosplenomegaly
     iii. Bradycardia
   - Transmitted
     i. In contaminated food
     ii. To the fetus via
       - Transplacental spread
       - Ascending infection
   - In the placenta causes
     i. Miliary granuloma
     ii. Focal necrosis
   - Fetal mortality rate from listeriosis is 50%
   - Treatment
     i. Amoxicillin or gentamicin
     ii. Duration 3 weeks

8. *Staphylococcus*
   - Is a genus of facultative anaerobes
   - Forms grape-like bunches
   - Classified on ability to form coagulase
   - Cause
     i.   Scalded skin syndrome
     ii. Toxic shock
     iii. Slime in i.v. cannulae
   - Meticillin-resistant *Staphylococcus aureus* (MRSA) is
     i.   Coagulase positive
     ii. DNAse positive
     iii. Catalase positive

9. *Actinomycetes israelii*
   - Is
     i. An anaerobe
     ii. A bacillus
   - Shows branching
   - Is slow growing
   - Occurs in
     i. Mouth
     ii. Intrauterine contraceptive devices (IUCDs)
   - Causes chronic granulomatous disease
   - Produces sulphur granules in tissues
   - Treatment
     i. Penicillin
     ii. Requires 6–12 months antibiotic therapy

Examples of Gram-negative/variable organisms

T. in
Obs
Gyn
Chpt 3.3

1. *Neisseria* family
   - Are diplococci

- Cause
  - i.   Meningitis (*N. meningitidis*)
  - ii. Gonorrhoea (*N. gonorrhoeae*)
- Are capnophilic (i.e. thrive in the presence of high CO_2)
- Treatment = cephalexin
- Multidrug resistance is growing

2. Gonorrhoea

- Infects mucous membranes of
  - i.   Urethra
  - ii. Endocervix
  - iii. Rectum
  - iv. Pharynx
  - v.   Conjunctiva
- Can infect Bartholin's gland
- Treatment
  - i.   IM ceftriaxone 250 mg stat
  - ii. Oral cefixime 400 mg
  - iii. IM spectinomycin 2 g
- A test of cure should be done 3 days after treatment
- 40% will also have concurrent *Chlamydia*
- Complications
  - i.   Gonococcal ophthalmia neonatorum
  - ii. Neonatal vaginitis, proctitis, and urethritis
  - iii. Disseminated gonococcal infection

3. *Gardnerella vaginalis*

- Is a facultative anaerobe
- Is Gram variable
- Is a bacillus
- Is a normal commensal organism of the vagina
- Is β-haemolytic

4. Bacterial vaginosis (BV)

Chpt 3.2

- Polymicrobial condition of the vagina characterized by
  - i.   Variable degrees of depletion of protective *Lactobacillus* species
  - ii. Marked increase in the population of other organisms especially anaerobes including *G. vaginalis*, *Mobincullus*, and *Atopobium vaginale*
- Over 60% of affected women are asymptomatic
- Aetiology is unknown
- Associated with mid-trimester miscarriage, preterm birth, rupture of membranes, endometritis
- More common in black women
- Amsel criteria for diagnosis (require 3 out of 4)
  - i.   Vaginal discharge
  - ii. Clue cells
  - iii. pH >4.5
  - iv. Fishy odour with alkali (10% KOH) on a wet mount (whiff test)
- Hay/Ison criteria (is based on Gram stain of vaginal discharge)
  - i.   Grade 1 = normal flora (predominantly lactobacilli)
  - ii. Grade 2 = mixed flora
  - iii. Grade 3 = BV and absent lactobacilli

- Clinical features
  - i.   Fishy smelling vaginal discharge (worse after intercourse)
  - ii.   White or grey vaginal discharge
- Treatment = metronidazole 400 mg b.d. for 7 days

5. **Syphilis**

Chpt 3.6

- Is caused by the spirochaete *Treponema pallidum*
- Classification
  - i.   Early – includes primary, secondary and early latent stages (i.e. < 2 years of infection)
  - ii.   Late – includes late latent and tertiary stages (i.e. > 2 years of infection)
- Stages
  - i.   Primary – chancre appears 10–90 days after initial exposure (persist 4–6 weeks before disappearing)
  - ii.   Secondary – occurs 1–6 months post primary infection
    - ▪ Symmetrical non-itchy rash on trunk and
    - ▪ Condylomata latum
    - ▪ Mucous patches around genitals or mouth
  - iii. Tertiary – occurs 1–10 years after initial infection
    - ▪ Characterized by the formation of gummas
    - ▪ Neurosyphilis – tabes dorsalis; generalized paresis of the insane; Argyll Robertson pupil
    - ▪ de Musset's sign
- Microbiological identification
  - i.   Cannot be cultured in lab
  - ii.   Serology is indistinguishable from
    - ▪ Yaw
    - ▪ Pinta
  - iii. Difficult to differentiate between active and treated past infection of syphilis
  - iv.   Non-specific test
    - ▪ Venereal Disease Research Laboratory (VDRL)
    - ▪ Rapid plasma reagin (RPR)
    - ▪ Wasserman's reaction
    - ▪ Hinton's test
  - v.   Specific tests
    - ▪ Fluorescent treponemal antibody-absorption test (FTA-ABS)
    - ▪ *Treponema pallidum* particle agglutination assay (TPPA)
  - vi.   Serology progress: IgM/FTA-ABS → IgG → TPPA → VDRL
  - vii. False positives in non-specific tests occur in
    - ▪ Viral infections
    - ▪ Lymphoma
    - ▪ Tuberculosis
    - ▪ Malaria
    - ▪ Chagas' disease
    - ▪ Pregnancy
- Causes endarteritis obliterans
- Treatment
  - i.   Penicillin G
  - ii.   Doxycycline
- The Jarisch–Herxheimer reaction is common post treatment

6. *Mycoplasma hominis*
- Present in 20% of sexually active women
- Can be either a primary or a co-pathogen in pelvic inflammatory disease (PID)

- Can cause postpartum pyrexia
- Can be a co-pathogen in chorioamnionitis
- Treatment
  i. Doxycycline
  ii. Clindamycin
  iii. Resistant to macrolides

7. *Chlamydia trachomatis*

Chpt 3.2

- Is an obligate intracellular gram negative organism
- Has 3 subgroups
  i. A–C (follicular conjunctivitis)
  ii. D–K (genital)
  iii. L1–L3 (lymphogranuloma venereum)
- Contains both DNA and RNA
- Grows on McCoy's culture
- Lifecycle
  i. Is 72 h
  ii. Elementary body → Reticular body → Inclusion body
- Treatment
  i. Azithromycin
  ii. Doxycycline
  iii. Erythromycin
  iv. Ofloxacin
  v. Rifampicin
- Test of cure is only recommended in pregnant or breastfeeding women

8. **Vaginal discharge in children can be caused by**

Chpt 2.5

- Foreign body (which is the commonest cause)
- *Streptococcus pyogenes*
- *Haemophilus influenza*
- *Shigella sonnei*
- Pinworms
- *Chlamydia*
- *Neisseria gonorrhoeae*

Wound infection

1. **Typically require 10^5 organisms to establish**

2. **In the presence of a foreign body 10^3 organisms are required**

Necrotizing fasciitis

1. **Consists of 2 types**

2. **Type 1**
   - Is associated with surgery/diabetes
   - Is due to polymicrobial infection
     i. Anaerobes
     ii. Facultative anaerobes
     iii. Obligate anaerobes

3. **Type 2 – due to Group A streptococcus**

4. **Treatment**
   - Surgical debridement
   - Antibiotic combination

   i.   Benzylpenicillin 1.2 g i.v. q.d.s.
   ii. Clindamycin
   iii. Ciprofloxacin
   ● Surgical re-exploration of the wound

PID

Chpt 3.9 1. **Clinical manifestations include**
   ● Pelvic and/or abdominal pain
   ● Dyspareunia
   ● Post-coital bleeding
   ● Discharge
   ● Cervical tenderness
   ● Fever

2. **Complications**
   ● Ectopic pregnancy
   ● Tubal infertility
      i.   12% after 1st episode
      ii. 20% after 2nd episode
      iii. 50% after 3rd episode
   ● Chronic pelvic pain
   ● Fitz–Hugh–Curtis syndrome (i.e. right upper quadrant pain and perihepatitis – occurs in 15% of women with PID)

3. **Causative organisms include**
   ● *Chlamydia*
   ● *Neisseria*
   ● *Mycoplasma*
      i. *hominis*
      ii. *ureaplasma*
   ● *Gardnerella*
   ● *Trichomonas vaginalis*
   ● GBS

4. **Treatments regimens (*Fig. 9.2*)**

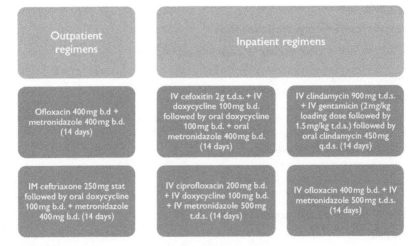

Figure 9.2 PID treatment regimens

Reiter's syndrome

1. Is a reactive arthritis caused by bacterial infection

2. Causative organisms include
   - *Salmonella*
   - *Yersinia*
   - *Shigella*
   - *Campylobacter*
   - *Chlamydia*
   - *N. gonorrhoeae*

3. Clinically manifests as a triad of
   - Urethritis
   - Arthritis
   - Uveitis

Fungi

1. Are multicellular eukaryotic organisms

2. Cell walls
   - Have no peptidoglycans
   - Contains ergosterol

3. Are eukaryotic (i.e. have membrane-bound organelles)

4. Contain
   - Fibrils
   - Chitins
   - Mannan
   - Glucan

5. Are aerobic

6. Reproduce via both asexual and sexual methods

7. Secrete keratinase

8. 4 main groups (*Box 9.5*)

Box 9.5 Fungal groups

Mould	True yeast	Yeast like	Dimorphic
• Multicellular • Grows as branching filament (hyphae/mycelia) • Reproduces by spores • Example: *Aspergillus*	• Unicellular • Reproduces by budding • Example: *Cryptococcus*	• Example: *Candida*	• Grows as yeast at 37°C • Grows as mycelia at 20°C • Example: *Histoplasma*

Protozoa

1. **Protozoa are unicellular, eukaryotic, free-living organisms**

2. **Consist of 2 types**
   - Protozoa
   - Helminths

3. **Include**
   - *Trichomonas vaginalis*
   - *Toxoplasma gondii*
   - *Giardia*
   - *Cryptosporidium*
   - *Plasmodium*

4. **Reproduction can either be asexual or sexual**

5. **Methods of asexual replication include**
   - Merogony (also known as schizogony)
   - Sporogony
   - Endodyogeny
   - Endopolygeny

6. **Form**
   - Trophozoites (the protozoon proliferative stage within the host cell)
   - Schizonts
   - Sporozoites (the cell form that infects new hosts)
   - Merozoites (result of merogony that occurs within the host cell)
   - Bradyzoites
   - Tachyzoites
   - Oocysts
   - Ookinetes (the fertilized zygotes capable of movement)

7. **Helminths are divided into 3 groups**
   - Fluke (trematode)
   - Tape (cessatode)
   - Ring (nematode)

T. in
Obs
Gyn
Chpt 3.3

8. ***T. vaginalis***
   - Is a flagellate protozoon
   - Transmission is venereal
   - Diagnosed via
     i. Wet prep
     ii. Polymerase chain reaction (PCR)
     iii. Culture
   - Symptoms include
     i. Discharge
     ii. Intense vulvo-vaginal itching and irritation
     iii. Strawberry cervix
     iv. Preterm delivery
   - Treatment is with metronidazole or tinidazole

T. in
Obs
Gyn
Chpt 8.26

9. ***T. gondii***
   - Is a zoonotic infection (predominantly via felines)
   - Diagnosis

    i.   IgM/A avidity
    ii. Serial samples taken 3 weeks apart
- Affects
    i.   Muscle
    ii. Neural tissue
    iii. Placenta
- Transmission in pregnancy
    i.   Is via transplacental in primary infection
    ii. Greatest risk = 26–40 weeks
    iii. Lowest risk = 10–24 weeks
    iv. The earlier the infection occurs in pregnancy the more severe the disease in the newborn
- Maternal risk
    i.   Chorioretinitis
    ii. Encephalitis
- Congenital infection causes
    i.   Stillbirth
    ii.   Cerebral calcifications
    iii. Microcephaly/hydrocephalus
    iv.   Choroidoretinitis
    v.   Cerebral palsy
    vi.   Epilepsy
    vii. Hepatosplenomegaly
    viii. Thrombocytopenia
- Treatment
    i.   Spiramycin
    ii. Sulfadiazine/pyrimethamine/folinic acid
- Toxoplasma IgM persist for 3 years after eradication

10. Malaria
- Is a mosquito-borne (female *Anopheles* mosquito) infectious disease
- Infects red blood cells
- Caused by *Plasmodium*
    i.   *falciparum*
    ii. *vivax*
    iii. *ovale*
    iv. *malariae*
    v.   *knowlesi*
- Severe malaria is defined as parasitaemia of more than 2%
- Maternal clinical features include
    i.   Fever
    ii.   Respiratory distress and pulmonary oedema
    iii. Arthralgia
    iv.   Retinal damage
    v.   Splenomegaly
    vi.   Hepatomegaly
    vii. Haemoglobinuria and renal failure
    viii. Biochemical abnormalities
        - Hypoglycaemia
        - Anaemia
        - Thrombocytopaenia

Box 9.6 Management of malaria

Vector control	Chemo-prophylaxis	Treatment
• Insecticides (DDT, permethrin)	• Mefloquine	• Quinine
• Mosquito nets	• Doxycycline	• Chloroquinine
• Skin repellents (50% DEET)	• Malarone	• Artemisinin
	• Quinine	

- ■ Acidosis
- ■ Hyperlactataemia
  ix. Coma
  x. Convulsions
  xi. Mortality (20% in non-pregnant women and 50% in pregnant women)
- Fetal effects of malarial infection include
  i. Miscarriage
  ii. Stillbirth
  iii. Premature labour
  iv. Low birth weight
  v. Placental parasitaemia
- Diagnosis is made via thin and thick blood films
- Management (*Box 9.6*)

Viruses

1. **General facts**
   - Viruses have no organelles
   - They depend on their host for
     i. Energy metabolism
     ii. Protein synthesis
   - Their genetic material is in the form of either (*Box 9.7*)
     i. RNA
     ii. DNA
   - Have a viral coat = capsid
   - Fetal transmission rate generally increases with gestational age
   - Incubation period for most viruses is approximately 21 days

Box 9.7 Examples of viruses according to genetic material type

RNA virus	DNA virus
• Rubella	• Herpes
• HIV	• Parvovirus
• Hepatitis A, C, D, E, G	• HPV
	• Hepatitis B
	• EBV
	• CMV
	• VZV

2. **Herpes is a virus family consisting of**
   - Cytomegalovirus (CMV)
   - Herpes simplex
   - Varicella

3. CMV

Chpt 8.24

- 50–80% women are seropositive
- Feto-maternal transmission rate = 40% (increases with gestational age)
- Causes symptoms in 10% of infected infants
- Causes congenital defects
  - i. Hearing loss – sensorineural
  - ii. Retinitis
  - iii. Cerebral palsy
  - iv. Hepatosplenomegaly
  - v. Hyperbilirubinaemia
  - vi. Intracranial calcification
  - vii. Thrombocytopenia
  - viii. Intrauterine FGR
  - ix. Microcephaly
- CMV IgM persists for months/years
- Diagnosis of maternal infection
  - i. Maternal IgG avidity
  - ii. High avidity means old infection
- Excreted in neonatal urine = 30%

4. Herpes simplex

Chpt 8.25

- 2 types
  - i. Type 1 – accounts for 30% of genital infections in the UK (50% in the USA)
  - ii. Type 2 – accounts for 70% of genital infections in the UK (50% in the USA)
- Fetal transmission
  - i. Is high if primary infection occurred in the last trimester with a rate ≥30%
  - ii. If there is a secondary episode during labour, the transmission rate is 1–3%
- Incubation = 21 days
- Affects
  - i. Skin
  - ii. Eyes
  - iii. Mouth
  - iv. CNS
- High fetal mortality
- Relative indication for caesarean section = presence of maternal lesions within 6 weeks of birth in the absence of
  - i. Ruptured membranes
  - ii. Spontaneous rupture of membranes (SROM) >6 h

5. Varicella zoster

Chpt 8.24

- Fetal transmission (congenital fetal varicella syndrome)
  - i. Limited to the 1st 20 weeks of gestation
  - ii. Overall rate = 1%
  - iii. Rate at 1–12 weeks = 0.4%
  - iv. Rate at 13–20 weeks = 2%
- Fetal varicella syndrome is characterized by
  - i. CNS anomaly
    - Microcephaly
    - Cortical atrophy
  - ii. Limb hypoplasia
  - iii. Cicatricial scarring
  - iv. Eye defects

- Microphthalmia
- Cataracts
- Chorioretinitis
- There is a risk of neonatal varicella if maternal infection occurs within 10 days of delivery
- Maternal complications include
  i. Pneumonitis (10%)
  ii. Encephalitis
  iii. Hepatitis
- Treatment
  i. If maternal infection occurs – aciclovir
  ii. If exposed to varicella – prevention of disease with VZIgG administration
  iii. VZIgG is not beneficial in a patient with chicken pox

6. Rubella

Chpt 6.6

- Is also known as German measles
- Is a togavirus
- Has a single-stranded RNA genome enclosed in a capsid
- Spreads via droplets
- Congenital defects (congenital rubella syndrome) if acquired during pregnancy include
  i. Eye manifestations
    - Cataract
    - Glaucoma
  ii. Heart defects
    - PDA
    - VSD
    - Pulmonary stenosis
  iii. Sensorineural hearing loss
  iv. Haematological manifestations
    - Thrombocytopenic purpura
    - Haemolytic anaemia
    - Lymphadenopathy
- Feto-maternal transmission rate
  i. 1st trimester = 90%
  ii. 2nd trimester = 30%
  iii. Risk of transmission is decreased after 16 weeks
- Causes defects in
  i. 1st trimester = 90% of infected fetuses
  ii. 2nd trimester = 20% of infected fetuses
  iii. >16 weeks = minimal risk of deafness only
  iv. >20 weeks = no increased risk

7. Parvovirus B19

Chpt 8.25

- Also known as
  i. Fifth disease
  ii. Slapped cheek syndrome
  iii. Erythema infectiosum
- 60% of women are immune to parvovirus B19
- Causes
  i. Miscarriage (overall risk of fetal loss = 6–12%)
  ii. Hydrops fetalis (3%) – due to fetal anaemia
- Does not cause congenital defects
- The virus attacks P blood group antigen (globiside) on RBCs and fetal heart

- Fetal transmission
  i. Mainly in 1st trimester
  ii. Rate = 30%
- Treatment = intrauterine fetal blood transfusion
- Not an indication for termination of pregnancy

T. in
Obs
Gyn

*Chpts 3.11
& 6.7*

8. **HIV**
   - Is a lentivirus (a member of the retrovirus family)
   - Primarily infects
     i. Th cells (particularly CD4)
     ii. Macrophage
     iii. Dendritic cells
   - Transmission
     i. Sexual – risk of transmission per act (in high risk countries) is
        - Female to male = 0.04%
        - Male to male = 0.08%
        - Receptive anal intercourse = 1.7%
     ii. (Latex condoms reduce this risk by 85%)
     iii. Blood products, i.e.
        - Intravenous drug users
        - Blood transfusion
     iv. Perinatal transmission
     v. (HIV have been found in low concentration in saliva, tears, and urine – potential for transmission from these is negligible)
   - Structure
     i. Spherical (120 nm diameter)
     ii. Composed of 2 copies of single-stranded RNA enclosed by a capsid
     iii. Capsid is
        - Composed of viral protein p24
        - Surrounded by a matrix composed of viral protein p17
     iv. Viral envelope
        - Surrounds the matrix
        - Composed of phospholipids and glycoprotein (i.e. gp120 and gp41)
     v. Glycoprotein enables the virus to attach to and fuse with target cells
   - Prevalence in the UK antenatal population
     i. Average is 0.17% (highest in London – 0.32%, and lowest in the North East and South West – 0.08%)
     ii. Approximately 1/3 of infections are due to HIV1 and 2/3 due to HIV2
   - Fetal transmission rate
     i. Without treatment = 15% (in European or North American countries)
     ii. With treatment ≤1%
   - Factors that increase vertical transmission rates
     i. High maternal viral load
     ii. Low CD4 count
     iii. Prolonged rupture of membranes
     iv. Chorioamnionitis
     v. Co-morbidity e.g. malaria, hepatitis C virus (HCV)
     vi. Breastfeeding
     vii. Preterm birth
   - Neonatal serology is of limited value as passively acquired maternal antibodies persist until 18 months of age
   - AIDS occurs when CD4 count is below 200/mm^3 blood

- Increases risk of
  i. Miscarriage
  ii. Pre-term delivery
  iii. Intrauterine FGR
- Complications include
  i. Kaposi's sarcoma
  ii. *Pneumocystis carinii* pneumonia
  iii. Non-Hodgkin's lymphoma
  iv. AIDS-related dementia

9. **Human papillomavirus (HPV)**
   - Consists of 5 groups
     i. α-papillomavirus
     ii. β-papillomavirus
     iii. γ-papillomavirus
     iv. Nu-papillomavirus
     v. Mu-papillomavirus
   - α-papillomaviruses consist of 2 subtypes
     i. Low risk – 6 and 11 (induce non-malignant changes)
     ii. High risk – 16, 18, 31, 33 and 45 (induce malignant changes)
   - Only infects epithelial cells
   - Structure
     i. Is made up of 75 capsomeres
     ii. Each capsomere consist of 5 molecules of L1 co-protein
     iii. Contains circular DNA
   - Genome is composed of
     i. Early proteins (E1, E2, E3, E4, E6, E7)
     ii. Late proteins (L1 and L2)
   - E6 and E7 are HPV proteins associated with cancer
   - Causes inactivation of
     i. p53
     ii. pRB
   - Incubation period is 2–8 months
   - Regresses spontaneously via cell-mediated immunity (70% regress within 1 year; 90% regress within 2 years)
   - Treatment
     i. Podophyllotoxin
     ii. Imiquimod
     iii. Cryotherapy

Chpts 3.10 & 6.7

10. **Hepatitis virus**
    - Types A–G
    - Hepatitis A – maternal-fetal transmission is rare
    - Hepatitis B (**Table 9.1**)
      i. Incubation = 6 weeks to 6 months
      ii. Progress of antigen detection with time
         - Surface → Core → e Antigen
      iii. Antibody production chronology (IgM)
         - Core → e Antigen → Surface
      iv. Immunity is confirmed by anti-surface IgM
      v. Prevalence among pregnant women in UK = 0.5%
      vi. Mother to child transmission

- Occurs via vertical transmission (includes pregnancy, labour and lactation)
- The transplacental route accounts for 5% of transmissions

vii. Feto-maternal transmission rate
- Transmission rates depend mainly on the viral load and on the antigen profile
- If mother is Hep B surface-antigen positive (HBsAg) = 20%
- If mother is Hep B e-antigen positive (HBeAg) = 90%
- Transmissions occurring during the 1st trimester = 10%
- Transmissions occurring during the 3rd trimester = 90%

viii. Treatment in pregnancy is possible with
- Interferon α
- Lamivudine

ix. Prophylaxis to a neonate of a Hep B e-antigen positive mother should be given at birth
- Hep B vaccine
- IgG

- Hepatitis C
  i. Prevalence in UK = 0.3–0.7%
  ii. Increases risk of obstetric cholestasis
  iii. Vertical transmission = 3–5%
- Hepatitis E
  i. Risk of maternal mortality = 5%
  ii. Risk of fulminant hepatic failure in pregnancy = 20%

Table 9.1 Hepatitis B serology

Stage of infection	HBsAg (surface Ag)	HBeAg (e Ag)	IgM anti-core Ab	IgG anti-core Ab	Hep B virus DNA	Anti-HBe Ab	Anti-HBs Ab
Acute (early)	+	+	+	+	+	–	–
Acute (resolving)	+	–	+	+	–	+/–	–
Chronic (high infectivity)	+	+/–	–	+	+	+/–	–
Chronic (low infectivity)	+	–	–	+	–	+/–	–
Immune (90%)	–	–	–	+	–	+/–	+/–
Post vaccination	–	–	–	–	–	–	+

11. HTLV

- Prevalence in UK = 0.25%
- Feto-maternal transmission is via breast milk
- Manifestations of congenital infection occur after 10–30 years
  i. T-cell leukaemia
  ii. Tropical spastic paraparesis

Chpt 8

CHAPTER 10

Pharmacology

CONTENTS

General principles

1. **Pharmacology comprises of 4 subdivisions**
   - Pharmacokinetics (i.e. what the body does to the drug)
     i. Absorption
     ii. Distribution
     iii. Metabolism
     iv. Excretion
   - Pharmacodynamics (i.e. what the drug does to the body)
   - Pharmacotherapeutics
   - Toxicology

2. **4 phases of human drug clinical testing**
   - Phase 1 – studied in normal volunteers
   - Phase 2
     i. In target population
     ii. Compared with a control drug
   - Phase 3
     i. Similar to phase 2, but in large groups
     ii. Compared with a control drug
   - Phase 4 – Post-marketing surveillance

3. **Distribution of a drug depends on**
   - Capillary permeability
   - Drug solubility (lipophilic drugs distribute across cell more easily)
   - Binding to plasma proteins

4. **Biotransformation**
    *   Makes drugs more polar (lipophilic properties of a drug hinder its elimination)
    *   Involves 2 phases
        i.   1 – metabolism
        ii. 2 – conjugation
    *   Metabolism includes
        i.   Oxidation
        ii. Reduction
        iii. Hydrolysis
    *   Conjugation occurs with
        i.   Glucuronate (e.g. paracetamol and morphine)
        ii. Glutathione
        iii. Sulphate (e.g. the contraceptive pill)
        iv. Acetic acid (e.g. hydralazine and isoniazid)
    *   Phase 1 occurs via the action of cytochrome P450
    *   Phase 2 occurs in the liver cytosol

5. **Volume of distribution (Vd)**
    *   Is the ratio of the amount of drug in the body to its plasma concentration
    *   Large Vd
        i.   Lipophilic drugs
        ii. Signifies that most of the drug is being sequestered in some tissue

6. **Drug interactions**
    *   Enzyme inductors (e.g. phenytoin)
    *   Enzyme inhibitors (e.g. sulfonamides)
    *   Enterohepatic circulation (reduced by ampicillin)
    *   GIT flora (reduced by ampicillin)

Pharmacology in pregnancy

1. **In pregnancy the following factors influence drug bioavailability**
    *   Increased circulating volume
    *   Increased renal blood flow (hence increased renal clearance of water-soluble drugs)
    *   Increased 3rd space
    *   Increased fat content
    *   Decreased albumin and binding proteins (hence free drug levels may not be low)
    *   Increased gastric emptying time
    *   Increased liver metabolism (hence increased clearance of drugs dependent on liver metabolism)
    *   Liver blood flow shows no change in pregnancy (hence no change in clearance of drugs whose elimination is dependent on liver blood flow, e.g. propranolol)

2. **Teratogens**
    *   Potential teratogens include all the 'A' drugs
        i.   Anticonvulsant
        ii. Antibiotics
        iii. Anticoagulants
        iv. Antimetabolites
        v.   Androgens

    vi. Alcohol

    vii. Antipsychotics

- Timing and defects (*Box 10.1*)

Box 10.1 Teratogenic effect of drugs according to timing of exposure

< Day 20	Day 20	Day 34	Day 36
• Limb defects	• Anencephaly	• Transposition of great vessels	• Cleft lip

Day 42	Day 84
• VSD • Syndactyly	• Hypospadias

3. **Most drugs cross the placenta except HIT**
   - **H**eparin
   - **I**nsulin
   - **T**ubocurarine

4. **Drugs that cause abortion (MET)**
   - **M**isoprostol
   - **E**rgotamine
   - **T**hrombolytics

5. The US Food and Drug Administration (FDA) pregnancy categories state the risk of a substance to a fetus (*Table 10.1*)

6. The FDA requires large amounts of data on a drug for it to be classified as pregnancy category A (thus many drugs that are category A in other countries are designated category C by the FDA)

Table 10.1 FDA pregnancy category

A	No fetal risk in pregnancy
B	Animal studies have failed to demonstrate a risk to fetus No adequate studies in pregnant women
C	Animal studies have shown adverse effect on the fetus No adequate studies in pregnant women Benefit of drug outweighs the potential risk
D	Evidence of risk of human teratogenicity Potential benefits outweigh potential risk
X	Evidence of risk of human teratogenicity Potential risk outweigh potential benefit of drug

Breastfeeding

1. **Most drugs enter the breast**

2. **Drugs not excreted in breast are**
   - Warfarin
   - Aminoglycosides

3. **Dopamine agonists (FDA pregnancy category B)**
   - Dopamine is a prolactin antagonist (increased dopamine causes a decrease in prolactin levels)
   - Reduces milk production
   - Used in
     i.   Pituitary tumours
     ii. Parkinson's disease
     iii. Inhibition of lactation
     iv. Hyperprolactinaemia
   - Includes
     i. Bromocriptine
     ii. Cabergoline

4. **Domperidone**
   - Is a dopamine antagonist
   - Is used to
     i. Stimulate lactation (by increasing prolactin secretion)
     ii. Increase gastric motility
   - Also used in treatment of
     i. Emesis
     ii. Parkinson's disease
   - Does not cross the blood–brain barrier

Analgesics

1. **Morphine (FDA pregnancy category C)**
   - Acts on μ-opioid receptors in
     i.   Brain
     ii. Substantia gelatinosa of spinal cord
     iii. GIT
   - Associated with
     i.   Analgesia
     ii.   Sedation
     iii. Euphoria
     iv.   Dependence
     v.   Respiratory depression
     vi.   Miosis (pinpoint pupil)
     vii. Constipation
     viii. Sphincter of Oddi spasm
   - Antidote
     i. Naloxone
     ii. NMDA (*N*-methyl-D-aspartic acid) antagonists (e.g. ketamine)
   - Metabolized in
     i.   Liver
     ii. Kidney
     iii. Brain

2. **Heroin (FDA pregnancy category X)**
   - Is diacetylmorphine (also known as diamorphine)
   - Is a prodrug of morphine
   - More lipophilic, hence crosses blood–brain barrier easily

- More potent than morphine
- Binds to μ-opioid receptors
- Side effects
  i. Euphoria
  ii. Drowsiness
  iii. CNS depression
- Fetal effects (if taken antenatally) are non-teratogenic and include
  i. Placental infection
  ii. FGR
  iii. Preterm birth
  iv. Fetal death
- Neonatal narcotics abstinence syndrome
  i. Incidence of narcotic use in the USA = 5%
  ii. Usually presents within 48 h of birth
  iii. Can occur up to 4 weeks after birth – this is because methadone is stored in fetal lung, liver, and spleen
  iv. Characterized by
    - CNS hyperirritability
    - High-pitched crying
    - Respiratory distress
    - Poor feeding
    - Seizures

3. **Fentanyl (FDA pregnancy category C)**
   - Is a μ-opioid agonist
   - Rapid onset
   - Short acting
   - 100 times more potent than morphine
   - Can cross the placenta

4. **Lidocaine (FDA pregnancy category B)**
   - Blocks voltage-gated sodium channels – prevents neurone depolarization
   - Is an antiarrhythmic
   - Half-life is 2 h
   - Metabolized by the liver
   - Toxicity symptoms
     i. Circumoral paraesthesia
     ii. Tinnitus
     iii. Blurred vision
     iv. Seizures
     v. Loss of consciousness
     vi. Cardiorespiratory compromise
     vii. ECG changes (widening PR interval and widening QRS)
   - Risk of cardiac toxicity is greatest in patients with underlying cardiac conduction problem (avoid giving in Wolff–Parkinson–White syndrome)
   - Maximum dose
     i. Without adrenaline = 3–5 mg/kg
     ii. With adrenaline = 7 mg/kg

5. **Cocaine (also known as benzoylmethylecgonine)**
   - Is obtained from the leaves of the coca plant
   - Acts as a

    i.   CNS stimulant

    ii. Appetite suppressant

    iii. Topical anaesthetic

    iv. Selective serotonin reuptake inhibitor (SSRI)

    v. Potent vasoconstrictor

- Is metabolized primarily in the liver
- Its metabolite can be detected in the urine

    i.   Within 4 h of intake

    ii. Up to 8 days post cocaine use

- Side effects

    i.   Tachycardia

    ii. Hallucinations

    iii. Bronchospasm

    iv. Crack lung syndrome

    v. Myocardial infarction

    vi. Tooth decay (due to breakdown of tooth enamel)

    vii. Bruxism (involuntary tooth grinding)

- Fetal effects (if taken antenatally) include

    i.   Vasoconstriction of uterine, placental, and umbilical artery leading to

       ■ FGR

       ■ Fetal death

       ■ Placental abruption

    ii. Prune-belly syndrome

    iii. Hydronephrosis

    iv. Reduced head circumference

    v. Gastroschisis

6. **Tramadol (FDA pregnancy category C)**
   - Is a centrally acting analgesic
   - Acts as a

    i.   Weak μ-opioid agonist

    ii. Serotonin releasing agent

    iii. Noradrenaline reuptake inhibitor

    iv. Nicotinic acetylcholine receptor antagonist

    v. M1 and M3 muscarinic acetylcholine receptor antagonist

   - Primary active metabolite is *O*-desmethyltramadol
   - Maximum dose is 400 mg/day

7. **Ethanol (FDA pregnancy category X)**
   - Is

    i.   An organic compound in which the hydroxyl functional group is bound to a carbon atom

    ii. A product of glucose fermentation

   - Chemical formula is C_2H_5OH
   - Boiling temperature = 78.4 °C
   - Acts as a

    i.   CNS depressant

    ii. γ-aminobutyric acid (GABA) receptor agonist

   - Metabolized

    i.   In the liver by alcohol dehydrogenase to acetaldehyde

    ii. Follows zero-order kinetics

   - Blood alcohol level of

    i.   0.05% (0.5 g/L) causes euphoria

ii. 0.08% (0.8 g/L) is the upper legal limit for driving
iii. 0.1% (1 g/L) causes CNS depression
iv. 0.4% (4 g/L) can cause death
- Recommended maximum consumption quantity is
  i.   For males = 140–210 g/week
  ii. For females = 84–140 g/week
- Complications of ethanol abuse (*Box 10.2*)

Box 10.2 Complications of ethanol abuse

Blood	Cardiac	GIT	Pregnancy
• Anaemia	• Cardiomyopathy	• Chronic gastritis	• Miscarriage
• Thrombocytopenia	• Hypertension	• Pancreatitis	• Aneuploidy
• Elevated triglycerides	• Stroke	• Liver cirrhosis and hepatitis	• Structural congenital anomalies
		• Fatty liver disease	
		• Oropharyngeal cancer	

Others
• Wernicke–Korsakoff syndrome
• Polyneuropathy
• Delirium tremens
• Fetal alcohol syndrome
• Dependence

- Fetal alcohol syndrome
  i.   Is a disorder of permanent birth defect in the offspring of women who drink alcohol in pregnancy
  ii. Incidence = 0.6 per 1000 live births in Canada
  iii. Features (*Box 10.3*)

Box 10.3 Features of fetal alcohol syndrome

Growth deficiencies	Craniofacial anomalies	CNS structural anomalies	Neurodevelopmental anomalies
• Low birth weight	• Smooth philtrum	• Microcephaly	• Epilepsy
• Short stature	• Thin vermilion	• Agenesis of corpus callosum	• Impaired fine motor skills
	• Small palpebral fissures	• Cerebellar hypoplasia	• Neurosensory hearing loss
			• Learning disabilities
			• Cognitive deficits

Antibiotics

General facts

1. **Bactericidal antibiotics**
   - Are antibiotics that target bacterial
     i.   Cell wall

    ii. Cell membrane

    iii. Enzymes

- Kill bacteria
- In low doses act as bacteriostatic

2. **Bacteriostatic antibiotics**
   - Inhibit bacterial growth and replication by inhibiting
     - i. Protein production
     - ii. DNA synthesis
     - iii. Cellular metabolism
   - High dose of bacteriostatics become bactericidal

3. **Drugs that interfere with folate metabolism**
   - Sulfonamides inhibits conversion of benzoic acid to folate
   - Dihydrofolate reductase inhibitors (inhibits conversion of folate to tetrahydrofolate) include
     - i. Trimethoprim
     - ii. Methotrexate
     - iii. Pyrimethamine

Example of antibiotics

1. **Penicillin**
   - Is a group of antibiotics derived from *Penicillium* fungi
   - Can be broadly divided into 5 groups
     - i. β-lactams
     - ii. β-lactamase resistant
     - iii. Broad-spectrum penicillins
       - Amoxicillin
       - Ampicillin
       - Co-amoxiclav (consists of amoxicillin with the β-lactamase inhibitor clavulanic acid)
     - iv. Antipseudomonal penicillins
       - Ticarcillin
       - Piperacillin
     - v. Mecillinams

2. **Sulfonamides**
   - Consist of 2 groups
     - i. Sulfonlyureas
     - ii. Thiazide diuretics
   - Acts as a competitive inhibitor of dihydropteorate synthetase (an enzyme involved in folate synthesis)
   - Side effects
     - i. Porphyria
     - ii. Stevens–Johnson syndrome
     - iii. Lyell syndrome (also known as toxic epidermal necrolysis)
     - iv. Blood dyscrasias
       - Agranulocytosis
       - Haemolytic anaemia
       - Thrombocytopenia

3. **Nitrofurantoin (FDA pregnancy category B)**
   - Is bactericidal
   - Is usually used to treat urinary tract infections
   - Is excreted mainly by the kidneys

Table 10.2 Antibiotics

Group	Mechanism	Cover	Side effect	Breastfeeding	Fetal risk
Bacteriostatic					
Lincosamide (clindamycin)	Binds to 50S ribosome	Anaerobes	Pseudomembranous colitis	Excreted in breast milk	FDA pregnancy cat. B No teratogenicity
Chloramphenicol	Binds to 50S ribosome	Broad spectrum Gram +ve Gram –ve MRSA Anaerobes	Aplastic anaemia	Excreted in breast milk	FDA pregnancy cat. C No teratogenicity Gray baby syndrome (↓ BP and cyanosis)
Macrolides (azithromycin, erythromycin, clarithromycin)	Binds to 50S ribosome Accumulate within leucocyte	Mycoplasma Mycobacteria Chlamydia Rickettsia Broad spectrum	Cholestatic jaundice Pseudomembranous colitis Diarrhoea Vomiting	Excreted in breast milk	FDA pregnancy cat. B
Macrolides (tacrolimus)			Cardiac damage Hypertension Blurred vision Hepatotoxicity Nephrotoxicity Posterior reversible encephalopathy syndrome Hyperkalaemia Hyperglycaemia Non-Hodgkin's lymphoma	Breastfeeding should be avoided	FDA pregnancy cat. C Hyperkalaemia Renal toxicity FGR Premature delivery

(continued)

Table 10.2 Continued

Group	Mechanism	Cover	Side effect	Breastfeeding	Fetal risk
Tetracycline	Binds to 30S ribosome	Broad spectrum	Pseudotumour cerebri (↑ intracranial BP) Maternal liver toxicity (if used antenatally)	Excretion in breast milk is low Compatible with breastfeeding	FDA pregnancy cat. D Adverse effects of fetal teeth and bone Congenital defects
Sulfonamides (trimethoprim)	Inhibits folate synthesis		Lupus Blood dyscrasias Kernicterus	Excretion in breast milk is low Compatible with breastfeeding	FDA pregnancy cat. D Jaundice Haemolytic anaemia Kernicterus
Bactericidal					
Ansamycin (rifampicin)	Inhibits DNA dependent RNA polymerase (inhibits mRNA synthesis) Lipophilic	Gram +ve	Hepatotoxic	Compatible with breastfeeding	FDA pregnancy cat. C Haemorrhagic disease of newborn
Glycopeptides (vancomycin, teicoplanin)	Inhibit cell wall synthesis; Inhibit peptidoglycan synthesis	Gram +ve	Nephrotoxic; Ototoxic; Neutropenia; Red man syndrome (due to histamine release)	Poorly absorbed from GIT (thus systemic absorption would not be expected)	FDA pregnancy cat. B
β-Lactams (penicillin)	Inhibit cell wall synthesis	Gram +ve	Neurotoxicity Seizures Urticaria	Excretion in breast milk is low Compatible with breastfeeding	FDA pregnancy cat. B

Drug	Mechanism	Spectrum	Adverse effects / notes	Breastfeeding	Pregnancy
β-Lactamase resistant (monobactams, carbapenems)		*S. aureus* Gram −ve			FDA pregnancy cat. C
β-Lactamase resistant (cephalosporin)			10% cross reactivity to penicillin	Excretion in breast milk is low; Compatible with breastfeeding	FDA pregnancy cat. B
Metronidazole	Inhibits nucleic acid synthesis; Is a prodrug (converted in bacteria to active form); Excreted via the kidney and bile	Anaerobes Protozoa	Black hairy tongue; glossitis; dark urine; peripheral neuropathy; leukopenia; disulfiram-like reaction		FDA pregnancy cat. B
Quinolone (ciprofloxacin, levofloxacin)	Inhibit bacterial DNA gyrase	Broad spectrum	Tendon damage; peripheral neuropathy; rhabdomyolysis; pseudomembranous colitis; ↑QT	Breastfeeding should be avoided	FDA pregnancy cat. C
Aminoglycosides (gentamicin, amikacin, tobramycin, neomycin)	Cell membrane lysis; Binds to 30S ribosomes	Gram −ve	Nephrotoxic; ototoxic; May impair neuromuscular transmission and should not be given to patients with myasthenia gravis	Compatible with breastfeeding	FDA pregnancy cat. C; 8th cranial nerve toxicity

- Has poor tissue penetration and thus should not be used to treat
  i. Pyelonephritis
  ii. Renal abscess
- Side effects
  i. Pulmonary fibrosis
  ii. Neonatal haemolysis (if used antenatally)

Antifungals

1. **General facts**
   - Fungal cell wall is composed of ergosterol (which is susceptible to antifungal medications)
   - Human cell membrane is composed of cholesterol (which is less susceptible to antifungal medications)
   - Side effects of antifungals include
     i. Nephrotoxicity
     ii. Hepatitis
     iii. Anaphylaxis

Antivirals

1. **Antiviral drugs do not destroy their target pathogens (they merely inhibit pathogen development)**

2. **Aciclovir (FDA pregnancy category B)**
   - Is a guanine analogue
   - Is a prodrug
   - Primarily used to treat herpes virus infections
   - Inhibits viral DNA polymerase

Table 10.3 Antifungals

Group	Drug	Mechanism of action	Fetal risk
Polyene	Nystatin Amphotericin B	Inhibits synthesis of ergosterol	FDA pregnancy cat. B
Imidazole	Ketoconazole Miconazole Clotrimazole Econazole Fluconazole	Inhibits synthesis of ergosterol	FDA pregnancy cat. C
Allylamines	Terbinafine Amorolfine	Inhibits squalene epoxidase action (an enzyme required for ergosterol synthesis)	FDA pregnancy cat. B
Echinocandins	Caspofungin	Inhibits cell wall glucan synthesis	FDA pregnancy cat. C
Griseofulvin		Binds to keratin and interferes with microtubule function in mitosis	FDA pregnancy cat. C
Pyrimidine analogue	Flucytosine	Inhibits fungal DNA/RNA synthesis	FDA pregnancy cat. C

- Is converted into active form
  i. In viral cell
  ii. By viral thymidine kinase
- Pharmacokinetics
  i. Poor water solubility
  ii. Poor oral bioavailability (15–30%)
  iii. Elimination half-life is 3 h
  iv. Renal excretion

3. **Neuraminidase inhibitors**
   - Is used in the treatment and prophylaxis of influenza virus A and B
   - Include
     i. Zanamivir (Relenza)
     ii. Oseltamivir (Tamiflu)
   - Zanamivir (FDA pregnancy category C)
     i. Dosing is limited to inhaled route
     ii. Pharmacokinetics
        - Oral bioavailability = 2%
        - Renal excretion
     iii. Could cause bronchospasm in asthmatic people
   - Oseltamivir (FDA pregnancy category C)
     i. Is a prodrug
     ii. Pharmacokinetics
        - Oral bioavailability = 75%
        - Metabolized in the liver to its active metabolite
        - Renal excretion
     iii. Side effects include
        - Stevens–Johnson syndrome
        - Neuropsychiatric disorders

4. **Ribavirin (FDA pregnancy category X)**
   - Primarily used to treat
     i. Respiratory syncytial virus infection
     ii. Hepatitis C
   - Is a prodrug
   - Is a purine analogue
   - Pharmacokinetics
     i. Oral bioavailability = 45%
     ii. Mean half-life = 12 days
     iii. Long half-life (RBCs concentrate the drug and are unable to excrete it; this pool is eliminated when RBCs are degraded in the spleen – a process that can take up to 6 months)
     iv. Renal and faecal (10%) excretion
   - Side effects
     i. Haemolytic anaemia
     ii. Teratogenic (in some animal species)

5. **Antiretroviral therapy (ART) (*Table 10.4*)**
   - Used for the treatment of retroviral infections (e.g. HIV)
   - Aim is to achieve a viral load of <50 HIV RNA copies/mL plasma
   - HAART (highly active antiretroviral therapy) includes combinations consisting of at least 3 drugs belonging to at least 2 classes of antiretrovirals

Table 10.4 Antiretrovirals

Class	Drug	Mechanism	Side effect	Fetal Risk
Nucleotide reverse transcriptase inhibitor (NtRTI)	Tenofovir	Inhibits reverse transcription (preventing synthesis of double-stranded viral DNA and thus viral multiplication)	Asthenia Hepatotoxicity Acute renal failure Fanconi syndrome	FDA pregnancy category B
Nucleoside reverse transcriptase inhibitor (NRTI)	Zidovudine Lamivudine Didanosine Emtricitabine		Myositis Lipodystrophy Peripheral neuropathy Pancreatitis Optic neuritis	FDA pregnancy category C FDA pregnancy category B
Non-nucleoside reverse transcriptase inhibitor (NNRTI)	Nevirapine Etravirine Efavirenz		Psychosis Insomnia Stevens–Johnson syndrome Toxic epidermal necrolysis Liver toxicity	FDA pregnancy category B (efavirenz is category D)
Protease inhibitor (PI)	Saquinavir Ritonavir Darunavir Indinavir Lopinavir	Inhibits protease activity (also found to have antiprotozoal properties)	Hyperlipidaemia Elevated hepatic transaminases	FDA pregnancy category B FDA pregnancy category C
Integrase inhibitors	Raltegravir	Inhibits the enzyme integrase		FDA pregnancy category C
Entry inhibitors	Maraviroc Enfuvirtide	Interfere with binding, fusion or entry of HIV-1 to host cells	Peripheral neuropathy Insomnia Depression Arthralgia Glomerulonephritis	FDA pregnancy category B

- HAART side effects include
  i. Lactic acidosis
  ii. Hyperglycaemia
  iii. Hepatitis
  iv. Pancreatitis
  v. Peripheral neuropathy
- Is used in the treatment of HIV
  i. When CD4 T-lymphocyte count is between 200 and 350 cells/mm^3 in asymptomatic patients
  ii. When viral load is greater than 10 000 HIV RNA copies/mL plasma
  iii. In severely symptomatic patients

6. **Drugs used in preventing HIV transmission from mother to fetus**
   - HAART is the treatment of choice if the woman is not on antiretroviral therapy prior to pregnancy
     i. Should commence between 20 and 28 weeks of gestation
     ii. Discontinued soon after delivery
     iii. Zidovudine is administered orally to the neonate for up to 6 weeks of life (within 4 h of birth)
     iv. Is known as START (short-term antiretroviral) therapy
   - Alternative to HAART is zidovudine monotherapy
   - Zidovudine is the only antiretroviral drug specifically indicated for use in pregnancy (excluding the 1st trimester)
   - Women who conceive on HAART should continue taking it throughout pregnancy

Antimalarial drugs

1. **There are 2 main groups of drugs**
   - Chemo-prophylaxis
   - Treatment

2. **Chemo-prophylaxis (Box 10.4)**
   - Is not 100% effective
   - Can be either
     i. Causal (i.e. directed against liver schizont stage – e.g. Malarone)
     ii. Suppressive (i.e. directed against the RBC stage of the malarial parasite – e.g. mefloquine)

Box 10.4 Safety of anti-malarial chemo-prophylaxis in pregnancy

Safe in pregnancy	Contraindicated in pregnancy
• Mefloquine	• Doxycycline (causes irreversible teeth discoloration and fetal bone growth disruption)
• Malarone (is a combination of atovaquone and proguanil)	• Primaquine (causes fetal haemolysis)

3. **Proguanil is a biguanide agent**

4. **Mefloquine (FDA pregnancy category C)**
   - Is the recommended chemo-prophylaxis in pregnant women (can be used in the first trimester)
   - Is the drug of choice in chloroquine-resistant falciparum malaria

- Trade name is Lariam
- Metabolized extensively in the liver
- Half-life = 2–4 weeks
- Excreted via
  i. Bile
  ii. Faeces
- Side effects include
  i. Depression
  ii. Insomnia
  iii. Hallucinations
  iv. Seizures

5. **Malaria treatment choices in pregnancy include**
   - Artesunate (not licensed for treatment in UK)
   - Quinine (FDA pregnancy category C)

Uterotonics

1. **Oxytocin (FDA pregnancy category A)**
   - Is synthesized in
     i. Supraoptic nucleus
     ii. Paraventricular nucleus
   - Stored and released by posterior pituitary gland
   - Non-neuronal sources of oxytocin include
     i. Retina
     ii. Thymus
     iii. Adrenal medulla
     iv. Pancreas
     v. Leydig cells
     vi. Corpus luteum
     vii. Placenta
   - Is a nanopeptide (consists of 9 amino acids)
   - Half-life is 6 minutes
   - Excreted in
     i. Bile
     ii. Urine
   - Acts on G-protein receptors which require
     i. Magnesium
     ii. Cholesterol
   - Inactivated/destroyed in the GIT
   - Regulates circadian rhythm
   - Peripheral functions of oxytocin include
     i. Letdown reflex
     ii. Uterine contraction
   - Maternal oxytocin triggers a transient inhibitory switch in GABA signalling (from excitatory to inhibitory) in the fetal brain during delivery
   - Route of administration of synthetic oxytocin
     i. Intranasal
     ii. Intramuscular
     iii. Intravascular
   - Side effects (*Box 10.5*)

Box 10.5 Side effects of oxytocin

CNS	CVS	GU	Biochemical
• Subarachnoid haemorrhage • Seizures	• Tachycardia • Hypertension • ↑ Cardiac output • Arrhythmia	• Pelvic haematoma • Uterine rupture	• Oliguria • Natriuresis • Hyponatraemia • Water intoxication

2. **Prostaglandins**
   • Are 20-carbon lipid molecules (including a 5-carbon ring) derived from fatty acids
   • They are produced at many sites throughout the body (produced by all nucleated cells except for lymphocytes)
   • Act as local messengers, hence are classified as paracrine hormones
   • They have many functions throughout the body, including contraction and relaxation of smooth muscle
   • In obstetric practice they are used for
     i.   Induction of labour
     ii. Termination of pregnancy
     iii. Management of postpartum haemorrhage (PPH)
   • Commonly used prostaglandins in obstetrics include
     i.   Prostaglandin E_1 (misoprostol is a synthetic form) – commonest use is for treatment of PPH and for termination of pregnancy
     ii. Prostaglandin E_2 (dinoprostone is a naturally occurring form) – commonest use is for induction of labour by ripening the cervix
     iii. Prostaglandin $F_{2\alpha}$ (dinoprost is naturally occurring, carboprost is synthetic) – commonest use is for induction of labour, termination of pregnancy, and treatment of PPH

3. **Misoprostol (FDA pregnancy category X)**
   • Is a synthetic prostaglandin E_1 analogue
   • Half-life is 40 minutes
   • Functions
     i. Prevention of non-steroidal anti-inflammatory drug (NSAID)-induced gastric ulcers
     ii. Labour induction
   • Mechanism of action in prevention of gastric ulcers
     i.   Inhibits secretion of gastric acid by the parietal cell via G-protein coupled receptor mediated inhibition of adenylate cyclase (leading to decreased intracellular cAMP)
     ii. Increases secretion of gastric mucus
     iii. Increases gastric mucosal blood flow
   • Side effects include
     i.   Uterine rupture
     ii. Uterine hyperstimulation
     iii. Amniotic fluid embolism
     iv. Diarrhoea
     v.   Vomiting
     vi. Headache

4. **Dinoprostone (FDA pregnancy category C)**
   • Is a prostaglandin E_2 analogue
   • Is associated with transient pyrexia (may be due to its effect on hypothalamic thermoregulation)
     i. Occurs within 15–45 min of administration

    ii. Return of temperature within 2–6 h after discontinuation of therapy

5. **Ergometrine (FDA pregnancy category X)**
   - Belongs to the group of ergot alkaloids
   - Chemically similar to lysergic acid diethylamide (LSD)
   - Works on the following receptors
     i. 5HT1
     ii. Dopamine
     iii. α-adrenergic
   - Functions
     i. Vasoconstrictor
     ii. Constricts intracranial extracerebral vessels
     iii. Uterine contraction
     iv. Relieves migraine
   - Side effects
     i. Ergotism or St Anthony's fire (prolonged vasospasm resulting in gangrene, hallucinations, abortions)
     ii. GIT (diarrhoea and vomiting)
   - Contraindications
     i. Induction of labour
     ii. 1st and 2nd stage of labour
     iii. Vascular disease
     iv. Severe cardiac disease
     v. Severe hypertension

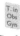

Tocolytics

Chpt 8.19

1. **There are 4 groups of tocolytics**
   - Oxytocin receptor antagonist (e.g. Atosiban)
   - β₂-agonists
     i. Salbutamol
     ii. Ritodrine
     iii. Terbutaline
   - Calcium channel blockers (e.g. nifedipine)
   - NSAIDs (e.g. indometacin)

2. **Atosiban**
   - Is an oxytocin receptor antagonist
   - Route of administration is intravenous
   - Contraindications
     i. Pre-eclampsia
     ii. Intrauterine death
     iii. Intrauterine infection
     iv. Antepartum haemorrhage
     v. Premature rupture of membranes after 30 weeks
   - Side effects
     i. Vomiting
     ii. Tachycardia
     iii. Hypotension
     iv. Headache
     v. Hot flushes

vi. Hyperglycaemia

vii. Fever

3. β₂-agonists (FDA pregnancy category B)
   - Side effects
     i.   Fluid retention secondary to decreased water clearance (pulmonary oedema)
     ii. Increased myocardial workload (myocardial ischaemia)
     iii. Increased heart rate
     iv. Increased gluconeogenesis of liver and muscle
     v.   Increased glycogenolysis
     vi. Hyperglycaemia
     vii. Hypokalaemia
     viii. Muscle cramps
     ix. Headaches
   - Include (*Box 10.6*)

Box 10.6 Examples of tocolytic β2-agonists

Ritodrine	Terbutaline	Salbutamol
• Half life = 2 h	• Half life = 6 h	• Half life = 2 h
• Route = oral	• Routes = oral, inhaled and subcutaneous	• Routes = oral, inhaled and i.v.

4. Nifedipine (FDA pregnancy category C)
   - Dihydropyridine calcium channel blocker
   - Is a vascular smooth muscle relaxant
   - Has no antiarrhythmic activity
   - Half-life is 2 h
   - Excretion via
     i. Urine
     ii. Bile
   - Unlicensed in pregnancy
   - Also used in treatment of
     i.   Hypertension
     ii. Angina
     iii. Raynaud's phenomenon
     iv. Pulmonary hypertension
   - Side effects
     i.   Hypotension
     ii. Vasodilatation
     iii. Tachycardia
     iv. Dependent oedema
     v.   Dyspnoea
   - Contraindications
     i.   Cardiogenic shock
     ii. Aortic stenosis
     iii. Acute porphyria
     iv. Within 1 month of myocardial infarction

Antihypertensive agents in pregnancy

T. in
Obs
Gyn

Chpt 8.12

1. **Hydralazine (FDA pregnancy category C)**
   - Vasodilator – arterioles > venules
   - Antioxidant
   - Metabolized by acetylation
   - Fast acting
   - Side effects
     - i.   SLE
     - ii. Tachyphylaxis
     - iii. Fluid retention
     - iv. Diarrhoea
     - v.   Headaches
     - vi. Blood dyskariasis
   - Dose = 25mg t.d.s. to 75mg q.d.s.

2. **Methyldopa (FDA pregnancy category B)**
   - Has dual mechanism of action
     - i.   Centrally acting α_2 agonist
     - ii. Competitive inhibitor of DOPA decarboxylase (i.e. the enzyme that converts L-DOPA into dopamine)
   - Prodrug
     - i.   Active metabolite is α-methylnorephinephrine
     - ii. Metabolized in liver
   - Half-life is 100 minute
   - Side effects are minimized if daily doses are below 1g
   - Side effects (**Box 10.7**)
   - Dose = 250mg b.d. to 1g t.d.s.

Box 10.7 Side effects of methyldopa

CVS	GIT	Neurological	Bone marrow suppression
• Rebound hypertension • Angina • Postural hypotension	• Dry mouth • Stomatitis • Sialadenitis • Hepatitis • Pancreatitis	• Bell's palsy • Parkinsonism	• Leukopenia • Thrombocytopenia • Haemolytic anaemia

↑ Prolactin	Autoimmune	Psychological
• Gynaecomastia • Amenorrhoea	• SLE	• Depression • Anxiety • Sexual dysfunction

3. **Labetalol (FDA pregnancy category C)**
   - Mixed $\alpha_1\beta$ blocker
   - Half-life is 8 h
   - Used only in 3rd trimester
   - Associated with

i.   FGR

ii. Neonatal hypoglycaemia

- Dose = 100mg b.d. to 600mg q.d.s.

4. Calcium channel blockers

- Two groups
  i.   Non-dihydropyridine
    - Verapamil (FDA pregnancy category C)
    - Diltiazem (FDA pregnancy category D)
  ii. Dihydropyridines (vascular selective calcium channel blockers)
    - Nimodipine (FDA pregnancy category C)
    - Nifedipine
- Nimodipine
  i.   Preferential action on cerebral arteries
  ii. Used in vasospasm post subarachnoid haemorrhage (SAH)

5. Antihypertensives to be avoided in pregnancy

- ACEis cause
  i.   Cardiovascular system (CVS) congenital malformations
  ii. Impaired fetal renal function – oligohydramnios
  iii. Skull defects
- Thiazide diuretics causes neonatal thrombocytopenia (if used in the third trimester of pregnancy)
- Statins (FDA pregnancy category X) results in CNS and limb defects

Antiepileptic drugs

Chpt 7.14

1. Epilepsy increases risk of teratogenicity regardless of antiepileptic therapy

- Background risk of teratogenicity is 2–3%
- If the mother has epilepsy and
  i.   Not on medication the risk is 4%
  ii. On medication the risk is 6–8%

2. In patients who are fit-free for 2 years the risk of recurrent seizures if therapy is withdrawn is <20%

3. General points about antiepileptic drugs in pregnancy

- Increase risk of teratogenicity by 3×
- Associated with
  i.   NTDs
  ii. Cleft lip/palate
  iii. Cardiac defects
  iv. Urogenital defects
  v.   Neonatal coagulopathies
- Mothers should be on folic acid 5 mg/day in pregnancy
- Vitamin K should be given at birth to neonates

4. Carbamazepine (FDA pregnancy category D)

- Is safest in pregnancy
- Fetal levels are approximately 50–80% of maternal serum levels
- Also used in treatment of
  i.   Bipolar disorder
  ii. Trigeminal neuralgia

5. **Valproate (FDA pregnancy category D)**
   - Drug of choice for primary generalized epilepsy
   - Has worst teratogenic profile among the antiepileptic medications
   - Fetal consequence include
     i. FGR
     ii. Hyperbilirubinaemia
     iii. Hepatotoxicity
     iv. Transient hyperglycaemia
     v. NTDs
     vi. Cardiac anomalies
     vii. Craniofacial defects
     viii. Urogenital defects (e.g. hypospadias)
     ix. Limb defects

6. **Phenytoin (FDA pregnancy category D)**
   - Lowers serum folate
   - Fetal consequence include
     i. Fetal anticonvulsant syndrome
     ii. Cleft lip/palate
     iii. Microcephaly
     iv. Cardiac abnormalities
     v. Mental retardation
   - Not associated with NTDs
   - Maternal side effects
     i. Nystagmus
     ii. Paraesthesia
     iii. Megaloblastic anaemia
     iv. Gingival hypertrophy
     v. Stevens–Johnson syndrome
     vi. Toxic epidermal necrolysis
   - Overdose causes
     i. Nystagmus
     ii. Diplopia
     iii. Slurred speech
     iv. Ataxia
     v. Hyperglycaemia

7. **Newer classes of antiepileptic drugs**
   - Lamotrigine (FDA pregnancy category C)
     i. Also used in the treatment of bipolar disorder
     ii. Excreted in breast milk
     iii. Crosses human placenta
   - Topiramate (FDA pregnancy category C)
   - Vigabatrin (FDA pregnancy category C)
   - Levetiracetam (FDA pregnancy category B)
   - Gabapentin (FDA pregnancy category B)

8. **Magnesium sulphate (FDA pregnancy category B)**
   - Used in
     i. Arrhythmias
     ii. Asthma
     iii. Eclampsia

- Side effects
  - i.   CNS depression
  - ii. Respiratory depression
- Antidote is 10ml 10% calcium gluconate

9. **Diazepam (FDA pregnancy category D)**
   - Is a benzodiazepine
   - Is a positive allosteric modulator of GABA
   - Used to treat status epilepticus
   - Also used to treat
     - i.   Insomnia
     - ii. Anxiety
     - iii. Restless leg syndrome
     - iv. Alcohol withdrawal
   - When taken in the 3rd trimester causes
     - i.   Neonatal benzodiazepine withdrawal syndrome (i.e. hypotonia, reluctance to suckle, cyanosis, impaired metabolic response to cold stress)
     - ii. Floppy infant syndrome
   - Antidote is flumazenil

Anticoagulants

Chpt 7

1. **Maternal risks of thromboprophylaxis in pregnancy include**
   - Bleeding (2%)
   - Wound haematoma (2%)
   - Allergic skin reaction (1.8%)
   - Osteoporosis (0.04%)

2. **Warfarin (FDA pregnancy category X)**
   - Is a synthetic derivative of coumarin
   - Interferes with synthesis of vitamin K-dependent clotting factors
     - i.   II
     - ii. VII
     - iii. IX
     - iv. X
   - Initial effects of warfarin are thrombogenic due to decrease in
     - i.   Protein S
     - ii. Protein C
   - Has high protein binding
   - Antidote is
     - i.   FFP
     - ii. Vitamin K
     - iii. Prothrombin complex concentrate
   - Teratogenic risk is an additional 2%
   - Maternal side effects
     - i.   Skin necrosis – due to decreased levels of protein C
     - ii. Purple toe syndrome (due to fat embolus)
     - iii. Purpura fulminans

3. **Warfarin embryopathy**
   - Occurs in 5% of fetuses if warfarin is administered between 6 and 12 weeks gestation

- Is dose dependent (higher incident noted in patients taking >5 mg/day)
- Features include
    i. Chondrodysplasia punctata
    ii. Midface hypoplasia
    iii. Pectus carinatum
    iv. Stippled epiphyses (leading to short proximal limbs and phalanges)
    v. Scoliosis
    vi. Laryngomalacia
    vii. Congenital heart defects
    viii. Ventriculomegaly

4. **Heparin – unfractionated (FDA pregnancy category C)**
    - Has the highest negative charge density
    - Weighs 8–15 kDa
    - One unit of heparin is
        i. The amount equivalent to 0.002 mg of pure heparin
        ii. The quantity required to keep 1 mL of cat's blood fluid for 24 h at 0 °C
        iii. Also known as Howell unit
    - Naturally occurring anticoagulant in
        i. Mast cells
        ii. Basophils
    - Activates antithrombin III, causing inactivation of
        i. Thrombin
        ii. Factor Xa
    - Side effects
        i. Heparin-induced thrombocytopenia
        ii. Osteoporosis
        iii. Alopecia
        iv. Hyperkalaemia
    - Antidote is protamine sulphate
    - Does not cross placenta
    - Not secreted in milk

5. **Heparin – LMWHs (FDA pregnancy category B)**
    - Average molecular weight is 4.5 kDa
    - Have a smaller risk of osteoporosis compared to unfractionated heparin
    - Include
        i. Enoxaparin (Clexane)
        ii. Tinzaparin (Innohep)
        iii. Dalteparin (Fragmin)
    - Effects of LMWH are monitored via anti-factor Xa activity
    - No need for monitoring APTT coagulation parameter
    - Doses of different types of LMWHs (**Table 10.5**)

Table 10.5 Doses of LMWHs

In Pregnancy	Enoxaparin	Dalteparin	Tinzaparin
Prophylactic dose	0.6 mg/kg o.d.	75 unit/kg o.d.	75 unit/kg o.d.
Therapeutic dose	1 mg/kg b.d.	100 unit/kg b.d.	175 unit/kg o.d.

6. **Tissue plasminogen activator (t-PA)**
   - Catalyses the conversion of plasminogen to plasmin
   - Plasmin is a fibrinolytic enzyme
   - Encoded by *PLAT* gene on chromosome 8
   - Streptokinase is a form of tPA
   - Recombinant t-PAs include
     i. Alteplase
     ii. Reteplase
   - Antidote is aminocaproic acid (an antifibrinolytic)

7. **Anticoagulants in patients who have contraindications to heparin include**
   - Danaparoid (is an inhibitor of activated factor X)
   - Lepirudin (is a direct thrombin inhibitor)
   - Fondaparinux (is an inhibitor of activated factor X)

Gastrointestinal agents

Gastro-oesophageal reflux disease drugs

1. **H$_2$ receptor blockers (FDA pregnancy category B)**
   - Are drugs that block the action of histamine on parietal cells in the stomach
   - Include
     i. Cimetidine
     ii. Ranitidine
   - Avoid cimetidine as it is an anti-androgen
   - Ranitidine is safest in pregnancy

2. **Proton pump inhibitors (PPIs)**
   - Act by irreversibly blocking H$^+$/K$^+$-ATPase of the gastric parietal cell
   - Reduces gastric acid secretion by up to 99%
   - Include
     i. Omeprazole (FDA pregnancy category C)
     ii. Pantoprazole (FDA pregnancy category B)
     iii. Lansoprazole (FDA pregnancy category B)
     iv. Rabeprazole (FDA pregnancy category B)
   - Vitamin B$_{12}$ deficiency may occur with long-term use
   - Avoid in pregnancy (reported cases of anencephaly)

3. **Antacids**
   - Are used to neutralize stomach acidity
   - Include
     i. Magnesium hydroxide (milk of magnesia)
     ii. Calcium carbonate (Rennie)
     iii. Aluminium hydroxide (Gaviscon)
   - Can result in milk-alkali syndrome (also known as Burnett's syndrome)
   - Gaviscon is safest in pregnancy

Antiemetics

1. **Most antiemetics are FDA pregnancy category B (prochlorperazine is FDA pregnancy category C) (*Table 10.6*)**

Table 10.6 Antiemetics

Antiemetics	Mechanism of action	Side effect
Cyclizine	H_1 receptor antagonist	Xerostomia Drowsiness
	Central anticholinergic action	Antimuscarinic effects Extrapyramidal effects
Metoclopramide	Dopamine D_2 receptor antagonist 5-HT$_3$ receptor antagonist 5-HT$_4$ receptor agonist Is also a gastroprokinetic agent	Extrapyramidal effects Hyperprolactinaemia Agranulocytosis Supraventricular tachycardia Neuroleptic malignant syndrome Tardive dyskinesia Oculogyric crisis (treated with procyclidine)
Ondansetron Granisetron	5-HT$_3$ receptor antagonist Reduces activity of vagus nerve	Constipation Headache
Prochlorperazine	Potent typical antipsychotic	Tardive dyskinesia Seizures Neuroleptic malignant syndrome

Laxatives and antidiarrhoeals

1. **Laxatives**
   - Can be divided into 4 main groups (*Box 10.8*)
   - Lactulose is FDA pregnancy category B
   - Senna is FDA pregnancy category C

Box 10.8 Groups of laxatives

Bulking agents	Stool softners	Osmotic agents	Stimulants
• Bran • Methylcellulose • Fybogel	• Docusate	• Lactulose • Sorbitol • Glycerine suppositories • Sodium phosphate	• Senna • Bisacodyl • Microlax enema • Castor oil

2. **Loperamide (FDA pregnancy category B)**
   - Is an antidiarrhoeal
   - Is a μ-opioid agonist
   - Acts only on opioid receptors in the large intestine
   - Does not cross the blood–brain barrier (thus does not have opioid effects in the CNS)

Anti-inflammatory and immune modulators

1. **NSAIDs**
   - Most NSAIDs are FDA pregnancy category D
   - Are non-selective inhibitors of cyclo-oxygenase (COX-1 and COX-2)
   - Have antipyretic activity
   - Include (*Box 10.9*)

2. **Indometacin (FDA pregnancy category C)**
   - Is an NSAID

Box 10.9 Types of NSAIDs

Acetic acid derivatives	Enolic acid derivatives	Fenamic acid derivatives	Propionic acid derivatives
• Indometacin	• Piroxicam	• Mefenamic acid	• Ibuprofen
• Diclofenac	• Meloxicam	• Flufenamic acid	• Naproxen
• Ketorolac			• Ketoprofen

Selective COX2 inhibitors
• Celecoxib
• Rofecoxib

- Inhibits synthesis of prostaglandin by inhibiting COX1 and COX2 enzymes
- Used to treat a PDA post natally
- Side effects if given antenatally
  i. Premature closure of ductus arteriosus
  ii. NEC
  iii. Neonatal pulmonary hypertension
  iv. Neonatal renal damage

3. **Aspirin (FDA pregnancy category D)**
   - Also known as acetylsalicylic acid
   - Is an
     i. Antipyretic
     ii. Anti-inflammatory
     iii. Antiplatelet (inhibits synthesis of thromboxane A_2 irreversibly)
   - Side effects
     i. Gastritis
     ii. Reye's syndrome (under the age of 12)
     iii. Metabolic acidosis (in overdose)
     iv. Neonatal haemorrhage if given within 5 days of delivery (hence stopped at 36 weeks gestation)
     v. Miscarriage (if used under 12 weeks gestation; although interestingly low dose aspirin is used in the treatment of recurrent miscarriage)

4. **Steroids – glucocorticoid group (FDA pregnancy category C)**
   - Include
     i. Prednisolone
     ii. Dexamethasone
     iii. Betamethasone
   - Antenatal corticosteroid treatment in preterm deliveries is associated with reduction in rates of
     i. RDS
     ii. Intraventricular haemorrhage
     iii. Neonatal death
   - Side effects include
     i. Hyperglycaemia
     ii. Leukocytosis
     iii. Cushing's
     iv. Peptic ulcers
     v. Osteoporosis

    vi. Psychiatric disturbances
- Hydrocortisone cover is needed to prevent adrenal crisis in patients (taking prednisolone dose >7.5 mg/day for >2 weeks) undergoing
  - i. Surgical procedures
  - ii. Starvation
  - iii. Labour

5. 5-aminosalicyclic acid (FDA pregnancy category B)
- Includes
  - i. Mesalazine
  - ii. Sulfasalazine
- Used in treatment of
  - i. Ulcerative colitis
  - ii. Crohn's disease
- Side effects
  - i. Agranulocytosis
  - ii. Hypospermia

6. Chemo-therapeutic agents include
- Alkylating agents (FDA pregnancy category D)
  - i. Cisplatin
  - ii. Carboplatin
  - iii. Cyclophosphamide
  - iv. Chlorambucil
- Antimetabolites (interfere with DNA production during the S-phase of the cell cycle)
  - i. Purine analogues (azathioprine)
  - ii. Pyrimidine analogues (5-fluorouracil)
  - iii. Antifolates (methotrexate)
- Alkaloids (block cell division by preventing microtubule function)
  - i. Vincristine (FDA pregnancy category D)
  - ii. Vinblastine (FDA pregnancy category D)
  - iii. Podophyllotoxin
  - iv. Paclitaxel
- Topoisomerase inhibitors (FDA pregnancy category D)
  - i. Topotecan
  - ii. Irinotecan
  - iii. Etoposide
- Antineoplastic (FDA pregnancy category D)
  - i. Doxorubicin
  - ii. Bleomycin

7. Azathioprine (FDA pregnancy category D)
- Interferes with purine synthesis
- Is a prodrug
  - i. Active metabolite is 6-mercaptopurine and 6-thioionosinic acid
  - ii. Metabolized by xanthine oxidase
- Side effects
  - i. Bone marrow suppression
  - ii. Carcinogenic

8. Mycophenolate mofetil (FDA pregnancy category C)
- Interferes with purine synthesis (by inhibition of inosine monophosphate dehydrogenase)
- Is a prodrug (active metabolite is mycophenolic acid)
- Less toxic that azathioprine

9. Methotrexate (FDA pregnancy category X) side effects (*Box 10.10*)

Box 10.10 Side effects of methotrexate

Bone marrow supression	GIT	Cardiorespiratory	Thrombosis
• Anaemia • Leukopenia • Thrombocytopenia	• Hepatitis • Pancreatitis • Pharyngitis • Gingivitis • Stomatitis	• Pericarditis • Pericardial effusion • Pulmonary fibrosis	• DVT • Retinal vein thrombosis • Cerebral thrombosis

Endocrine agents

Table 10.7 Endocrine agents

Drug	Mechanism of action	Side effects	Fetal risk
Carbimazole	Prodrug Active form = methimazole Prevents thyroid peroxidase enzyme from coupling and iodinating tyrosine residues on thyroglobulin Reduces production of T3 and T4	Bone marrow suppression (agranulocytosis)	FDA pregnancy cat. D
Propylthiouracil (PTU)	Inhibits thyroperoxidase enzyme Inhibits peripheral conversion of T4 to T3 by inhibiting tetraiodothyronine 5′ deiodinase enzyme	Agranulocytosis	FDA pregnancy cat. D (preferred over carbimazole as has lower placental transfer and excretion in breast milk)
Metformin	Is a biguanide agent Suppresses hepatic gluconeogenesis (via activation of AMP-activated protein kinase) Increases insulin sensitivity Enhances peripheral glucose uptake Increases fatty acid oxidation Is not metabolized and excreted unchanged in the urine Reduces overall mortality by 30% when compared to insulin Reduces LDL cholesterol and triglycerides	Hypoglycaemia Lactic acidosis Gastrointestinal upset	FDA pregnancy cat. B
Glibenclamide	Is a sulfonylurea class of drug Stimulates insulin release by inhibiting ATP-sensitive K+ channels in the pancreatic β cells Metabolized by the liver	Hypoglycaemia Cholestasis	FDA pregnancy cat. B

(continued)

Table 10.7 Continued

Drug	Mechanism of action	Side effects	Fetal risk
Rosiglitazone	Is a thiazolidinedione agent Decrease insulin resistance and leptin levels by binding to peroxisome proliferator-activated receptors (PPAR) in the fat cell nucleus	Increased risk of myocardial infarction (by 43%) Stroke Bone fractures Macular oedema Hepatotoxic	FDA pregnancy cat. C
Repaglinide	Is a meglitinide agent Stimulates insulin release by inhibiting ATP-sensitive K+ channels in the pancreatic β cells	Hypoglycaemia Weight gain	FDA pregnancy cat. C
Acarbose	Reduces the rate of digestion of complex carbohydrates by inhibiting α-glucosidase enzyme in the small intestines Inhibits pancreatic amylase Metabolized in the GIT	Flatulence Diarrhoea	FDA pregnancy cat. B
Vildagliptin	Is a dipeptidyl peptidase-4 (DPP-4) inhibitor	Pancreatitis	FDA pregnancy cat. B
Exenatide	Is an incretin Is a glucagon-like peptide agonist Increases pancreatic insulin secretion Suppresses pancreatic release of glucagon	Pancreatitis Possible increase in thyroid cancer risk	FDA pregnancy cat. C

Drugs used in gynaecology

1. **Mifepristone (FDA pregnancy category X)**
   - Is a competitive progesteronic receptor antagonist
   - Causes
     i. Cervical softening and dilatation
     ii. Decidual degeneration
     iii. Release of endogenous prostaglandins
     iv. Increased sensitivity of myometrium to prostaglandins
   - Is an
     i. Anti-glucocorticoid
     ii. Anti-androgen
   - Used in
     i. Emergency contraception
        ■ Delays ovulation
        ■ Prevents implantation
     ii. Medical termination (600 mg)
        ■ Up to 9 weeks gestation
   - Contraindications
     i. Severe asthma
     ii. Chronic adrenal failure

iii. Ectopic pregnancy

iv. Acute porphyria

v. Hepatic impairment

vi. Renal impairment

2. **Cyproterone acetate (FDA pregnancy category X)**
- Is an anti-androgen
  i. Suppresses action of testosterone and DHT on tissues
  ii. Suppresses LH
- Used in
  i. BPH
  ii. Prostate cancer
  iii. Priapism
  iv. Hirsutism
- Has a weak progestogenic activity (can be used to treats hot flushes)
- Suppresses synthesis of
  i. Cortisol
  ii. Aldosterone
  iii. Oestrogen
- Side effects
  i. Hepatotoxicity
  ii. Low cortisol
  iii. Low aldosterone
     - Loss of sodium
     - Hyperkalaemia
  iv. Gynaecomastia
  v. Galactorrhoea
  vi. Osteoporosis
  vii. Thrombosis (only if given with oestrogen)

T. in
Obs
Gyn

*Chpts 2.10
& 2.11*

Hormone therapy

1. **Tibolone**
- Also known as Livial
- Is a selective tissue oestrogenic activity regulator (STEAR)
- Used as
  i. HRT
  ii. Osteoporotic prevention
- Has oestrogenic, progestogenic, and androgenic properties
- Functions
  i. Relives climacteric symptoms
  ii. Prevents osteoporosis
  iii. No endometrial stimulation
  iv. Non-oestrogenic effects on breast tissue

2. **SERMs**
- Include
  i. Raloxifene
  ii. Tamoxifen
  iii. Clomifene (acts via blocking oestrogen leading to an increase in FSH)
- Have both oestrogen and anti-oestrogen activity
- Excreted via faeces

- Used for
  - i. Prevention of osteoporosis
  - ii. Decreasing risk of breast cancer
- Side effects
  - i. Thrombosis
  - ii. Endometrial carcinoma (tamoxifen)
  - iii. Hot flushes

3. **Danazol**
   - Is derived from a synthetic ethisterone, which is a modified testosterone
   - Has a weak androgenic activity
   - Is a gonadotrophin antagonist
   - Acts on the pituitary gland and inhibits LH and FSH causing inhibition of ovarian steroidogenesis, resulting in decreased secretion of oestradiol
   - Does not affect pituitary hormones
   - Used to treat
     - i. Endometriosis
     - ii. Uterine fibroids
     - iii. Menorrhagia (induces amenorrhoea)
   - Does not cause osteoporosis
   - Can masculinize a female fetus
   - Side effects
     - i. Fluid retention
     - ii. Weight gain
     - iii. Masculinizing side effects

4. **Buserelin**
   - Is a GnRH agonist
   - Acts on the pituitary
     - i. Initially causes increase of LH and FSH levels
     - ii. Eventually after 21 days
       - Receptor downregulation occurs
       - LH and FSH levels decrease
   - Used to treat
     - i. Prostate and breast cancer
     - ii. Endometriosis
     - iii. Uterine fibroids
   - Maximum duration of treatment is 6 months
   - Side effects
     - i. Menopausal symptoms
     - ii. Osteoporosis

Contraceptives

Chpt 4

General facts about contraceptives

1. **Pregnancies in the UK**
   - Unplanned = 30%
   - Unplanned pregnancies due to contraceptive method failure = 10%
   - Termination rate = 2%

2. **Methods of contraception include**
   - Combined oral contraceptive pill (COCP)

- Progesterone only
  i.   Progesterone only pill (POP)
  ii. Injection (Depo-Provera)
  iii. Implant (Implanon)
- Intrauterine coils
  i.   Devices (IUCD; copper based)
- ii. Systems (IUS; progesterone based)
- Barrier plus spermicide
  i.   Condom
  ii. Femidom
  iii. Diaphragm
  iv. Sponge
- Coitus interruptus (withdrawal method)
- Sterilization
- Thermo-regulation (Billings' method)
- Lactational amenorrhoea method

3. **The pearl index is the number of unwanted pregnancies per 100 women using the method of contraception for 1 year (*Table 10.8*)**

Table 10.8 Pearl indexes for different contraceptive methods

Contraceptive methods		Pearl Index
Oral	COCP	0.1–1.5
	POP	1.5–3
Intra-uterine	IUS	0.1
	IUCD	<3
Implanon		<0.1
Depo-Provera		0.3–1
Barriers	Condom	4–10
	Diaphragm	8–20
Sterilization		<0.5
Withdrawal		10–20
Thermo-regulation		20–30

COCP

1. **Mechanism of action**
   - Inhibits ovulation (by suppressing FSH and LH)
   - Increases viscosity of cervical mucus

2. **Contraindications**
   - Pregnancy
   - Post partum
     i.   Breastfeeding <6 weeks post partum
     ii. Non-breastfeeding <3 weeks post partum
   - Smoking >15/day above the age of 35
   - BMI >35

- Arterial disease
  - i. >2 risk factors for cardiovascular disease
  - ii. Ischaemic heart disease
  - iii. Stroke
- Hypertension
  - i. Systolic BP >160 mmHg
  - ii. Diastolic BP >95 mmHg
- Valvular heart disease with
  - i. Pulmonary hypertension
  - ii. Subacute bacterial endocarditis
- Venous thromboembolism
- Migraine with aura
- Cancer
  - i. Breast
  - ii. Malignant hepatoma
- Cirrhosis
- Raynaud's disease
- SLE

3. **COCPs can be used in the following cancers**
   - Cervical
   - Endometrial
   - Ovarian
   - Gestational trophoblastic disease

4. **Generations of COCPs**
   - First (contain high dose of oestrogen 50 µg)
     - i. Ovran
     - ii. Norinyl
   - Second (contains standard dose of oestrogen 30–35 µg)
     - i. Cilest
     - ii. Loestrin
     - iii. Logynon
     - iv. Microgynon
     - v. Microgynon ED
     - vi. Norimin
   - Third (contains new forms of progesterone)
     - i. Femodene
     - ii. Femodene ED
     - iii. Marvelon
     - iv. Mercilon

5. **Oestrogen content in COCPs**
   - Low = 20 µg
   - Standard = 30–35 µg
   - High = 50 µg

6. **Progesterone content in COCPs**
   - First and second generation
     - i. Levonorgestrel
     - ii. Norethisterone
   - Third generation
     - i. Desogestrel

ii. Gestodene

iii. Norgestimate

7. **Third generation progesterones**
   - Increase risk of venous thrombosis
   - Reduce the incidence of
     i. Acne
     ii. Headache
     iii. Weight gain
     iv. Breast symptoms
     v. Breakthrough bleeding

8. **Missed pill rule**
   - If missed <3 pills (2 if taking a low oestrogen content COCP)
     i. Take missed pill
     ii. No need extra precaution
   - If missed >3 pills (2 if taking a low oestrogen content COCP)
     i. Take missed pill
     ii. Extra precaution for 7 days
     iii. If in third week omit pill-free interval
     iv. If in first week use emergency contraception

9. **Risk of venous thromboembolism**
   - Background risk is 5 in 100 000
   - On COCP
     i. Second generation is 15 in 100 000
     ii. Third generation is 25 in 100 000
   - In pregnancy is 60 in 100 000

10. **Decreased risk of**
   - Ovarian cancer by 40–80% in user >10 years
   - Endometrial cancer
     i. By 50%
     ii. Benefit last for 20 years after discontinuing COCP

11. **Increased risk of**
   - Breast cancer
     i. Risk falls to normal after 10 years of discontinuing COCP
     ii. No increased risk with oestrogen alone
   - Cervical cancer (unclear at the moment)

Progesterone-only contraception

1. **Mechanism of action**
   - Inhibits ovulation
     i. Low-dose progesterones inconsistently inhibit ovulation in 50% of cycles
     ii. Intermediate-dose progesterones (Cerazette and Implanon) inhibit ovulation in 97–99% of cycles
     iii. High-dose progesterones (Depo-Provera) completely inhibit ovulation and follicular development
   - Increases viscosity of cervical mucus

2. **Side effects**
   - Irregular bleeding
   - Weight gain

- Breast discomfort
- Depression
- Acne

3. **Can be used within 3 weeks of delivery without any extra precautions**

4. **Oral progesterone-only contraception**
   - Includes
     i.   Etynodiol diacetate (Femulen)
     ii. Norethisterone (Micronor)
     iii. Levonorgestrel (Norgeston)
     iv. Desogestrel (Cerazette)
   - Contraindications
     i.   Pregnancy
     ii. Undiagnosed vaginal bleeding
     iii. Liver tumour
     iv. Acute porphyria
     v.   History of breast cancer (can be used after 5 years of disease remission)
   - Safety window is 3 h except for Cerazette where it is 12 h

5. **Missed pill rule**
   - POP has a short time frame (3 h) except for Cerazette (12 h)
   - After a missed pill
     i. Take the missed or late pill
     ii. Extra precaution should be used for 48 h

6. **Bleeding patterns on POP**
   - Amenorrhoea in 20%
   - Regular bleeding in 40%
   - Erratic bleeding in 40%

7. **Parental progesterone-only contraception**
   - Includes
     i.   Medroxyprogesterone acetate i.m. injection (Depo-Provera)
     ii. Norethisterone enantate i.m. injection – lasts 8 weeks
     iii. Etonogestrel-releasing implant (Implanon) – effective up to 3 years
   - Reliably inhibits ovulation

8. **Medroxyprogesterone acetate (Depo-Provera)**
   - Is given i.m.
   - Lasts for 12 weeks
   - Timing of injections
     i. Given 5 days post partum in non-breastfeeding women
     ii. If given <6 weeks post partum, risk of menorrhagia increases
   - Side effects
     i.   Weight gain (2 kg/year) in 70%
     ii. Osteoporosis (hence avoid use for more than 2 years)
     iii. Delay in return to fertility by 6–18 months
   - Bleeding patterns with Depo-Provera
     i.   Irregular bleeding
     ii. Amenorrhoea in 55% at 12 months
     iii. Amenorrhoea in 68% at 24 months
   - 60% conceive within 12 months of discontinuation
   - 84% conceive within 24 months of discontinuation

- Decreases serum oestrogen level due to its complete inhibition effect on ovulation
- Associated with reduction in bone density within the first 2 years of use
- Reduces risk of endometrial cancer by 80%

9. **Implanon**
   - Contains etonogestrel 68 mg
   - Lasts for 3 years
   - Serum levels of progesterone
     i.   Reach ovulation-inhibiting levels within 24 h of insertion
     ii. Reach peak levels within 1–13 days
     iii. Decline within 1 week of implant removal
   - 90% start to ovulate within 3 weeks of removal
   - Bleeding patterns on Implanon
     i.   Amenorrhoea in 20%
     ii. Prolonged bleeding in 20%
     iii. Infrequent bleeding in 5%

Intrauterine coils

1. **Two types**
   - Devices (copper based)
   - System (progesterone based)

2. **Insertion**
   - Immediately after first or second trimester abortion
   - From 4 weeks post partum
   - At any time in the menstrual cycle
   - Extra precaution is not needed for
     i.   Copper coil (is effective immediately)
     ii. Mirena if inserted on day 1 of cycle (otherwise will need 7 days precaution)

3. **Complications**
   - Risk of expulsion is
     i.   5%
     ii. Common in the first year (especially within the first 3 month)
   - Risk of uterine perforation is 1 in 1000
   - Risk of pelvic infection is greatest in the 20 days post insertion

4. **Intra-uterine coil device**
   - Contains copper
   - Mode of action
     i.   Copper is toxic to ovum and sperm
     ii. Inhibits fertilization
     iii. Inhibits implantation
   - Irregular or heavy bleeding is common in the first 3–6 months
   - Licensed for 7–10 years' use depending on brand

5. **Intrauterine coil system (Mirena)**
   - Contains a compartment which gradually releases levonorgestrel
   - Mode of action
     i.   Mediated via progestogenic effect on endometrium
     ii. Endometrial atrophy occurs within 1 month of insertion
     iii. Increase in endometrial phagocytic cells
     iv. Increase cervical mucus viscosity
     v.   75% still continue to ovulate

- Lasts for 5 years
- Bleeding patterns
  i.   Irregular bleeding is common in the first 6 months
  ii. Amenorrhoea in 65% at 12 months

Emergency contraception

1. **Emergency contraception methods include**
   - Levonorgestrel 1500 µg (within 72 h of unprotected sexual intercourse)
   - Yuzpe's regimen
   - Copper intrauterine device (within 5 days of unprotected sexual intercourse or within 5 days of ovulation)
   - EllaOne

2. **Levonorgestrel 1500 µg**
   - Efficacy of use
     i.   Within 24 h = 95% effective
     ii. 24–48 h = 85% effective
     iii. 49–72 h = 58% effective
   - Inhibits ovulation for 5–7 days if taken prior to ovulation
   - Women taking liver enzyme inducers should take 3000 µg of levonorgestrel within 72 h
   - Side effects
     i.   Nausea in 14%
     ii. Bleeding within 7 days of taking levonorgestrel in 16%
   - Timing of next menses
     i.   Within the expected date = 80%
     ii. Within 7 days after the expected date = 95%

3. **EllaOne**
   - Contains ulipristal acetate 30 mg
   - Is a selective progesterone receptor modulator (SPRM)
   - Can be used up to 120 h after unprotected sexual intercourse
   - Mode of action
     i.   Inhibits ovulation
     ii. Suppresses growth of follicles
     iii. Delays endometrial maturation

Intrapartum science

CONTENTS

Labour

General facts

Chpt 9.1
1. **Labour is also known as parturition**

2. **Is diagnosed retrospectively by detection of**
   - Cervical dilatation
   - Cervical effacement

3. **Labour is divided into 3 stages**
   - Stage 1 (effacement and dilatation of the cervix up to full dilatation – 10 cm) – divided in to
     i. Latent phase (dilatation up to 4 cm)
     ii. Active phase (dilatation from 4 cm onwards)
   - Stage 2 (from full cervical dilatation to delivery of the fetus) – divided into
     i. Propulsive phase
     ii. Expulsive phase (delay is defined if the expulsive phase last > 2 h in nulliparous and > 1 h in multiparous women)
   - Stage 3 (delivery of placenta)

4. **The angulation of the birth canal is known as the curve of Carus**

5. **Mechanism of labour**
   - Engagement
     i. The transverse or oblique diameter of the fetal head enters the pelvic brim
     ii. Asynclitism occurs prior to engagement
   - Descent of fetal head to below the ischial spines and flexion
   - Fetal head rotation to the occipito-anterior position, shoulders enter pelvis
   - Extension and delivery of fetal head
   - Restitution
   - Delivery of shoulders and rest of body

Disorders of labour

Chpt 9.4
1. **Labour dystocia**
   - 3 patterns have been described

  i.   Prolonged latent phase
  ii. Primary dysfunctional labour
  iii. Secondary arrest
- Prolonged latent phase
  i.   Incidence = 3.5% in nulliparous women
  ii. Relates to delayed cervical ripening
  iii. Augmentation with oxytocin is not beneficial
- Primary dysfunctional labour
  i.   Is cervical dilatation slower than 1 cm/h during the active phase of stage 1 of labour
  ii. Incidence = 26% in nulliparous women and 8% in multiparous women
- Secondary arrest
  i.   Incidence = 6% in nulliparous women and 2% in multiparous women
  ii. Usually linked with fetal malposition

T. in
Obs
Gyn
Chpt 8.27
& 9.11

2. **Breech presentation**
- Incidence at
  i.   28 weeks = 30%
  ii. Term = 3%
- Aetiology (**Box 11.1**)

Box 11.1 Aetiology of breech presentation

Pregnancy related	Fetal structural abnormality	Fetal growth abnormality	Placental abnormality
• Increased parity • Multiple pregnancy • Prematurity	• Hydrocephalus • Myelomeningocoele	• FGR • Oligohydramnios • Polyhydramnios	• Placenta praevia • Short umbilical cord

Uterine abnormality	Pelvic abnormality
• Bicornuate uterus	• Contracted pelvis

- Types of breech
  i.   Extended (or frank breech) = 60–70%
  ii. Flexed (or complete breech)
  iii. Footling
- Fetal risks of vaginal breech delivery
  i.   Intracranial haemorrhage
  ii. Brachial plexus injury
  iii. Limb fractures
  iv. Spinal cord injury

3. **Reasons for predominance of cephalic presentation**
- Piriform shape of uterus
- Calcification of fetal skull (increased skull density)

T. in
Obs
Gyn
Chpt 10.4

4. **Shoulder dystocia**
- Occurs when there is failure of the shoulders to deliver with gentle downwards traction on the fetal head
- Incidence = 0.6%
- Anterior shoulder is commonly involved

- Signs
  - i.   External rotation failure
  - ii. Turtle necking
- Can cause fetal distress due to a reduction in O_2 supply caused by
  - i.   Uterine contraction
  - ii. Fetal chest compression
- Fetal complications
  - i.   Asphyxia
  - ii. Brachial plexus injury
  - iii. Fracture of clavicle (in 15%) and humerus (in 1%)
- Brachial plexus injury
  - i.   Occurs in 10% of shoulder dystocia
  - ii. Permanent neurological damage occurs in 10% of brachial plexus injury
  - iii. Caesarean section does not eliminate the risk of brachial plexus injury
- Risk factors
  - i.   Conventional risk factors predict 15% cases of shoulder dystocia
  - ii. Fetal macrosomia (but note that 48% of shoulder dystocia cases occur in fetuses <4 kg)
  - iii. Maternal diabetes
  - iv. Maternal obesity
  - v.   Previous shoulder dystocia
  - vi. Prolonged labour
  - vii. Instrumental delivery
- 2300 caesarean sections need to be performed to prevent 1 permanent neurological injury from shoulder dystocia
- Recurrence rate = 15%
- Fetal pH drops at a rate of 0.04/min

Electronic fetal monitoring

General facts

1. **Fetal physiology in labour**
   - Maternal placental blood flow
     - i.   Is 500 mL/min
     - ii. Stops when uterine contraction exceeds 30 mmHg
   - Fetus needs 60–90 s between contractions to regain normal blood gases
   - Umbilical cord circulation
     - i.   Is not affected by contractions in first stage of labour
     - ii. Stops during active stage of pushing (especially in the umbilical vein)
   - Cell metabolism
     - i.   Fetal glycogen stores are generated in the third trimester (therefore the preterm fetus has less glycogen stores)
     - ii. In hypoxic conditions the fetus undergoes anaerobic metabolism, utilizing blood glucose and stored glycogen to produce energy
     - iii. The energy produced via anaerobic metabolism is 1/20th of that produced via aerobic metabolism

2. **Fetal response to**
   - Hypoxaemia (decrease in the O_2 content of arterial blood with normal cell and organ function) (**Fig. 11.1**)
   - Hypoxia (O_2 deficiency which affects peripheral tissues) (**Fig. 11.2**)

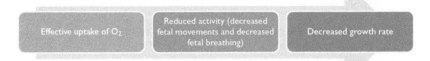

Figure 11.1 Fetal response to hypoxaemia

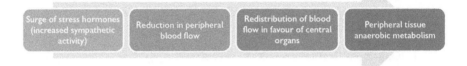

Figure 11.2 Fetal response to hypoxia

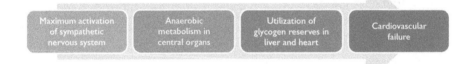

Figure 11.3 Fetal response to asphyxia

- Asphyxia (when the cellular energy production is no longer sufficient to meet the fetal demands) (*Fig. 11.3*)

3. **Criteria for diagnosis of acute intrapartum hypoxia causing brain damage**
   - Evidence of metabolic acidosis in umbilical arterial vessels
     i.   pH <7
     ii. Base excess >12
   - Early onset of severe or moderate neonatal encephalopathy in term babies
   - Cerebral palsy of spastic quadriplegic or dyskinetic type

4. **Spalding sign on X-ray represents overlapping of fetal skull bones in advanced maceration of fetal tissues**

T. In
Obs
Gyn

Chpt 9.6–9.8

Cardiotocography (CTG)

1. **CTG records**
   - Fetal heart rate (by recognizing R-R interval on the ECG)
   - Uterine contractions

2. **Consists of 2 transducers**
   - Heart ultrasonic sensor
   - Tocodynamometer

3. **Speed of recording is usually 1 cm/min**

4. **CTG has a high false-positive rate (about 50%)**

5. **Baseline heart rate**
   - Is defined as a fetal heart rate recorded between contractions over a period of at least 10 min
   - Tachycardia is defined as a baseline fetal heart rate >160 bpm
   - Bradycardia is defined as a baseline fetal heart rate <110 bpm

6. **Variability**
   - Is the beat-to-beat variation of the fetal heart beat
   - Normal variability is 5–25 bpm
   - Variability >25 bpm is known a saltatory pattern
   - Reduced variability (i.e. <5 bpm) is seen in
     i. Sleep cycle
     ii. Preterminal pattern
   - Sinusoidal pattern
     i. Seen in fetal anaemia or feto-maternal haemorrhage
     ii. Has a frequency of 3–5 cycles/min
     iii. Seen as a smooth undulating sine wave pattern

7. **Accelerations**
   - Defined as an intermittent increase in heart rate of more than 15 beats lasting for more than 15 s
   - A reactive CTG should contain 2 acceleration in a 20-min period
   - Sign of adequate oxygenation

8. **Decelerations**
   - Defined as a drop in heart rate of more than 15 beats lasting for more than 15 s
   - Consist of 3 types
     i. Early
     ii. Late
     iii. Variable
   - Early decelerations
     i. A reflex generated drop in heart rate that occurs during a contraction
     ii. The nadir of the drop in heart rate corresponds to the peak of the uterine contraction
     iii. Are not related to hypoxia
     iv. Are due to mechanical forces acting on the fetus
   - Late decelerations
     i. Often signify hypoxia
     ii. May be associated with placental insufficiency
   - Variable decelerations
     i. Are classified as uncomplicated or complicated
     ii. Account for 80% of all decelerations
     iii. Uncomplicated variable decelerations last for <60 s
     iv. Are due to cord compression
     v. Risk of hypoxia increases if decelerations last for >60 s

9. **CTG is classified according to the National Institute for Health and Clinical Excellence (NICE) guidelines into 3 categories (*Box 11.2*)**
   - Normal (when all 4 features are reassuring)
   - Suspicious (when 1 feature is non-reassuring)
   - Pathological (when 1 feature is abnormal or >2 features are non-reassuring)

Box 11.2 CTG features

Reassuring	Non-reassuring	Abnormal
• Baseline = 110–160 bpm • Variability = 5–25 bpm • No decelerations • Accelerations present	• Baseline = 100–109 or 161–180 bpm • Variability <5 bpm for >40 min but <90 min • Early decelerations • Variable decelerations with over 50% of the contractions occuring for 90 min • Single prolonged deceleration up to 3 min	• Baseline <100 or > 180 bpm • Sinusoidal pattern for >10 min • Variability <5 bpm for 90 min • Late or atypical variable decelerations with over 50% of the contractions occuring for 30 min • Single prolonged deceleration over 3 min

10. **There are 4 patterns of hypoxic changes on the CTG**
   • Acute (when there is a sudden acute drop in baseline) – fetal pH drops by 0.01/ min
   • Subacute (when the fetal heart rate stays below the baseline during the majority of the time) – fetal pH drops by 0.01 every 2–3 min
   • Evolving – shows the following sequence of changes (**Fig. 11.4**)
   • Chronic

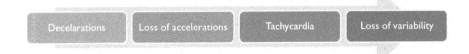

Figure 11.4 Sequence of CTG changes in evolving hypoxia

11. **Acute Hypoxia aetiology**
   • Unknown (50%)
   • Placental abruption
   • Scar dehiscence/rupture
   • Cord prolapse
   • Uterine hyperstimulation
   • Epidural top-up

12. **Evolving hypoxia has 3 stages**
   • Stress stage (is the presence of decelerations without a rise in baseline)
   • Distress stage
      i.   Reaches maximum tachycardia (usually 20–30 bmp above baseline)
      ii. Marked reduction in baseline variability (< 2 bpm)
   • Collapse stage
      i.   Is the sudden decline in fetal heart rate in a step-wise manner to terminal bradycardia
      ii. Is usually short (20–60 min from the onset of fetal heart decline)
      iii. Also known as Hon's step-ladder pattern to death

ST analysis (STAN)

1. **Is based on the concept that the ST interval of the fetal ECG reflects the function of the fetal myocardium during stress**

2. It combines fetal heart rate interpretation along with ST interval analysis

3. The analysis takes into account 30 ECG complexes at a time and calculates the T/QRS ratio

4. **Physiology of ST interval changes in hypoxia**
   - Hypoxia causes fetal adrenaline surge and myocardial anaerobic metabolism
   - Adrenaline surge activates glycogenolysis
   - Increased glycogenolysis causes increased K^+ release
   - Increased plasma K^+ leads to an increase in T-wave amplitude
   - Rate of increase in T-wave amplitude depends on the amount of glycogen the fetus needs to utilize to maintain its myocardial energy balance

5. **There are 3 types of STAN event**
   - Biphasic ST
   - Baseline rise in T/QRS ratio
   - Episodic rise in T/QRS ratio

6. **Biphasic ST events**
   - Seen
     i.   In initial phase of hypoxia
     ii. When fetus is not capable of responding to hypoxia
     iii. In myocardial dysfunction, due to cardiac malformation or infections
   - There are 3 grades
   - Repeated grade 2 and 3 events should be regarded as a sign of abnormality

7. **Baseline rise in T/QRS ratio**
   - Occurs when there is a rise in the T/QRS ratio lasting for more than 10 min
   - Reflects fetal response to hypoxia with anaerobic metabolism
   - If it is more than 0.05 it is significant

8. **Episodic rise in T/QRS ratio**
   - Occurs when the rise in the T/QRS ratio returns to baseline within 10 min
   - Reflects fetal distress
   - If it is >0.10 it is significant
   - Corresponds to short-lasting hypoxia

Medical physics and clinical applications

Ultrasound

General facts of ultrasound

1. **Physics of sound**
    *   The human ear can detect frequencies between 20 and 20 kHz
    *   Ultrasound frequencies are those above 20 kHz
    *   Range normally used in medical imaging is between 2 and 15 MHz
    *   Ultrasound waves are longitudinal compression waves
    *   Speed of sound in all tissues is assumed to be 1540 ms^{-1}
    *   C = fλ (where c = speed of sound; f = frequency; λ = wavelength)
    *   Ultrasound imaging uses the pulse echo principle

2. **Ultrasound probes consist of 2 elements**
    *   Transducer (made from materials that exhibit piezoelectric behaviour; e.g. quartz or ceramic)
    *   Receiver

3. **Acoustic intensity**
    *   Is the measure of energy flux over a certain time period
    *   Is defined as sound power per unit area
    *   The SI unit is watts per square meter (W/m^2)

4. **Frame rate**
    *   Is the frequency at which an imaging device produces unique consecutive images (frames)
    *   Is expressed in frame rates per second
    *   The higher the resolution the longer it takes for the ultrasound probe to generate an image limiting the maximum achievable frame rate. Hence, there is a trade-off between resolution and frame rate (relevant when imaging fast moving objects such as the heart)

5. **Interaction of ultrasound wave with tissue (Figs 12.1 and 12.2)**
    *   Reflection
        i.   Is the change in direction of a wavefront at an interface between two different media so that the wavefront returns into the medium from which it originates

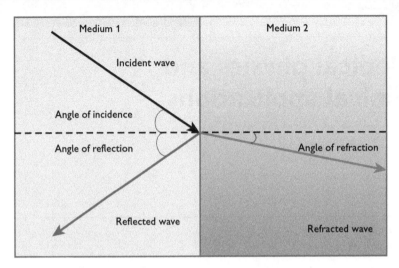

Figure 12.1 Wave reflection and refraction

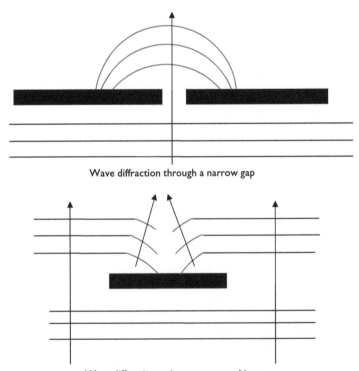

Wave diffraction through a narrow gap

Wave diffraction as it goes past an object

Figure 12.2 Wave diffraction

    ii. The law of reflection states that the angle at which the wave is incident on the surface equals the angle at which it is reflected

    iii. Strength of reflection from an object depends on its acoustic impedance

- Refraction is the change in direction of a wave due to a change in its speed as it passes from one medium to another
- Diffraction
  - i. Is the apparent bending of waves around small obstacles and the spreading out of waves past small openings
  - ii. Occurs when a wave encounters an obstacle that has a diameter comparable to its wavelength
  - iii. Higher frequency waves are rarely diffracted
  - iv. Only changes the direction in which the wave is travelling
- Scatter
- Absorption is defined as the direct conversion of sound energy into heat as it travels though a medium

6. **Ultrasound can produce biological effects in 3 ways**
   - Cavitation (i.e. the growth, oscillation and decay of small gas bubbles under the influence of an ultrasound wave)
   - Microstreaming (is the formation of small local fluid circulations and can be both intra- and extracellular)
   - Heating

7. **Ultrasound is limited by its inability to image through**
   - Air
   - Bone

8. **3-dimensional ultrasound imaging consists of a sweep of multiple 2-dimensional scans in parallel and then reconstruction of a third Z-plane, creating a volume box containing 3-dimensional voxels instead of 2-dimensional pixels**

9. **4-dimensional ultrasonography is 3-dimensional ultrasonography with the 4th dimension being time**

General facts about Doppler

1. **Physics of Doppler ultrasonography**
   - The Doppler effect is based on the fact that reflected or scattered ultrasound waves from a moving interface will undergo a frequency shift
   - Doppler shift is the change in frequency of a wave for an observer moving relative to the source of the wave
   - Used in medicine to detect and measure blood flow (RBCs are the major reflectors)
   - Doppler shift is dependent on the
     - i. Insonating frequency
     - ii. Velocity of moving blood
     - iii. Angle between sound beam and direction of moving blood
   - Doppler shift frequency is the difference between the transmitted and received frequencies

2. **There are 3 types of Doppler mode in ultrasound machines**
   - Pulse
   - Power
   - Colour

3. **Factors affecting the displayed Doppler image in ultrasound machines**
   - Transmitted power

- Doppler gain (influences the overall sensitivity)
- Frequency (the higher the frequency, the higher the resolution and the lower the penetration)
- Velocity (also known as pulse repetition frequency)
- Sample gate
  i. Influences axial resolution of Doppler signal
  ii. The higher the sample gate the higher the resolution is but at the expense of a lower frame rate
- Wall filter

4. **Pulse Doppler**
   - Allows a sampling gate to be positioned over a vessel visualized on the grey-scale image. The amplitude of the signal is approximately proportional to the number of moving RBCs
   - Provides information on
     i. Direction of blood flow
     ii. Velocity of blood flow
     iii. Flow characteristics
   - Is angle dependent (flow perpendicular to transducer is difficult to detect)

5. **Power Doppler**
   - Also known as energy or amplitude Doppler
   - Allows detection of a larger range of Doppler shifts and thus better visualization of small vessels, but at the expense of directional and velocity information
   - Advantages
     i. Free from aliasing
     ii. No angle dependences
     iii. Higher sensitivity to detect low flow or small blood vessels
     iv. Better penetration
   - Disadvantages
     i. No directional information
     ii. No velocity information

6. **Colour Doppler**
   - Provides an estimate of the mean velocity of flow within a vessel by colour coding the information and displaying it superimposed on the grey-scale image
   - The flow direction is arbitrarily assigned the colour red or blue, indicating flow toward or away from the transducer, respectively.
   - Also provides information on
     i. Overall view of flow in an organ
     ii. Direction of flow
     iii. Velocity of flow
   - Disadvantages
     i. Poor temporal resolution
     ii. Is angle dependent

Ultrasound imaging measurements in non-pregnant pelvis

1. **Endometrial thickness**
   - During the reproductive age it ranges between 5 and 14mm
   - In postmenopausal women it is <4mm

2. **Ovarian follicles**
   - Are simple anechoic areas within the ovaries with clear and well-defined walls

- Grow at a rate of 2 mm/day
- Reach a maximum diameter of 20–25 mm before ovulation

3. **Corpus luteum can be**
   - Solid
   - Cystic
   - Haemorrhagic

4. **Ultrasound imaging is used in all stages of *in vitro* fertilization (IVF) treatment to monitor oocyte development, retrieval, and transfer**
   - Stage 1 (pituitary desensitization)
     - i. Patient is given GnRH agonist
     - ii. This stage of treatment lasts for 2 weeks
   - Stage 2 (ovarian superovulation)
     - i. Achieved with daily injections of gonadotrophin
     - ii. hCG is given prior to oocyte collection when the largest follicle is 18 mm and endometrial thickness is 6 mm
   - Stage 3 (oocyte collection)
     - i. Oocytes are retrieved 36 hours after hCG injection
   - Stage 4 (embryo transfer)
     - i. Performed 2–3 days after oocyte collection
   - Stage 5 (post embryo transfer)
     - i. Progesterone supplements are given to support corpus luteal function

Ultrasound imaging measurements in early pregnancy

1. **Gestational sac**
   - Detected transvaginally from 31 days (4^{+3} weeks) of gestation when it measures 2–3 mm
   - Detected transabdominally from 5^{+3} weeks
   - Grows 1 mm/day in diameter
   - Consist of 2 fluid-filled compartment
     - i. Inner amniotic cavity
       - From 8 weeks gestation it expands rapidly within the chorionic cavity such that it soon occupies most of the gestational sac
     - ii. Outer chorionic cavity
       - Dominates in early pregnancy
     - iii. Fusion of chorionic and amniotic membrane
       - By the end of the first trimester
       - Obliterates chorionic cavity
   - Used to calculate gestational age before embryo is visible

2. **Yolk sac**
   - Becomes visible in chorionic cavity transvaginally at 5 weeks gestation (when it measures 3–4 mm)
   - Should be seen in all pregnancies with a gestation sac diameter >12 mm
   - Grows until it reaches a maximum diameter of 6 mm (at 10 weeks gestation)

3. **Embryonic pole**
   - Is usually visible when gestational sac diameter is >18 mm
   - Can be visualized transvaginally at 37 days gestation (usually measuring 2–3 mm)
   - Crown rump length (CRL) is used as a measure of gestation before 12 weeks but is unreliable after this (as the fetus is more likely to be in a flexed position)
   - Biparietal diameter (BPD) is used for measuring gestational age after 12 weeks gestation

4. **Heart action**
   - Is detectable at 5^{+2} weeks gestation
   - Should be visualized in all embryos of crown–rump length (CRL) >6 mm in length

5. **Fetal spine can be identified from 9 weeks gestation**

6. **Nuchal translucency**

Chpt 6.12
   - Is increased in chromosomal abnormality (e.g. trisomy 21, 18, Turner's syndrome) between 11 and 14 weeks of gestation
   - Nuchal thickness >6 mm – linked to
     i. Chromosomal abnormalities
     ii. Cardiac anomalies
     iii. Fetal viral infection
     iv. Rhesus incompatibility

7. **Risk of miscarriage based on ultrasound findings of**
   - Empty gestation sac = 12%
   - CRL
     i. <5 mm = 7%
     ii. >10 mm = 1%

8. **Early pregnancy ultrasound imaging findings for**
   - Embryonic death (based on the Royal College of Obstetrics and Gynaecologists guidelines)
     i. Absence of cardiac activity in an embryo with a CRL >6 mm
     ii. Absence of yolk sac/embryo in a gestation sac with a diameter >20 mm
   - Complete miscarriage
     i. Thin and regular endometrium
   - Incomplete miscarriage
     i. Endometrial thickness >5 mm
     ii. Hyperechoic tissue within the uterine cavity

9. **Ectopic pregnancy**

Chpt 5.7
   - Is defined as implantation of a fertilized ovum outside the uterine cavity
   - Incidence in UK = 9.6/1000 pregnancies
   - Ultrasound imaging findings
     i. Pseudosac within the uterus
        - In 10–29% of ectopic pregnancies
        - Appears avascular on Doppler examination
     ii. 78% of ectopic pregnancies are ipsilateral to the corpus luteum
     iii. Free fluid in pouch of Douglas in 20–25% of ectopic pregnancies
     iv. 'Sliding organs' sign
   - Management
     i. Expectant (has a failure rate of 40–50%)
     ii. Medical (has a success rate with methotrexate of 74–94%)
     iii. Surgical (includes salpingectomy or salpingostomy)
   - There are 6 types of ectopic pregnancy (***Box 12.1***)

10. **Placenta praevia**

Chpt 8.3
   - Term used to describe the placental position in relation to the uterine lower segment after 28 weeks of gestation
   - Implies that the leading edge of the placenta lies within 5 cm of the internal cervical os
   - Statistics
     i. At 22 weeks gestation – 5% of women will have a low-lying placenta
     ii. 25% of women with low-lying placenta will have placenta praevia

Box 12.1 Types of ectopic pregnancy

Tubal	Interstitial	Cervical	Ovarian
• Occurs in 93% of all ectopic pregnancies	• Occurs in 1.1–6.3% of all ectopic pregnancies	• Occurs in 0.15% of all ectopic pregnancies	• Occurs in 1 : 4,000 to 1 : 7,000 deliveries

Abdominal	Heterotopic
• Occurs in 1 : 3,400 to 1 : 8,000 deliveries	• Occurs in 1 : 6,000 deliveries • Is the combination of an intrauterine and ectopic pregnancy

Box 12.2 Causes of polyhydramnios

Increased fetal production	Decreased fetal swallowing	Idiopathic
• Maternal diabetes mellitus • Constitutional fetal macrosomia • Fetal hyperdynamic circulation which is due to • Fetal anaemia (e.g. Rhesus disease or parvovirus infection) • AV fistula • Structural fetal abdnormalities (e.g. open NTDs, teratomas)	• Upper GIT obstruction • Fetal neurogenic disease	

- Is broadly classified into
  i. Minor (i.e. placenta encroaches into the lower segment of the uterus)
  ii. Major (i.e. placenta encroaches to, or covering the internal cervical os)

Use of ultrasound in assessing fetal well being

Chpt 6.10 **1. Amniotic fluid index (AFI)**
- Is the sum of measurement of the depth of the largest cord-free vertical pool in each of the 4 uterine quadrants
- AFI <5 cm = oligohydramnios
- AFI >25 cm = polyhydramnios

2. Polyhydramnios
- Is defined as an AFI >25 cm or when the largest pocket of amniotic fluid is more than 8 cm in vertical depth
- There are 3 main causes of polyhydramnios (*Box 12.2*)

3. Oligohydramnios
- Is defined as an AFI <5 cm or when the largest pocket of amniotic fluid is <2 cm in vertical depth
- Causes of oligohydramnios (*Fig. 12.3*)

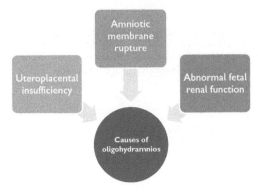

Figure 12.3 Causes of oligohydramnios

4. **FGR**
   - Is defined as birth weight <10th centile for gestation
   - Types of FGR
     i.   Symmetrical
     ii. Asymmetrical

5. **Symmetrical growth restriction**
   - Occurs when there is equal reduction in growth velocity of both the fetal head circumference and the abdominal circumference
   - Due to
     i.   Constitutionally small fetus
     ii. Pathologically small fetus (due to early-onset uteroplacental insufficiency or triploidy)

6. **Asymmetrical growth restriction**
   - Describes when there is deferential reduction in growth velocity of the fetal head to the abdominal circumference
   - Is a consequence of uteroplacental insufficiency

7. **Doppler high resistance patterns**
   - Bilateral notches with mean resistance index (RI) >0.55
   - Unilateral notch with mean RI >0.65
   - Total pulsatility index (PI) >2.5

8. **Doppler findings in uteroplacental insufficiency**
   - Uterine artery notches
   - Umbilical artery – absent end-diastolic blood flow
     i.   Occurs only when over 75% of placental bed has been obliterated
     ii. Associated with 85% chance of fetal hypoxaemia
     iii. Associated with 50% chance of fetal acidaemia
   - Umbilical artery – reversed end-diastolic blood flow
     i.   Carries a 10-fold increase in perinatal mortality compared with those with normal umbilical artery waveforms
   - Fetal arterial redistribution
     i.   Is reported when the ratio of the middle cerebral artery (MCA) PI to umbilical artery (UA) PI is increased above the 95th centile
   - Abnormal fetal ductus venosus Doppler
     i.   Is associated with severe fetal acidaemia
     ii. Normal fetal ductus venosus Doppler in a growth-restricted fetus indicates that there is adequate fetal compensation

9. **Fetal biophysical profile**
   - Is used to assess fetal well being
   - It has 5 criteria, each scoring a maximum of 2 points
     i. Fetal tone (assessed over 30 min)
     ii. Fetal movements
     iii. Breathing movements
     iv. Amniotic fluid volume
     v. Fetal heart rate
   - Score
     i. Range from 0 to 10
     ii. <6 = abnormal
     iii. 7–8 = suspicious

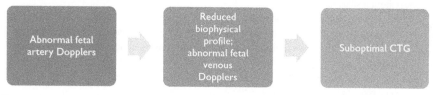

Figure 12.4 Chronology of fetal growth restriction

Examples of fetal abnormalities detected by ultrasound imaging

1. **NTDs**
   - Incidence in the UK is 2–5/1000 births
   - Signs on ultrasound imaging
     i. Lemon sign – describes the abnormal scalloping of the frontal bones (used as a marker between 16 and 24 weeks gestation)
     ii. Banana sign – describes a crescent or banana-shaped cerebellum that produces an abnormally small transcerebellar diameter
     iii. Cisterna magna is reduced in size

2. **Types of NTD**
   - Spina bifida occulta (unfused vertebral arch)
   - Spina bifida cystica
     i. Neural tubes and their coverings protrude through the vertebral arch
     ii. Meningocoele
        - Neural tube lies in its normal position
        - Cyst formed by protruding subarachnoid membrane and space
     iii. Meningomyelocoele – neural tube lies ectopic in the cystic space
     iv. Associated with hydrocephalus
   - Rachischisis
     i. No neural tube
     ii. Neural tissue is fused with skin
   - Anencephaly

3. **Anterior abdominal wall defects**
   - Consist of 2 types
     i. Omphalocele
     ii. Gastroschisis
   - Associated with raised maternal serum AFP
   - Incidence is 1 : 4000 births

4. **Renal pelvic dilatation**
   - Is associated with postnatal uropathies
     i. Pelviureteric junction obstruction
     ii. Duplex kidney
     iii. Reflux
   - Upper limit of normal of fetal renal pelvic diameter at
     i. Second trimester = 5 mm
     ii. Third trimester = 10 mm

Invasive procedures

Chpt 6.14 1. **Invasive procedures performed under ultrasound guidance include**
   - Amniocentesis
   - Chorion villus sampling
   - Intrauterine fetal blood transfusion
   - Fetoscopic surgery (e.g. shunt insertions, aiding primary port insertion for use in laser ablation for twin-to-twin transfusion syndrome or oesophageal occlusion for diaphragmatic hernia)
   - Amnioreduction
   - Fetal reduction/intracardiac K^+ injections

2. **Amniocentesis**
   - Is usually performed at 16 weeks gestation
   - Procedure-related risk of miscarriage is $\approx 1\%$

3. **Chorion villus sampling**
   - Is usually performed at 10–14 weeks of gestation
   - Procedure-related risk of miscarriage is ≈ 1–2%

Ionizing radiation

Radiation

1. **Radiation can be broadly divided into**
   - Ionising radiation
   - Non-ionizing radiation

2. **Ionization**
   - Is the process of converting an atom or molecule into an ion by adding or removing charged particles
   - A positive charged ion is produced when an atom or molecule releases an electron
   - A negative charge ion is produced when an atom receives an electron

3. **Radioactive decay**
   - Is the process by which an unstable atomic nucleus spontaneously loses energy by emitting ionizing particles and radiation
   - Is a stochastic process (i.e. it is impossible to predict when a given atom will decay)
   - Becquerel
     i. Is the SI unit of radioactive decay activity
     ii. 1 Bq is defined as 1 decay/s
     iii. 1 curie (Ci) = 3.7×10^{10} Bq
   - Half-life is the time taken for the activity of a given amount of a radioactive substance to decay to half of its initial value

4. Ionizing radiation
- Occurs in radioactive decay
- Includes
  i.   Alpha radiation
  ii. Beta radiation
  iii. Gamma radiation

5. Alpha particles
- Are emitted from the nucleus of an atom
- Are similar to helium-4 nucleus
- Consist of 2 neutrons and 2 protons
- Are heavily ionizing
- Have a
  i.   High mass
  ii. Low penetration depth
  iii. High energy
- Can be stopped with a sheet of paper
- Alpha decay is responsible for 99% of helium production on earth
- Applications include
  i.   Smoke detectors
  ii. Power source for cardiac pacemakers

6. Beta particles
- Divided in to
  i.   Beta minus
  ii. Beta plus
- Can be shielded by few centimetres of metal
- Beta minus
  i.   Is an electron
  ii. Arises from beta minus decay of a neutron (*Fig. 12.5*)

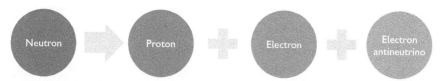

Figure 12.5 Beta minus decay

- Beta plus
  i.   Is a positron
  ii. Has a high energy
  iii. Arises from beta plus decay (where energy is used to convert a proton) (*Fig. 12.6*)

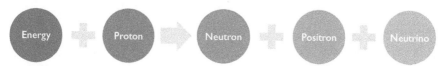

Figure 12.6 Beta plus decay

7. **Gamma rays**
   - Are electromagnetic radiation of high frequency (i.e. above 10^{19} Hz)
   - Produced by
     i.   Radioactive decay
     ii. Fusion
     iii. Fission
   - Consist of photons emitted by the nucleus of an atom
   - Have short wavelength
   - Applications include
     i.   Sterilizing medical equipment
     ii. Removing decay-causing bacteria from foods or preventing fruit and vegetables from sprouting to maintain freshness and flavour
     iii. Gamma knife surgery
     iv. Gamma emitting radioisotopes in nuclear medicine (technetium-99m)
   - Ionization occurs via 3 main processes
     i.   Photoelectric effect
     ii. Compton scattering
     iii. Pair production
   - Shielding from gamma rays requires large amount of mass (e.g. lead, aluminium, concrete)

8. **Geiger–Nuttall law states that short-lived isotopes emit more energetic alpha particles than long-lived ones**

9. **Radiation poisoning (Box 12.3)**
   - Is also known as radiation sickness or acute radiation syndrome
   - Is due to exposure to excessive ionizing radiation
   - Is associated with acute exposure
   - There is no treatment to reverse the effects of irradiation
   - Drugs used to mitigate the effects of radiation poisoning
     i.   5-androstenediol – was introduced as a radiation countermeasure by the US armed forces
     ii. Potassium iodide – to protect the thyroid gland from ingested radioactive iodine

Box 12.3 Radiation poisoning

Mild (exposure to 1 - 2 Gy)	Moderate (exposure to 2 - 3.5 Gy)	Severe (exposure to 3.5 - 5.5 Gy)	Very severe (exposure to 5.5 - 8 Gy)
• Vomiting within 48 h of exposure	• Vomiting within 24 h of exposure	• Vomiting within 1 h of exposure	• Vomiting within 30 min of exposure
• Depression of immune system	• Fever	• Symptoms of moderate radiation	• Symptoms of severe radiation
• Stillbirth	• Hair loss	• Diarrhoea	• Disorientation
• Spontaneous abortion	• Infection	• 50% fatality after 30 days	• Dizziness
• 10% fatality after 30 days	• Haematemesis		• Hypotension
	• Maelena		
	• 30% fatality after 30 days		

X-radiation

1. **X-radiation (or X-ray)**
   - Is a form of electromagnetic radiation
   - Is emitted by electrons (either in orbitals outside of the nucleus, or while being accelerated to produce Bremsstrahlung-type radiation)

- Also known as Roentgen radiation
- Has a wavelength in the range of 10–0.01 nm

2. **Exposure**
   - Is the measure of an X-ray's ionizing ability
   - Roentgen
     i. Represents the amount of radiation required to create 1 electrostatic unit of charge of each polarity in 1 cm³ of dry air
   - Coulomb per kilogram (C/kg)
     i. Is the SI unit of ionizing radiation exposure
     ii. It is the amount of radiation required to create 1 C of charge of each polarity in 1 kg of matter

3. **Absorbed dose is the measure of energy absorbed**
   - Gray (Gy)
     i. Is the SI unit of absorbed dose
     ii. Is the amount of radiation required to deposit 1 J of energy in 1 kg of any kind of matter
   - Rad
     i. 100 rad = 1 Gy

4. **Equivalent dose**
   - Is the measure of biological effect of radiation on human tissue
   - The SI unit is Sievert (Sv)
   - Roentgen equivalent man (rem)
     i. 1 Sv = 100 rem

5. **General facts**
   - Ionising Radiation Regulations (IRR) 1999 dose limit for pregnant personal working with ionizing radiation state that fetal exposure dose should be below 1 mGy
   - Background ionizing radiation levels in the UK
     i. Ranges from 1 to 100 mSv/year
     ii. Average is 2.7 mSv/year (which equates to 1 mGy for a fetus *in utero* for 9 months)
   - Childhood cancer (i.e. in the first 15 years of life)
     i. Risk
        - Background risk = 1 in 500
        - Additional risk after fetal exposure to 1 mGy of ionizing radiation *in utero* after 3 weeks gestation is below 1 in 10 000
     ii. Most common types are
        - Leukaemia
        - Brain tumours (gliomas and medulloblastomas)
        - Sarcomas (rhabdomyosarcoma and osteosarcoma)
        - Wilms' tumour
   - Ionizing radiation threshold dose for fetal malformation is 100–200 mGy
   - Ionizing radiation dose for permanent sterility in
     i. Males = 3500–6000 mGy
     ii. Females = 2500–6000 mGy
   - Fetal CNS is particularly sensitive to radiation at 25 weeks of fetal life
   - Maximum fetal dose from
     i. Abdominal X-ray = 4.2 mGy
     ii. Chest X-ray = <0.01 mGy
     iii. Intravenous urogram (IVU) = 10 mGy
     iv. Pelvic CT = 80 mGy
   - Absorption of fetal iodine, often used as contrast in imaging, increases from 11 weeks of gestation

Table 12.1 Additional lifetime risk of cancer (per examination) due to fetal radiation exposure caused by maternal imaging studies

Imaging study	Additional risk of cancer	Equivalent to natural background radiation exposure of
Abdominal X-ray	1 in 30 000	4 months
Chest X-ray (posteroanterior film)	1 in 1 000 000	3 days
IVU	1 in 8000	14 months
Lung ventilation	1 in 200 000	2.4 weeks
Lung perfusion	1 in 20 000	6 months
Bone scan	1 in 5000	2 years
Myocardial perfusion study	1 in 1100	8 years

6. **Pulmonary embolism (PE)**
   - Deep vein thrombosis (DVT) is found in 70% of patients with PE
   - Computed tomography pulmonary angiography (CTPA)
     i.   Negative predictive value is over 99%
     ii. Fetal radiation exposure varies from 3.3 to 130 µGy
     iii. Increased lifetime risk of maternal breast cancer by 13.6%
     iv. Additional increase in childhood cancer risk of 1 : 1 000 000 above baseline rate
   - V/Q scan
     i. Fetal radiation dose is 100–370 µGy (i.e. ×3 greater than CTPA)
     ii. Additional increase in childhood cancer risk of 1 : 280 000 above baseline rate

Radiotherapy

1. **Radiotherapy is the use of ionizing radiation for the management of both malignant and non-malignant conditions**

2. **Examples of non-malignant conditions managed with radiotherapy include**
   - Trigeminal neuralgia
   - Thyroid eye disease
   - Prevention of keloid scarring

3. **Radiotherapy for the management of malignancy can be**
   - Curative
   - Adjunct
   - Palliative

4. **Mechanism of action – radiation causes DNA damage via direct or indirect ionization of the atoms which make up the DNA chain**

5. **Limitations – tumour cells in hypoxic environments are more resistant to radiation damage**
   - Oxygen is a potent radiosensitizer
   - Solid tumours can outgrow their blood supply and thus be in a hypoxic environment

6. **Dose for**
   - Solid epithelial tumour ranges from 60 to 80 Gy
   - Lymphoma is 20–40 Gy

7. **Fractionation**
   - Allows normal cells time to recover between treatments

- Allows tumour cells in radio-resistant phase of the cell cycle during treatment to cycle into a more sensitive phase for the next treatment dose
- Allows time for reoxygenation of hypoxic tumour cells between treatments
- Schedule in adults is
  i. 2 Gy/day
  ii. 5 days per week

8. **Types of tumour and their radiosensitivity**
   - Sensitive – leukaemia, lymphoma, and germ cell tumours
   - Resistant – renal cell cancer and melanoma

9. **Radiosensitizing drugs include**
   - Cisplatin
   - Nimorazole
   - Cetuximab

10. **Types of radiotherapy**
    - External beam radiotherapy
    - Brachytherapy

11. **Side effects**
    - Oedema
    - Infertility
    - Fibrosis
    - Epilation
    - Dryness
    - Cancer
      i. Rate is 1 in 1000
      ii. Usually occurs 20–30 years following treatment

Nuclear medicine and radioisotopes

1. **Nuclear medicine**
   - Principles
     i.   Uses radioactive isotopes (taken internally)
     ii. Based on radioactive decay
     iii. Emissions captured by gamma camera
   - Is used for
     i. Imaging
     ii. Treatment
   - Imaging includes
     i.   Scintigraphy
     ii. Positron emission tomography
     iii. Gallium scans
     iv. Indium white blood cell scans
     v.   Octreotide scans
   - Treatment includes
     i.   Iodine-131 for hyperthyroidism
     ii. Strontium-89 for palliation of bone pain
     iii. Brachytherapy
   - Nuclear medicine imaging shows physiological function of a system rather than anatomical imaging

2. **Radionuclide**
   - Is an atom with an unstable nucleus

- Emits ionizing radiation
- Commonly used in medical practice
  - i.   Barium-133
  - ii. Thallium-201
  - iii. Strontium
  - iv. Technetium-99m
  - v.   Iodine-131
  - vi. Gallium-67
  - vii. Cobalt-60
  - viii. Indium-111
  - ix. Xenon-133
  - x.   Krypton-81

Non-ionizing radiation

1. **Non-ionizing radiation refers to any type of electromagnetic radiation that does not carry enough energy per quantum to ionize atoms or molecules**

2. **This includes**
   - MRI
   - Light amplification by stimulated emission of radiation (LASER)

MRI

1. **General facts about magnetism**
   - Faraday's law states that any change in the magnetic environment of a coil of wire will cause a voltage to be induced in the coil
   - Tesla (T)
     - i.   Is the SI unit for magnetic field
     - ii. $1\,T = 1$ weber per square meter (Wb/m^2)
     - iii. $1\,T = 10\,000$ gauss
   - Weber (Wb)
     - i.   Is the SI unit for magnetic flux
     - ii. A change in magnetic flux of $1\,Wb/s$ will induce an electromotive force of $1\,V$
   - Magnets in MRI produce $0.5\text{–}3\,T$
   - Typical values of magnetic fields
     - i.   Human brain $= 10^{-9}$ to 10^{-8} gauss
     - ii. Earth $= 0.31$ to 0.58 gauss
     - iii. Refrigerator magnet $= 50$ gauss
     - iv. The surface of a neutron star $= 10^{12}$ to 10^{13} gauss

2. **MRI uses**
   - Magnetic fields to align atomic nuclei (usually hydrogen protons) within body tissues
   - Radiofrequency fields
     - i.   To systematically alter the alignment of this magnetization, causing the hydrogen nuclei to produce a rotating electromagnetic field
     - ii. After the field is turned off, the protons decay to their original spin-down state and the difference in energy between the two states is released as a photon. It is these photons that produce the signal which is detected by the scanner

3. **Types of MR image**
   - T_1-weighted images
     - i.   Also known as spin-lattice (longitudinal) relaxation time

   ii. Is the decay constant for the recovery of the z component of the nuclear spin magnetization

   iii. Water- and fluid-containing tissues are dark

   iv. Fat-containing tissues are bright

   v. Provides good white matter/grey matter contrast in the brain

- T_2-weighted images
  - i. Also known as spin-spin (transverse) relaxation time
  - ii. Water- and fluid-containing tissues are bright
  - iii. Fat-containing tissues are dark
  - iv. Less dependent on field strength than T_1 values
  - v. Is sensitive to water content
- Fluid attenuated inversion recovery (FLAIR) sequence
  - i. Free water is dark
  - ii. Oedematous tissue remains bright
- In most situations T_1 time is greater than T_2
- T_1/T_2-relaxation time is long in fluids (e.g. $T_1 = 1350\,ms$ and $T_2 = 200\,ms$ for blood)
- T_1/T_2-relaxation time is short in solid organs (e.g. $T_1 = 490\,ms$ and $T_2 = 40\,ms$ for liver)

LASER

1. **Is a type of electromagnetic radiation**

2. **Laser beams are**
   - Spatially coherent
   - Narrow low-divergent beam
   - Monochromatic
   - Highly collimated (i.e. being parallel diverging)

3. **Physics of light**
   - Light
     - i. Is electromagnetic radiation of a wavelength that is visible to the human eye
     - ii. Velocity in vacuum is $299\,792\,458\,ms^{-1}$
     - iii. Exhibits polarization
   - Electromagnetic spectrum includes
     - i. Radiowaves
     - ii. Microwaves
     - iii. Infrared
     - iv. Visible light
     - v. Ultraviolet
     - vi. X-rays
     - vii. Gamma rays
   - Photon
     - i. Is the basic unit of light
     - ii. Is governed by quantum mechanics
     - iii. Exhibits wave-particle duality
     - iv. Is mass-less
     - v. Has no electric charge
     - vi. Does not decay spontaneously in empty space
     - vii. Has 2 possible polarization states
   - Wavelength of a light is inversely proportional to the energy of a quantum
     - i. Short wavelengths have high energy (e.g. blue light – 470 nm)
     - ii. Long wavelengths have low energy (e.g. red light – 670 nm)

4. **Physics of laser**
   - Laser consists of
     - i. An optical resonator
     - ii. A gain medium
   - An electron can transit to other energy levels by absorbing or releasing energy
     - i. Transition from a lower to higher energy level requires absorption of photons
     - ii. Transition from higher to lower energy levels requires photons to be released
   - Energy of the photon absorbed or released as the electron transits between energy levels governs the wavelength of light absorbed or emitted
   - Each wavelength in the electromagnetic spectrum has an individual colour
   - The transitions of the electron are divided into 3 types
     - i. Spontaneous absorption (i.e. electron transits from a lower to a higher energy level by absorbing a proton)
     - ii. Spontaneous emission (i.e. an electron excited to an upper energy level will drop to a lower energy level and a photon will be emitted)
     - iii. Stimulated emission (i.e. photon is emitted from an excited atom when it is stimulated by other photons)
   - Laser is produced by stimulated emission
   - Laser can be of any state (*Box 12.4*)

Box 12.4 Types of laser

Gas	Liquid	Solid	Plasma
• Helium-neon • CO_2 • Argon (used for coagulation)	• Coumarin 102 • Stibene • Rhodamine 6G	• Ruby • Neodymium : yttrium aluminium garnet (Nd : YAG) • Titanium sapphire • Neodymium glass	

Semiconductor
• Diode

5. **Interaction of laser beam with living tissue**
   - Thermal effect – leads to denaturation of tissue and depends on
     - i. Laser wavelength
     - ii. Laser power
     - iii. Time duration to exposure
     - iv. Tissue optical coefficient
   - Mechanical effect – results from creation of
     - i. A plasma
     - ii. An explosive vaporization
     - iii. Cavitation
   - Photoablative effect
   - Photodynamic effect

6. **Thermal effects of laser on living tissue**
   - Hyperthermia
   - Coagulation
     - i. Produced by desiccation, blanching, and a shrinking of the tissues by denaturation of proteins and collagen
     - ii. Responsible for haemostasis
   - Volatilization
     - i. Various constituents of tissue disappear in smoke at above 100 °C
     - ii. Coagulation necrosis occurs at the edges of volatilization zone
     - iii. Cutting effect is obtained when the volatilization zone is narrow

7. **Applications in medicine**
   - Gynaecology
     - i. Treatment of cervical intraepithelial neoplasia (CO_2 laser)
     - ii. Treatment in endometriosis
     - iii. Laparoscopic surgery
   - Obstetrics
     - i. Selective laser photocoagulation in treatment of twin-to-twin transfusion syndrome (Nd : YAG or diode laser)
   - Urology
     - i. Lithotripsy
     - ii. Photoselective vaporization of the prostate
     - iii. Laser ablation of the prostate
   - Laser eye surgery
   - Laser hair removal
   - Laser skin treatments

8. **Nd : YAG laser**
   - Is a solid state laser
   - Emits light with a wavelength of 1064 nm (infrared spectrum)

9. **CO_2 laser**
   - Is the highest power continuous wave laser
   - Emits infrared light (wavelength of 10 μm)

Microwaves

1. **Are electromagnetic waves with frequency ranging from 0.3 to 300 GHz**

2. **Includes ultra high frequency (UHF) and extremely high frequency (EHF) electromagnetic waves**

3. **Microwave energy is produced by**
   - Klystron tubes
   - Magnetron tubes
   - Solid state diodes

4. **Are absorbed by molecules that have a dipole moment in liquids**

5. **Applications**
   - Domestic
     - i. Wi-Fi
     - ii. Bluetooth
     - iii. Microwave ovens
   - Broadcasting, telecommunications, and satellite communications

- Radar
- Global navigation positioning system
- Medical
  i.   Microwave ablation for atrial fibrillation
  ii. Endometrial ablation
  iii. Treatment of benign prostatic hyperplasia

Electrosurgery

1. **Electrosurgery**
   - Is the application of high frequency electric current (in the frequency of 100 kHz to 5 MHz) to tissue as a means to cut, coagulate, desiccate, or fulgurate
   - Uses alternating current to directly heat (Ohmic heating) the tissue
   - Common electrode configurations
     i.   Monopolar (high-power unit (400 W) generates high frequency current)
     ii. Bipolar (low-power unit – 50 W)
     iii. Tripolar
   - Generates smoke plumes which contain
     i.   Chemical by-products (e.g. formaldehyde, hydrogen cyanide, toluene)
     ii. Intact cells
     iii. Intact viral DNA
     iv. Viable bacteria

2. **Electrosurgical modalities**
   - Cutting
     i.   High-power density is applied to vaporize tissue water content
   - Coagulation
     i.   Uses waveforms with lower average power
   - Desiccation
   - Fulguration
     i.   Electrode held away from the tissue
     ii. The air gap between the electrode and tissue becomes ionized
     iii. An electric arc is discharge
     iv. Superficial tissue burning occurs

3. **Electrocautery**
   - Is the process of destroying tissue using heat conduction
   - Used mainly for cauterization
   - Uses direct current to produce heat

4. **Physics of electrosurgery**
   - Electric current is the flow of electrons (in metal and semiconductors) or ions (in liquid)
   - Electric conduction in biological tissue is due to interstitial fluid
   - Ohm's law states that voltage is the product of electric current and resistance
   - Electric current at 50 Hz produces intense muscle and nerve activation
   - Sensitivity of neural and muscle cells to electric current is inversely proportional to its frequency (i.e. the higher the frequency the lower the sensitivity)

5. **Diathermy**
   - Is dielectric heating
   - Is a process in which radiowave or microwave electromagnetic radiation heats a dielectric material
   - Produced by rotation of molecular dipoles in high frequency alternating electric field

CHAPTER 13

Research tools

CONTENTS

Research methodology

Study design

All research follows a similar framework

1. **Plan the study**
    - Decide the field to be examined
    - Literature review to
        i.   Ascertain the existing state of knowledge
        ii. Identify specific areas requiring investigation

2. **Design the study**
    - Define the variables to be controlled and observed
    - State a hypothesis
    - Decide which type of study should be utilized
    - Identify the appropriate population
    - Design the details of the experimental methodology to be used
    - Calculate the sample size

3. **Consider ethical issues and apply for ethical committee approval if required**

4. **Sample the population, perform the study, and collect the data**

5. **Use descriptive and inferential statistics to summarize the population characteristics and draw conclusions about the hypothesis tested**

6. **Interpret the study findings in the context of already existing knowledge**

7. **Present the study**
    - Conference
    - Scientific publications

Types of epidemiological studies

1. **Epidemiological studies can be divided into**
   - Interventional studies – individuals or groups are observed after they are subjected to an intervention
   - Observational studies – individuals or groups are only observed
     i.   At a single time point – cross-sectional studies
     ii. Over a period of time – longitudinal studies

2. **Interventional studies can be**
   - Randomized controlled trials – individuals or groups are randomly assigned to either a control or an intervention group
     i.   Double-blinded – neither the participants nor the researcher are aware at the time of the study being conducted as to which participants are receiving the intervention
     ii. Single-blinded – only the researcher is aware at the time of the study as to which participants are receiving the intervention
     iii. Non-blinded – both the participants and the researcher are aware as to which participants are receiving the intervention
   - Non-randomized (also called quasi-experiments) – there is no random allocation. Useful when randomization is not possible or unethical. Examples of this design include
     i.   Interrupted time series analysis – one or more observations are made on the individuals (or groups) several times before and after an intervention
     ii. Case (intervention or outcome of interest)–control (no intervention or negative for the outcome)

3. **Observational studies include**
   - Ecological
     i.   Populations rather than individuals are studied
     ii. Susceptible to confounding factors ('ecological bias')
   - Cohort
     i.   Cohort is a group sharing common characteristics
     ii.   An outcome (e.g. disease)-free cohort sharing a common exposure is followed over time and monitored for how many will develop the outcome compared with a similar but unexposed cohort
     iii. Can be prospective or retrospective
     iv.   The effect of rare exposures and multiple outcomes can be observed
     v.   Can calculate incidence and relative risk
     vi.   Expensive and time consuming
     vii. Typically high drop-out rates
     viii. Prospective cohort studies are considered the highest quality epidemiological observational type of study
   - Cross-sectional
     i.   Characteristics of a population, or sample, are observed at a single point in time
     ii. Provide data on the entire population studied
     iii. Can calculate prevalence, absolute, and relative risks but not incidence
   - Case–control
     i.   Studies association of disease with past exposure
     ii. Exposure of cases (individuals with the disease) is compared with that of controls (individuals without the disease)
     iii. Can calculate odds ratios and absolute risk but not relative risk
     iv. Useful for rare diseases

v. Can be relatively quick and inexpensive

vi. Susceptible to 'recall bias' since information obtained retrospectively

4. **The strength, or degree of trust, ascribed to evidence depends on the source and type of study it was derived from. In general, in ascending order, this is (Fig. 13.1)**

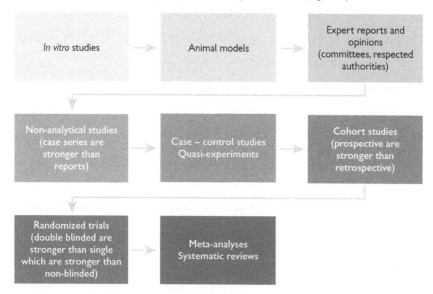

Figure 13.1 Strength of evidence (in ascending order)

5. **Statistical bias occurs when there is a systematic distortion of the collected data. There are many types of bias. Some common ones are**
   - Selection (which also includes sampling) bias
   - Systematic bias
   - Recall bias
   - Bias of an estimator (or experimenter expectancy bias)
   - Measurement bias

Medical statistics

Variables and sampling

1. **Variable is a characteristic being measured**

2. **Data are a collection of information about one or more variables**

3. **Population is the entire set of values or subjects of interest under study**

4. **Sample is a subset of values or subjects derived from the population**

5. **Data from samples are analysed in order to extrapolate to the population, using statistics:**
   - Descriptive statistics utilize observations made in the sample to describe a population and estimate its properties (e.g. a sample mean gives an estimate of the population mean)
   - Inferential statistics study patterns and relationships between variables in the sample to generalize results to the population (e.g. hypothesis testing, correlations, interpolation)

6. The estimates and conclusions drawn from the sample about the population may carry an estimation error (known as a sampling error) because different samples from the same population will produce different results. This leads to statistical uncertainty

7. How accurate the estimates and conclusions are depends on:
   - How representative the sample is of the population (a sample not representative of the population leads to bias error)
   - The sample size (n) is related to the power of a study (sampling error reduces with larger sample size)

8. Sampling can be:
   - Random – every individual unit has the same probability of being selected from the population
   - Stratified
     i. Parameters of interest differ between non-overlapping groups (strata) but not within groups
     ii. Only an appropriate number of individual units need to be randomly selected from each stratum
   - Cluster
     i. Parameters of interest differ within non-overlapping groups (clusters) but not across them
     ii. An appropriate number of individual units need to be randomly selected from only a few clusters
   - Multi-stage
   - Multi-phase

9. Variables can be
   - Categorical – data can only be one of a finite number of values or categories
     i. Nominal (there is no ranking within the categories, e.g. male or female)
     ii. Ordinal (there is ranking within the categories or values, but the difference between these is not relevant or to a scale, e.g. Apgar scores)
   - Quantitative – data are numerical, either continuous (e.g. blood pressure) or discrete (e.g. number of pregnancies)
     i. Interval (as for ordinal, but the intervals between the values are equally spaced)
     ii. Ratio (as for interval, but a value of 0 denotes that the variable is absent)

10. Analysis of 1 variable is termed univariate analysis

11. Analysis of the association between 2 or more variables is termed multivariate

Distributions

1. Probability distribution refers to the relative frequency of occurrence of the possible values that a variable can take

2. There are many types of distribution. Those encountered in medicine include
   - Normal
   - Positively or negatively skewed
   - Bimodal
   - J-shaped or reversed J-shaped
   - Uniform

3. Values characterizing a distribution
   - Measures of location within the distribution (useful mainly when the distribution of the variable is unimodal)
     i. Mean ($\bar{x}$)

- The average of the values (x)

$$\bar{x} = \frac{x1 + \cdots + xn}{n}$$

- Sensitive to outliers (extreme values)
- Cannot be calculated for nominal or ordinal types of variables

ii. Median
- The middle value of a sample after arranging the values in an increasing order
- Robust to outliers
- Cannot be calculated for nominal types of variables

iii. Mode
- The most frequently occurring value
- Can be used to describe all types of variable

- Measures of spread of the distribution (not possible to calculate these for nominal or ordinal types of variables)
  i. Standard deviation (s)
  - Measure of the average distance that individual values are from the sample mean
  - The mathematical formula is

$$s = \sqrt{\frac{\sum (x - \bar{x})^2}{(n-1)}}$$

  ii. Coefficient of variation (CV)
  - Ratio of the standard deviation to the mean

$$CV = \frac{s}{\bar{x}}$$

  - It has no units
  iii. Range
  - The difference between the lowest and the highest value

$$Range = X\,max - X\,min$$

  - Sensitive to outliers
  iv. Interquartile range = The range between the first (Q1) and third (Q3) quartile (each quartile contains 25% of the values, hence, the boundaries of the above quartiles are the numbers below which 25% and 75% respectively of the values occur; the interquartile range includes all the values in between)

4. **Normal distribution (also known as Gaussian distribution)**
- Is bell shaped
- The mean, median, and mode are the same
- 68% of values lie within 1 standard deviation of the mean
- 95% of values lie within 1.96 standard deviations of the mean (also known as the 'normal range')
- 99% of values lie within 2.57 standard deviations of the mean
- Standard error of the mean (SE)
  i. Is an estimate of how far away from the true (unknown) population mean a sample mean is. In other words, it is the standard deviation of the sample mean with respect to the population mean

   ii.   It depends on
   - The variability of the individual values (i.e. the standard deviation of the sample)
   - The sample size (decreases with increasing sample size)
   iii. The mathematical formula is

$$SE = \frac{s}{\sqrt{n}}$$

- Confidence interval (or region) is the area likely to include the true value of the parameter (or parameters) in question (e.g. population mean, difference between the mean of 2 populations)
   i.   The 95% or 99% confidence interval (CI) is commonly used
   ii. It signifies that there is a 95% or 99% chance that the interval contains the true value
   iii. The mathematical formula for the 95% CI of a mean is

$$CI = \bar{x} \pm 1.96 \times SE$$

   iv. For the 99% CI substitute 1.96 with 2.57
   v.   The level of confidence of the interval (i.e. 95% or 99%) is a measure of its accuracy
   vi. The width of the CI is a measure of its precision. It is related to
   - The chosen level of confidence
   - The sample size. Whilst the sample mean remains the same, the CI width decreases as the sample numbers increase, implying that the precision of identifying correctly where the population mean lies increases
   vii. If the CI for a difference of the mean of 2 populations crosses 0 then
   - The finding is not significant, since this implies that it is possible that the true mean difference could be 0 even if the 2 samples mean difference is not
   - In such a situation, if the sample size is made larger then it is possible that the CI width will become smaller and will not cross 0, hence, for the same mean difference the result will become significant

Statistical hypothesis testing

1. **Hypothesis testing involves stating a null hypothesis about a population variable along with an alternative hypothesis which can be either one- or two-sided (i.e. that the difference can be in one or in both directions)**

2. **A hypothesis can only be rejected but never accepted**

3. **Significance level is the evidence required to reject the null hypothesis and conclude that an event has not arisen by chance**

4. **P-value**
   - It is the probability of obtaining a statistic result as the one that was observed while accepting the null hypothesis as true. In other words, the p-value is the probability of obtaining a false-positive result
   - By convention a p-value of <0.05 is accepted as the significant level of evidence (i.e. the observed result would have arisen by chance every 1 in 20 times the study was performed)
   - Another commonly used p-value is <0.01

5. **There are 2 types of error**
   - Type I (also known as α error or false positive)
     i. Occurs when the null hypothesis is wrongly rejected (i.e. falsely detecting a difference)
     ii. Related to the significance level and consequently the p-value
   - Type II (also known as β error or false negative)

i.   Occurs when we wrongly fail to reject the null hypothesis (i.e. failing to detect a true difference)
ii.   Related to the power of a study

6. **Power (sensitivity) of a study**
   - The probability that the test applied will correctly reject the null hypothesis
   - The higher the power, the lower the probability of a type II error
   - Power $= 1 - \beta$
   - For a power calculation, two components need to be established first
     i.   The desired clinical difference to be detected
     ii.   The variability of the measured parameter
   - Power calculations can be used to
     i.   Reflect the minimum sample size needed to reject the null hypothesis at a particular significance level
     ii.   Predict the minimum detectable difference of the studied effect which is likely to be observed for a particular sample size
   - The sample size needed for a study is not related to the population size but to the magnitude or frequency of the effect or event studied
   - The larger the effect or more frequent the outcome, the fewer the numbers needed in a sample to prove a statistically significant difference
   - In medical practice, the power of a study is usually set at 80–90% (i.e. the probability of detecting a significant difference, and rejecting the null hypothesis, by doing the study is 80–90%) and the significance level is usually set at 1% or 5% (i.e. the probability of the detected significant difference having been achieved by chance is 1% or 5%)

7. **Statistical hypothesis tests can be**
   - Parametric
     i.   Assumptions are made about the characteristics of the probability distribution of the variables
     ii.   Have a higher statistical power than non-parametric tests, leading to a lower chance of a type II error
   - Non-parametric
     i.   Make no assumptions about the probability distributions of the variables
     ii.   Are more robust than parametric tests, leading to a lower chance of a type I error

8. **It is important to ascertain if a distribution of quantitative variables is normal in order to decide what statistical hypothesis test should be performed on the sample**

9. **Normality of a sample distribution can be ascertained**
   - Visually (by utilizing a plot)
   - By a goodness-of-fit test for normal distribution
     i.   Shapiro–Wilk
     ii.   Kolmogorov–Smirnov

10. **Non-normally distributed samples can be converted to a normal one by transforming the data (e.g. logarithmic transformation)**

11. **If a sample (and by inference the population) is normally distributed, parametric statistical hypothesis tests can be utilized such as**
   - t-test
     i.   Can be
        - Independent – used when comparing 2 unpaired distributions
        - Paired – used when comparing 2 paired distributions (effectively each pair acts both as a case and control)
     ii.   Can be

- One sample – observations are drawn from a single sample
- Two sample – observations are made on two different samples
- ANOVA (analysis of variance)
  i. Very similar to t-test
  ii. Used when multiple distributions are compared
  iii. Apart from normality, it also assumes that the variance (amount of spread) in each distribution is the same
  iv. Because multiple comparisons are made and some might be significant by chance, the Bonferroni correction can be applied. This tests each individual comparison separately at a smaller significance level (which is equal to what it would be if only 1 hypothesis was tested at a time over the number of comparisons made) thus maintaining the overall significance level

12. **For non-normally distributed quantitative data and for categorical data, non-parametric statistical hypothesis tests can be utilized such as**
   - Wilcoxon's signed rank test (which is the non-parametric equivalent of the paired t-test)
   - Mann–Whitney U (which is the non-parametric equivalent of the independent t-test)
   - Kruskal–Wallis one way analysis of variance (which is the non-parametric equivalent of ANOVA)
   - Friedman two-way ANOVA

13. **χ^2 test**
   - Tests if there is an association between categorical variables
   - It is a measure of the difference (distance) between the expected count in each study group (as predicted by the null hypothesis) to the experimentally observed ones
   - Prerequisite is that each group should have sufficiently enough data
     i. Smallest group should have ≥ 1 expected counts
     ii. $\geq 80\%$ of groups should have ≥ 5 expected counts
   - It does not give information on the type or degree of the association

Quantifying the association between categorical data

1. **Statistical hypothesis tests, such as the χ^2, can only show an association between categorical variables but cannot quantify the strength and direction of this association. For this, several methods can be employed**

2. **The difference in frequency of occurrence of categorical variables (events) between two groups (e.g. control and intervention, exposed and non-exposed) can be expressed in terms of**
   - Risk estimation
     i. Deals with proportions
     ii. Risk can show either reduction or increase, depending on the direction of the association
   - Odds calculations – deals with probabilities (see *Fig. 13.2*)

3. **Risk is the chance of the event being investigated occurring**
   - The risk in a given group (control or observed) = the number of events occurring in that group divided by the total population (with or without the event) in the group
   - Absolute risk difference (AR) is the difference in risk between the two groups
   - AR = risk observed group – risk control group
   - Relative risk (RR) is the risk of 1 group relative to the other (i.e. the ratio of the risk of the 2 groups)
   - RR = risk observed group/risk control group

i.   RR of 1 means that there is no difference between the groups

ii. RR of >1 means that there is greater risk in the observed group compared with the control group

iii. RR of <1 means that there is lower risk in the observed group compared with the control group

4. **Odds is the probability of an event occurring versus the probability of the event not occurring**
   - The odds in a given group (control or observed) = the number of subjects with the event occurring in that group divided by the number of the subjects without the event in the group
   - Odds ratio (OR) is the odds of an event occurring in one group divided by the odds of it occurring in the other group (meaning it quantifies how much more likely it is for an event to occur in one group versus the other)
   - OR = odds observed groups/odds control group

5. **CIs can be calculated for RRs, ARs, and ORs**

6. **If a CI for RR crosses 1, then the risk difference between the two groups is not significant**

7. **The advantages of utilizing ORs are**
   - ORs from different studies can be compared and combined
   - They are amenable to logistic regression
   - They can be calculated in case–control studies (RRs cannot since the number or ratio of cases to controls in the population is not known)

8. **If an event is rare in the control group then the OR is approximately equal to the RR**

Number of subjects with event occurring in observed group = a	Number of subjects without event occurring in observed group = b	Total number of subjects in observed group $= a + b = e$	Risk for event occurring in observed group $= \dfrac{a}{e}$	Odds (probability) of event occurring in observed group $= \dfrac{a}{b}$
Number of subjects with event occurring in control group $= c$	Number of subjects without event occurring in control group $= d$	Total number of subjects in control group $= c + d = f$	Risk for event occurring in control group $= \dfrac{c}{f}$	Odds (probability) of event occurring in control group $= \dfrac{c}{d}$
			Absolute risk $= \dfrac{a}{e} - \dfrac{c}{f}$ **Relative risk** $= \dfrac{a/e}{c/f}$	**Odds ratio** $= \dfrac{a/b}{c/d}$

Figure 13.2 Summary of risk and odds calculations. For ease of identification, each individual calculation included is derived from the boxes with the same colour or border

9. **Number needed to treat (NNT)**
   - A measure of the effectiveness of an intervention

- It corresponds to the number of subjects needed to receive an intervention for one event to occur (or be prevented, depending on the direction of the association)
- The lower the NNT the more effective the intervention
- By definition

$$NNT = \frac{1}{AR}$$

10. **In summary, when comparing categorical variables**
   - A statistical hypothesis test (e.g. χ^2 test) will show if there is an association
   - ORs will quantify this association
   - CIs for the ORs will indicate how precise this quantification of association is

Correlation and regression

1. **Variables can be assigned as being dependent or independent**
   - Independent variables are not altered by other variables, are taken as given and are selected or controlled in order to study their relationship to the dependent variables
   - Dependent variables are observed and are altered by the independent variable. Evidence is sought to prove if, and how, their values are influenced by the alteration of the independent variables

2. **Covariance occurs when variables change together**

3. **Correlation**
   - Is the degree of association between variables
   - It has no units
   - Expressed by using correlation coefficients
     - i. Pearson's correlation coefficient r
       - Most commonly used parametric test of correlation
       - Accesses linear associations only
       - r values range from −1 to +1
       - $r = 0$ implies no association between variables
       - $r = +1$ implies perfect positive linear correlation
       - $r = -1$ implies perfect negative linear correlation
       - Its calculation includes the use of the standard deviation, hence, making it susceptible to outliers
     - ii. Spearman's rank correlation coefficient
       - Non-parametric equivalent of Pearson's r test
       - The values of each variable are ranked in ascending order
       - Pearson's r is then calculated utilizing the ranks for the variables
       - Robust to outliers

4. **Correlation does not imply causation because there might be confounding variables**

5. **Confounding variables**
   - Are variables that correlate with both the dependent and the independent variables
   - Cause spurious relations
   - Lead to type I error

6. **Regression**
   - A set of methods to establish the relationship between variables in order to
     - i. Explain the acquired data or
     - ii. Predict other values of a variable based on those collected experimentally
   - When the relationship between an independent (regressor or predictor) and dependent (regressand or response) variable is linear, then the method of linear regression in employed

- Linear regression is a parametric method, therefore the variables need to be quantitative and with a normal distribution
- Transformation
  i. A mathematical function is applied to all the values of a variable
  ii. Non-linear relations can be transformed to linear (e.g. via squaring the values)
  iii. If the variables are not normally distributed, it may be possible to transform them into a normal distribution (e.g. via logarithmic transformation) and then study the relationship with linear regression
- A regression equation is generated which describes the average linear relationship between the variables
- Regression parameters include
  i. The slope of the line
  ii. The intercept of the line along the y (dependant) axis
  iii. The SEs for the above
  iv. The p-value of the statistical test for rejecting the null hypothesis that there is no association between the regressor and regressand
- The regression equation describes the average relationship between the variables (i.e. the slope of the line) but does not give information about the closeness of the association (i.e. how close the points are to the line). Since the regression line is an average one, it can be generated both with points closely positioned around the line and with points widely scattered and at a distance from the line.
  i. The regression coefficient is the slope of the line (i.e. the relation)
  ii. The coefficient of correlation measures the closeness of the association
- Not all values (points) affect the slope of the fitted line equally
  i. Points at either end have a greater effect in pulling the line (and hence altering the slope) towards them compared with those in the middle
  ii. Leverage is a measure of this effect
  iii. Residual is a measure of how good the fit of the line is to a point
  iv. Therefore, outliers or omission of values at the edges will affect the slope more than those situated in the middle of the regressor's range
- Using the regression model, values for the dependant variable can be ascertained for any value of the regressor
  i. Interpolation is the use of regressor values from within the range used to construct the model
  ii. Extrapolation is the use of values from outside the range used to construct the model. This relies more heavily on the regression assumptions and can more readily lead to erroneous dependant values
- Multiple linear regression is applied to describe the linear relationship between 1 dependent and many independent variables (co-variates)
- Logistic regression
  i. Studies an independent variable in order to predict the probability of a dependent (categorical) variable occurring
  ii. Despite using categorical data, it is a parametric test since in the analysis the association between the 2 variables is expressed in terms of ORs – these are transformed logarithmically and then a linear model is constructed
  iii. Multiple logistic regression
     - Studies the effect of many independent variables (co-variates) in predicting the probability of an event occurring
     - Must first demonstrate that the co-variates are independent of each other
- There are numerous non-linear regression models which try to best fit a given set of data to a predefined equation instead of a line (e.g. quadratic regression fits the equation of a parabola)

- Various non-parametric regression methods exist for ascertaining the relations between variables which do not have a predetermined shape (structure)
  - i. The structure of the relationship is constructed based on the data
  - ii. Larger sample numbers are needed since both structure and parameters of the resulting model need to be derived

Clinical testing

Diagnostic test performance

1. In ascertaining the usefulness of a test, several parameters can be calculated

2. These can be derived from studies where the cases and controls are known and the test under investigation is studied for its ability to correctly or incorrectly detect those subjects with or without the condition

3. Definitions
   - True positive (TP) is a subject with the condition who is correctly identified as having it by the test
   - True negative (TN) is a subject without the condition who is correctly identified as not having it by the test
   - False positive (FP) is a subject without the condition who is incorrectly identified as having it by the test
   - False negative (FN) is a subject with the condition who is missed by the test

4. True positive rate (TPR) = sensitivity = Power = $1 - \beta$

5. True negative rate (TNR) = specificity = $1 - \alpha$

6. False positive rate (FPR) = type I error = $\alpha = 1 -$ specificity

7. False negative rate (FNR) = type II error = $\beta = 1 -$ sensitivity

8. Likelihood ratio (LR) is a measure of the effectiveness of a test
   - LR usually refers to the LR of a positive result which measures how many times more likely a positive test is in someone that has the condition tested for compared to finding a positive test in someone that does not have it = TPR/FPR = sensitivity/(1 – specificity)
   - LR = 1 means that the post-test probability of the subject being positive for the condition tested is no different from the pretest probability
   - LR = >1 means that the post-test probability is higher than the pretest probability
   - LR = <1 means that that the post-test probability is lower
   - LR of a negative result measures how many times more likely a negative test is in subject who does not have the condition tested for compared with finding a negative test in subject who does have it = TNR / FNR = specificity / (1-sensitivity)

9. Positive predictive value (PPV) is the probability that a subject with a positive test has the condition = TP/(TP + FP)

10. Negative predictive value (NPV) is the probability that a subject with a negative test does not have the condition = TN/(TN + FN)

11. Accuracy is a measure of how many correct results the test gives in relation to all the tests performed = (TP + TN)/all tests performed

12. For screening tests, it is desirable to have a high sensitivity, thus minimizing missed cases

13. For diagnostic tests, it is desirable to have high specificity, thus minimizing misdiagnoses

14. Since the specificity and sensitivity are inversely related, which one will be of more importance depends on the consequences of a missed diagnosis versus a misdiagnosis. The cut-off value for a test can be chosen using a receiver operator characteristic (ROC) curve

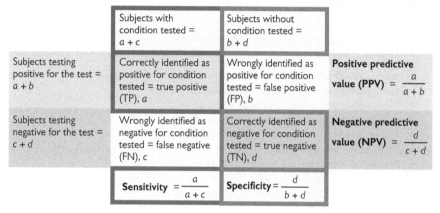

Figure 13.3 Summary of calculations for clinical test performance. For ease of identification, each individual calculation included is derived from the boxes with the same colour or border

15. ROC curve
   - It is a graphical plot
   - Can be a plot of
     i. Sensitivity versus (1 − specificity)
     ii. TPR versus FPR (also called relative operating characteristic curve)
   - It essentially depicts the trade-offs between true and false positives

16. Incidence of an event is the risk of the event occurring per unit time

17. Prevalence of an event = total number of events in the population (often at a specified time) divided by the population size
   - Represents how common an event is
   - Can calculate what the prior odds of an event (or condition) occurring is

18. Bayes' theorem states that: the prior odds of having a condition x, the LR derived from the test utilized = posterior odds

19. In practice, this means that tests with the same sensitivity and specificity may have very different predictive values depending on the background odds (prevalence) of a condition occurring. This is especially true when comparing the predictive value of the same test for a condition in a low- and in a high-risk population. Mathematically, sensitivity and specificity will remain the same however, the PPV for the low-risk population will be lower than that for the high-risk population due to the absolute differences in the TP and FP for the 2 populations caused by the different prevalence. Hence, the usefulness of a test depends on the population it is used on

20. Other useful measures of a test include
   - Precision (reproducibility) – a measure of the test's ability to produce the same result every time it is repeated on the same subject
   - Intra-observer variability – a measure of how precise a test is if the same operator repeats it

- Inter-observer variability – a measure of how precise a test is if different operators perform it

Screening programmes

1. **A screening programme is an attempt to detect a condition in individual members of a population who are not exhibiting its symptoms or signs**

2. **Screening can be**
   - Universal – all members of a population are screened
   - Targeted – only members with a high prior odds of having the condition are screened

3. **In 1968 the WHO published a report called** *Principles and practice of screening for disease* **(by Wilson and Jungner). The conclusions are summarized here**
   - The condition screened for should be an important health problem
   - The natural course of the condition must be known
   - A latent or early symptomatic stage of the condition must exist
   - There should be treatment and this should be more effective if commenced early
   - Facilities for diagnosis and treatment must be available
   - A test for the condition must exist
   - The test must be acceptable to the screened population
   - There should be agreement on who to treat
   - The cost of diagnosing and treating cases found should be cost-effective in comparison with the possible medical cost as a whole
   - The process of finding cases should be continuous and not just 'once only'

Index

extrapyramidal pathway 98
extravasation 228
extra-villous trophoblast 170, 281
exudation 228, 230
eye development 49–50

face and neck development 46–9
factor V Leiden 246
fallopian tubes 87
false negative 374–5, 380, 381
false positive 374–5, 380, 381
Faraday's law 364
fasciae 63–4
fat 187–8, 225
fatty acids 187
female genital tract 82–9
female reproductive system 144–50
    folliculogenesis 144–5
    menarche 148–9
    menopause 149–50
    oogenesis 145–6
    reproductive cycle 146–8
femoral arteries 91–2
femoral nerve 101
femoral ring 56
femoral sheath 55, 56
femoral triangle 55
fenamic acid derivatives 329
fentanyl 307
Ferguson reflex 224
fetus/fetal:
    abnormalities detected with
        ultrasound 357–8
    acid-base changes 115
    adrenal development 171, 226
    alcohol syndrome 309
    arterial redistribution 356
    arterial values 114
    biophysical profile 357
    calcium 122
    cells 281
    circulation 168–9
    compartment and proteins 222
    development in 1st week of life 16
    development in 3rd week of life 17
    development from week 4 to 7 18
    development from week 7 to 20 18
    development from week 25 to 37 19
    ductus venosus Doppler, abnormal 356
    endocrine system 226
    erythrocytes 169

erythropoiesis 169
    gonadal development 226
    growth restriction 356, 357
    immunology 280
    lung 167–8
    maternal gas values 135
    membranes 22–4, 166–7
    monitoring, electronic 343–7
    movements (quickening) 171
    oxygen transport 134–6
    parathyroid development 226
    pituitary development 226
    respiratory system 134–6, 167
    skull 109–10
    swallowing 166
    thyroid development 226
    tissues 165–9
    urine 165
    weight 172
fibrinoid deposits 22
fibrinolytic cascade 246–7
fibrinolytic system 176
fibroblast growth factor (FGR) 355–6
fibroma-thecomas 261
Fick's law 131
FIGO classification:
    cervical cancer 257, 260
    ovarian carcinoma 263
first breath following delivery 167
flow phase of injury 236
fluids 111–13
folate metabolism 310
follicles 145
follicle stimulating hormone (FSH) 151, 205–6
folliculogenesis 144–5
fontanelles 27, 109, 110
Food and Drug Administration (FDA)
        pregnancy category 305
foramen caecum 47
foramen ovale 30
foregut 34–5
fossae 54–7, 59
fractionation 362–3
functional residual capacity 133
fungi 293

gall bladder 35, 74
gamma rays 360
Gardnerella vaginalis 289
gaseous exchange 131